Stories in the Time of Cholera

Stories in the Time of Cholera

Racial Profiling during a Medical Nightmare

CHARLES L. BRIGGS WITH
CLARA MANTINI-BRIGGS

University of California Press

BERKELEY   LOS ANGELES   LONDON

This material is based upon work supported by the National Science Foundation under Grant No. 9408820. Any opinions, findings, and conclusions or recommendations expressed in this material are those of the authors and do not necessarily reflect the views of the National Science Foundation.

Parts of this book previously appeared in different form and are reprinted here courtesy of their publishers: Charles L. Briggs, "Lessons in the Time of Cholera," *Infectious Diseases and Social Inequality in Latin America,* Working Paper Series, no. 239 (Washington, D.C.: Latin American Program, Woodrow Wilson International Center for Scholars, 1999): 1–30; and Charles L. Briggs, "Modernity, Cultural Reasoning, and the Institutionalization of Social Inequality: Racializing Death in a Cholera Epidemic in Venezuela," *Comparative Studies in Society and History* 43, no. 4 (2000): 665–700, reprinted with the permission of Cambridge University Press.

University of California Press
Berkeley and Los Angeles, California

University of California Press, Ltd.
London, England

Library of Congress Cataloging-in-Publication Data

Briggs, Charles L., 1953–.
    Stories in the time of cholera : racial profiling during a medical nightmare / Charles L. Briggs with Clara Mantini-Briggs.
        p.   cm.
    Includes bibliographical references and index.
    ISBN 0-520-23031-0 (alk. paper)
        1. Cholera—Venezuela—Epidemiology.   2. Cholera—Social aspects—Venezuela.   I. Mantini-Briggs, Clara, 1956–   II. Title.

    RA644.C3 B685   2003
    614.5'14'0987—dc21   2002016552

Manufactured in Canada

12 11 10 09 08 07 06 05 04 03
10 9 8 7 6 5 4 3 2 1

The paper used in this publication meets the minimum requirements of ANSI/NISO Z39.48–1992 (R 1997) *(Permanence of Paper).* ⊗

We dedicate this book to compañeros
and compañeras *all over the world
who struggle to place health
at the center of struggles for social justice
rather than turn disease into a tool
for making social inequality seem just.*

It is easy to overwhelm what people *know* with what they *fear.*
Existing stereotypes quickly amalgamate with misrepresentations
of medical and sociological knowledge. . . . Cultural narratives
of perversion and contagion seem endlessly capable of turning
apparently interpretation-proof facts into ammunition for media
hysteria and individual discrimination.

Cindy Patton, *Fatal Advice*

Contents

Illustrations

xi

FIGURES

MAPS

TABLES

Preface

Writing this book has been painful, sometimes downright depressing. It relates stories of the epidemic of cholera that took place in eastern Venezuela in 1992–1993 and the violent, uncanny deaths that resulted. This research project seemed to come looking for us, rather than the other way around. Clara Mantini-Briggs had been working as a public health physician in Tucupita, the capital of Delta Amacuro state, for only four months when the epidemic began. Having studied cholera firsthand earlier in 1992 in Apure and Zulia states, she took a major role in directing efforts to end the epidemic. She was right in the middle of the bodies, IVs, buckets of diarrhea, and tireless community leaders that we describe in this book. Charles Briggs had worked in the delta since 1986, and in November 1992 he discovered the epidemic during a short visit to Tucupita. He returned in June 1993 to assist in setting up health education and treatment programs that centered on cholera prevention. That's when we met. That summer we inaugurated a pilot program in Mariusa, the area in which Charles had worked intensely and which had been severely affected by the disease.

By 1994 it was apparent that little was being done to prevent future epidemics. "The Warao," as the indigenous population is known, had been blamed for the outbreak. In 1994 and 1995, we traversed virtually the entire fluvial area. In addition to giving talks on how to prevent cholera and other infectious diseases, we asked who had died in each community and explored perceptions of the causes and effects of the epidemic. We came to believe that trying to figure out why so many people had died from a preventable and easily treated disease and then making our conclusions widely available constituted one of the most important means of trying to keep the cycle of death and inaction from being repeated. Cholera narratives circulated far beyond the delta, so we traveled to Caracas, Washington, D.C.,

Atlanta, Georgia, Geneva, Dhaka (Bangladesh) and elsewhere, interviewing public health officials about the Latin American epidemic.

This book breaks new ground in a number of ways. First, we have been able to document the mechanisms through which denigrating images are generated through specific institutional practices and in response to concrete organizational crises, presented for public consumption, used in creating widely shared perceptions of people and events, and made the center of public policy. The epidemic provides a powerful site to explore these questions. Caught off guard by cholera, public health authorities, politicians, and patients needed to come up with explanations that would enable them to figure out what to do—and fast. At the same time, since the disease was cholera, the images that were called into service were powerful depictions of the social inequality that lies at the heart of the modernist project. Making sense of this situation can provide particular clarity about how denigrating images are produced and how they shape conditions of life and death.

Second, it points forcefully to the pervasive and far-reaching impact of this process on people's lives. We introduce the term *medical profiling* to suggest that, just as police officers in the United States single out people of color for traffic stops and searches, clinicians and public health authorities sometimes assume that members of particular communities are natural targets for particular diseases and are less likely to be capable and "cooperative" patients. The effects of this process extend far beyond questions of medicine and public health per se. We introduce the term *sanitary citizens* in drawing attention to the way that some people are credited with understanding modern medical concepts and behaving in ways that make them less susceptible to disease. Others get branded as *unsanitary subjects;* they are deemed to be incapable of helping themselves or taking advantage of medical services—and even presented as threats to the health of the body politic. The dramatic case that we describe shows not just the fallacies and injustices associated with designating people as unsanitary subjects but the way this label can justify denials of basic social and political rights.

Third, this book goes beyond the examination of different locations on a global stage to detail the processes by which stories, images, policies, manuals, and statistics circulate among different sites and how they are transformed as they take up residence in different spaces. Social inequality does not take the same form in Geneva that it does in Caracas or Tucupita, but the circulation of representations that link cholera to poverty and cultural difference helps to sustain the legitimacy of social inequality in each place. This book points to the need to grasp how people and institutions located in very different sites are tied together, and it provides a model for documenting and analyzing these connections.

Finally, we think this book shows that using cultural reasoning or other strategies to blame individuals and populations with little access to power and resources really doesn't work for anyone. Strategies for coping with institutional vulnerabilities actually render institutions and their employees less capable of doing their jobs—and thus eventually more vulnerable. Our goal is not to add a new chapter to the old game of passing along the blame. Rather, we hope to provide everyone who is affected by social inequality, stigma, and disease—that is, all of us—with new tools for figuring out how institutions can be run, studies carried out, and lives lived without resorting to a denigrating process that ultimately denigrates us all.

From start to finish, the research that has gone into this book has been collaborative. We discussed nearly every aspect of the data and interpretation, juxtaposing the perspectives of the physician and public health practitioner and the anthropologist. We had anticipated drafting the book collaboratively as well, but the professorial life of the academic provides much more space for writing than does that of a public health physician. Moreover, memories of her intense participation in scenes of death and misery frequently made the task of writing about the epidemic too painful for Clara. She wrote chapter 5, which poignantly describes the feel of a cholera epidemic and details the demanding work needed to bring it to an end, and contributed to chapter 3. The first-person singular voice in chapter 5 is thus Clara's, and the "we" that appears in chapter 3 belongs to both of us. The "I" that inhabits the others is Charles Briggs's.

Our determination to speak is a response not simply to the need to cry out against the silence that surrounds the periodic return of cholera and everyday death in the delta, where half of the children still die today. It is also a response to a deeper problem: social inequality and infectious diseases are on the rise worldwide. Assertions regarding cultural difference—the idea that poor people and individuals representing marginalized communities think and act differently and cannot embrace modern hygiene and medicine—increasingly shape institutional practices that permit or even multiply unnecessary and unconscionable deaths from disease. Silencing the stories that challenge dominant views embeds inequality more powerfully and invisibly in the work of even the best and most high-minded practitioners.

Specifics may place this narrative in Venezuela in 1992 and 1993, but the general problem has a great deal to say about tuberculosis in Peru or New York, or about AIDS in Zimbabwe, Haiti, or San Francisco. This is, in the end, a story about all of us, about the ways that we are implicated in the resurgence of "old diseases" as well as the emergence of new plagues. It is, in the end, a story about finding ways to deal with disease and inequality that avoid blaming others, a paralyzing defensive reaction that precludes a deeper search for answers that could avert a dumbfounding return to disease patterns that resemble those of the nineteenth century. We believe that it is possible to practice medicine and public health on the basis of a shared sense of responsibility and justice.

In this book we discuss the work of people we respect and admire, individuals who have offered us friendship, collegiality, and often shelter. During recorded interviews, some public health officials and practitioners talked about the epidemic in ways that stereotype the populations in which cases were concentrated, sometimes in a subtle way, sometimes blatantly. These interviews placed us in a deep quandary. Quoting their words and exploring their significance would risk placing these individuals in a bad light, which is not what we intend. We adopted two means of coping with this problem. First, we use pseudonyms for all people interviewed in the course of the study. The only individuals who are referred to by their real names are people we encountered only through their written words or their statements to the press. Second, making moral judgments about individuals—naming heroes and villains—does not figure among our goals. Our point is to detail ideologies, institutions, and practices that contribute, however indirectly, to denigrating people's lives and endangering their health. Pinning the blame on particular individuals, communities, and nations was precisely the strategy used by dominant institutions to shield themselves from blame for the epidemic; we argue that this tendency is widespread and pernicious and that it has fatal results. It is more interesting and productive to see how well-trained professionals who are working hard to improve health conditions can contribute to the very forms of suffering they seek to counter.

Nonetheless, these events and the stories that people told about them do reveal some unflattering actions and attitudes. It would be possible simply to leave these out of the story, but we believe it is necessary to weigh the possibility of embarrassing some individuals against the likely effects of erasure. When attitudes and actions endanger lives by unwittingly turning stereotypes into institutional practices, remaining silent would be, in our estimation, the most ethically irresponsible position. We would rather err on the side of offending dedicated professionals than of collaborating in the suppression of narratives and perspectives that are generally denigrated or silenced by the press and a range of institutional actors. We ask readers who identify with the people whom we quote to conduct their own assessment of the risks of leaving hard words out of the story. We ask readers not to take the easy way out by erroneously asserting that we have judged able public health practitioners and clinicians as harboring evil intentions or as being engaged in conspiratorial efforts to kill helpless people.

One final word of warning. We focus on the period from January 1991 to June 1993. Levels of poverty and social inequality have not improved in Venezuela since that time, but the political context of health policy has altered radically. The two political parties that dominated the political scene in 1992 have largely lost their hold on power. President Carlos Andrés Pérez was impeached in 1993, and the current president, Hugo Chávez Frías, has criticized institutional practices that foster social inequality, including globalization, neoliberal economic policies, and practices that increase the vulnerability of poor Venezuelans. A new Bolivarian constitution, adopted in December 1999, transformed the Ministerio de Sanidad y Asistencia Social (Ministry of Health and Public Assistance) into the Ministerio de Salud y Desarrollo Social (Ministry of Health and Social Development). The new ministry instituted a Plan de Salud Integral (Comprehensive Health Plan) that focuses specifically on using new ideas and resources to challenge social inequality and to improve the health of the most vulnerable populations. The World Health Organization and the Pan American Health Organization have also undergone changes in perspectives and institutional structures. We offer these pages as a contribution to these efforts to generate less fatal means of linking health and social inequality.

Acknowledgments

Expressing the many debts we accumulated over the course of eight years of research is a daunting task. We have asked hundreds of people to tell us about what were often the most difficult days of their lives. One example: In Wakanoko, a small community near Guayo, nearly a third of the population died from cholera in a single night, and another third left the community shortly thereafter, stricken by fear and grief. The community's two vernacular healers, or *wisidatu*, a father and son, lived in one household. We spoke with the survivors, the elder man's two wives and the one remaining son. Their memories were so strong and immediate that they honestly believed that the two men had died no more than a month before we spoke with them in 1994, even though about two years had elapsed. The words spoken by the younger widow and her son-in-law were so filled with pain and grief that they seemed to transport us to a different world, one far from the clear blue sky, brown river, and dense green forest that met the eye. How do you thank someone for this type of gift? In the months that we spent traveling from community to community in the delta, we often slept in the homes of the people we had met only as darkness appeared. We shared the rice, spaghetti, flour, and medicine that we had brought with us and the fish, crabs, coffee, and hospitality they offered us, renewing old friendships and creating myriad bonds of amazing intensity. Clara provided free medical care.

It would be satisfying to thank each person personally in these pages. But to do so would violate their privacy. It would attach their names to stories and could lead to unforeseeable consequences. We promised not to reveal names. We can state here only that we deeply appreciate how difficult it was to tell these stories and that we feel honored to have heard them. We hope that when people read what we have written or hear these words relayed by relatives and friends, they will believe that their trust was well placed. Most of all, we hope that this book will help bring about changes, so that the sorts of horrendous health conditions they now face—even outside of times of cholera—and the insidious, denigrating racism that shapes many people's lives will soon exist only in the pages of this book.

A similar problem renders it impossible to thank adequately the many physicians, nurses, public health and other officials, politicians, businesspeople, taxi drivers, and others we interviewed. They often recounted statements and actions that had placed their jobs and institutions on the line, taking real professional risks. Sometimes, when officials in Delta Amacuro wanted to erase the word *cholera* from public consciousness, just speaking with us—period—constituted an act of bravery. We thank them for taking time from busy schedules and for deeming the potential professional risks to be less important than collectively trying to figure out why the epidemic was so catastrophic and how such disasters can be prevented. We appreciate their candidness and their willingness to reflect on what they perceived as their failures as well as their successes. We offer this book as a contribution to their efforts to better the lives of the people they serve. In particular, we thank physicians, nurses, and other health workers and officials in public health institutions from Pedernales to Tucupita to Caracas to Washington to Geneva. We also thank the director of the Regional Health Service and the Malarial Institute in Tucupita for giving Clara permission to undertake this research in the delta and for providing assistance with gasoline and medical supplies. This work has been greatly enriched by friendships and frank exchanges of ideas with individuals in the Ministerio de Sanidad y Asistencia Social in Caracas, Tucupita, Maturín, Maracay, and elsewhere; the Pan American Health Organization; the Centers for Disease Control; UNICEF; the World Health Organization; and the International Centre for Diarrhoeal Disease Research, Bangladesh. In particular, this study would not have been possible if employees of the Regional Health Service of the Ministerio de Sanidad y Asistencia Social in Tucupita, the Pan American Health Organization in Washington, D.C., and the World Health Organization in Geneva had not displayed so much professionalism, patience, and generosity in allowing us to return again and again for interviews, to copy documents, and to observe daily activities and the way crises were handled.

One of our deepest debts is to the people who lived at the time of the epidemic where the Mariusa River hits the Caribbean coast, including those who now are most often found on the mainland in Barrancas, Puerto Ordaz, Caracas—or just about anywhere else in Venezuela. The long-time head of this community, one of the first people to be killed by cholera in the delta, was one of Charles's oldest and dearest friends in the delta. He is still much missed. His son, whom we have called José Rivera in this book, has taken his father's place as leader. We have shared many struggles with him and other Mariusans since 1992, responding to requests for assistance in their attempts to obtain the health and educational rights to which all Venezuelans are entitled. The time that José Rivera and so many other Mariusans took to narrate a host of different aspects of the epidemic's story has shaped the human core of this book. These stories of death, flight, and confinement are the quintessential embodiment of the fear, bitterness, and oppression that Mariusans have experienced in recent decades. The Mariusans have long been envisioned as the "least civilized" or the "real Indians" in the delta, and the cholera epidemic deepened these stereotypes and heightened their social and political effects. We salute them for their willingness to revisit these painful memories, and we hope that our relationship provides them with additional resources for advancing their struggle.

This book could not have assumed its present form without the assistance of Tirso Gómez. He accompanied us on nearly every trip into the delta, using his extraordinary memory and knowledge of the delta and its people to locate communities. His intelligence and sense of humor sustained us on many days when exhaustion and the emotional impact associated with this work made it difficult to go on. His skill in helping us hone our health education presentations in such a way as to empower community members and render the information memorable is much appreciated. We also enjoyed the company of Surdelina Gómez and their children and grandchildren in the family house in Hubasuhuru. We are able to thank them by name because we have not quoted them in this work.

Rosalino Fernández, Esperanza Jiménez de Fernández, Elizabeth Gómez, and Estrella Mantini Amundaray played just as crucial a role through years of painstaking work in transcribing some 180 hours of recordings. We never could have completed the project if they had not been willing to turn these sounds, including raucous meetings in which everyone seemed to be talking at once, into a vast quantity of text. We were fortunate to be able to engage a number of able research assistants on the project, and the participation of Mauricio Albrizio, Dolores Calderón, Tania Granadillo, and Jesse Mills is deeply appreciated.

We owe a particular debt of gratitude to activists Catalina Herrera, Librado Moraleda, Arnoldo Solares, and Dalia Herminia Yanez. They have dared to stage massive protests on the streets of Tucupita, displacing the notion of exotic, pre-modern *indígenas* by drawing attention to land expropriation, environmental degradation, labor exploitation, and institutional racism. We have learned a great deal through hundreds of conversations with them, joining them in protests and other actions. Leaders of the Consejo Nacional Indígena de Venezuela (CONIVE), including José and Tito Pollo and Jesús González, inspired us and offered valuable insights and critiques, as did Saul Rivas and Noelis Pocatierra.

Our *compadres* Hector Romero and Belkis Ruíz provided two of the most sustained and satisfying friendships that we have ever known. Hector—sociologist, lawyer, statesman, and intellectual—helped us deepen our understanding of delta politics and Marxist theory through discussions often powered by salsa dancing and tasty *parrilla* (barbecue). Anthropologist Noreye Guanire has also stood for many years as friend and interlocutor.

We have grown greatly through conversations with Venezuelan colleagues. Yolanda Salas has x-rayed the way that Venezuelan nationalism has been multiply refracted in popular narrative. She generously read the manuscript. María Eugenia Villalón's critique of the ideologies that shape programs of bilingual conversation—along with her friendship and conversation over the years—has made our work more stimulating and fruitful. She also passed along a health education pamphlet that crucially aided our analysis. The Department of Anthropology of the Instituto Venezolano de Investigaciones Científicas provided an institutional home for several years, and we value our conversations with colleagues there, including Nelly Arvelo-Jiménez, H. Dieter Heinen, and Werner Wilbert. Johannes Wilbert shared his deep knowledge of the delta and friendship. Bernarda Escalante of the Instituto Caribe de Antropología y Sociología was also generous. Officials in the Regional Office of Indigenous Affairs and the national Office of Indigenous Affairs provided support in a number of ways.

It is impossible to repay the kindness of Dain Borges, Steve Epstein, Paul Farmer, Ramón Gutiérrez, Patricia Márquez, Larry Palinkas, James Trostle, and Greg Urban in reading the manuscript, or of Victor Pablo White, who indexed it. We hope that they can see the benefit of their wisdom reflected in the final pages. Feliciana Briggs and Kathy Mooney turned their meticulous vision to the task of proofreading parts of the manuscript. Stan Holwitz's editorial skill in locating insightful readers, shepherding the manuscript through the review process, and both challenging and supporting its authors is exemplary. The amount of time and energy that Rebecca Frazier, Laura Harger, and Marian Schwartz devoted to editing the manuscript is simply astounding, and our gratitude runs deep. The support of all of these individuals helped turn the often lonely task of writing into a collective enterprise.

Papers presented at a variety of institutions and meetings afforded crucial criticism, and reactions by Iain Boal, Fernando Coronil, Veena Das, Steven Epstein, Ludmilla Jordanova, Elaine Lawless, Mark Nichter, Randall Packard, and Charles Rosenberg on these occasions and in other conversations proved to be particularly helpful. Colleagues in the Department of Ethnic Studies at the University of California, San Diego, helped to shape our thinking about economies of race and racism, as did friends in other departments, particularly Aaron Cicourel, Steven Epstein, Lisa Lowe, Tanya Luhrman, Jim Holston, Vince Rafael, and Kit Woolard. Charles Briggs's collaboration over many years with Dick Bauman has greatly shaped his sense of the politics of discourse and narrative.

This research was funded by the John Simon Guggenheim Memorial Foundation, the National Science Foundation, the Social Science Research Council, the National Endowment for the Humanities, the Wenner-Gren Foundation for Anthropological Research, Inc., Vassar College, and the Academic Senate of the University of California, San Diego. Charles Briggs was afforded an ideal environment in which to write about the epidemic by the Latin American Program of the Woodrow Wilson International Center for Scholars; the stimulating conversations with staff and fellows there, especially Akhil Guptz, Michael Katz, and Luise White, were most helpful. Several chapters were presented in a seminar on postcolonial writing there, and the readings offered by Akhil Gupta, Jim Hevia, Doug Howland, David Gilmartin, and Luise White helped to focus questions of voice and audience. The final phases of the editing process took place while he was a Fellow at the Center for Advanced Study in the Behavioral Sciences at Stanford University. Some parts of this book appeared in different form in the Working Paper Series, number 239, Latin American Program, Woodrow Wilson International Center for Scholars, Washington, D.C. (1999), and in *Comparative Studies in Society and History.*

The research for this book has been woven deeply into the lives of Feliciana Briggs and Gabriel Fries-Briggs, from constant conversations about cholera to months spent in delta communities. Their forbearance and good nature has helped sustain us, and their acute observations informed our perspectives. We thank Clara's parents, Guerino Mantini and Elba Amundaray de Mantini, and her siblings, Leopoldo, Estrella, Italo, Guerino, Miguel, Sol, Alba, and Julio. Their energy and bravery have reminded us always of what is at stake and of the possibility to dream even amid seemingly insurmountable obstacles. Our marvelous nephews and nieces, Nancy, Matthew, José Miguel, Oriana, Rachel, Leopoldo, Carla, Hernán, Guerino, Italo, Gabriel, Orietta, Jean Carlos, María Giselle, Michelle Claret, Fiorella, Pierinna, Patricia,

Lionel, and Monica de los Angeles, fill our lives with activity, energy, and a sense of purpose.

Finally, we hope that this book contributes directly to the struggle for health and social justice of Venezuelans classified as *indígenas*, both directly and indirectly. We could not profit financially from other people's suffering, and the authors' proceeds from the book will thus be used to develop programs through the Fundación para las Investigaciones Aplicadas Orinoco aimed at bettering the health and well-being of *indígenas*.

Introduction
Death in the Delta

In 1992 and 1993 some five hundred persons died in the maze of rivers and thousands of large and small islands that form the delta region of the Orinoco River in eastern Venezuela (see map 1).[1] The disease that killed so many so quickly was cholera. I (Charles Briggs) stumbled onto the epidemic in November 1992 during a two-week visit to Tucupita, a city of some forty thousand inhabitants and the capital of Delta Amacuro state. Many of my friends from the delta were living on the streets of Tucupita and nearby Barrancas del Orinoco, another small city on the edge of the delta, begging and performing odd jobs to survive, sleeping in shelters constructed of stray pieces of plastic and surplus lumber. Nine of my closest friends had died. The survivors were terrified.

Cholera is nearly unrivaled in terms of the speed with which it kills. Healthy adults can die in as little as three to twelve hours after the first symptoms appear. Humans absorb water, sodium, and chloride through the intestines. The toxin produced by the *Vibrio cholerae* bacteria paralyzes the gut in such a way that intestinal cells secrete water and electrolytes, resulting in diarrhea and extremely rapid dehydration. Persons who are acutely symptomatic suddenly begin to expel an unbelievable volume of diarrhea and vomit—10 percent of a person's body weight can be lost in a matter of hours. The stench of diarrhea and vomit becomes overwhelming. The rapid dehydration leaves cholera patients weak and thirsty, their arms and legs grow cold and clammy, and powerful cramps seem to shrivel their limbs and tie them in knots. The tips of their tongues and their lips turn blue, their eyes sink back into their sockets, and their skin hangs limply on their bodies. A fifteen-year-old can be mistaken for a person of seventy.

Unless the lost fluid is replaced, consciousness fades rapidly. If not treated with rehydration therapy, as many as 70 percent of symptomatic patients

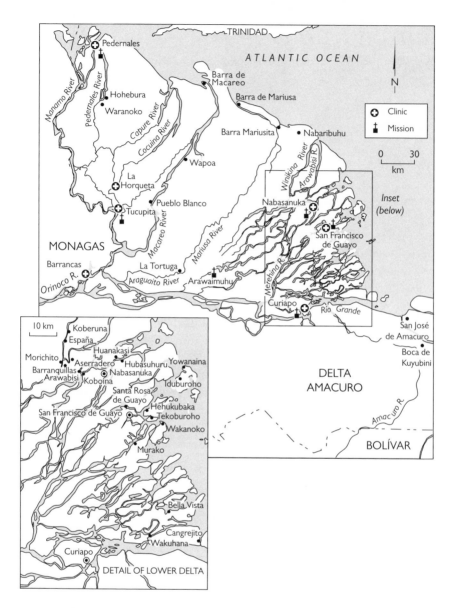

Map 1. Delta Amacuro, showing principal places mentioned in the text. Inset shows lower-central delta area.

can die.[2] What is most appalling is that cholera is easy to prevent and treat. Uncontaminated food and water are all that is needed to keep the disease at bay. Most patients can be saved by drinking a commonly available solution containing sugar, salt, and electrolytes, and even severely dehydrated, nearly unconscious patients can be brought back to life through intravenous rehydration. The disease also responds readily to antibiotic treatment.

Two of my friends, Salomón Medina—known as "Comando"—and José Rivera, related the horrors induced by the epidemic. Both are from the delta community of Mariusa. I had known Medina for many years. Previously a stocky, round-faced man of some sixty years of age with a distinguished demeanor, he now looked thin and beleaguered, and his movements were uncertain and jerky. Rivera, a serious, hard-working young man in his twenties who possessed great warmth and a fine sense of humor, seemed to have aged at least two decades in the two years since I had seen him. Now thin and pale, and red-eyed from lack of sleep, he bore the weight of several worlds on his shoulders. He was a favorite son of Santiago Rivera, who had been the *kobenahoro* (governor), the political leader of Mariusa, for about thirty years, as well as a great storyteller and a respected—even feared—healer. Lacking age, experience, and authority, José Rivera had been thrust into a leadership role by his father's death in some of the most precarious circumstances his community had ever faced.

Medina and José Rivera were on the Mariusa River at the point where it reaches the Caribbean when they first witnessed the effects of cholera. This area is deemed to be one of the most "remote" parts of the vast matrix of forested, often swampy islands that make up the 40,000-square-kilometer Orinoco delta, in which some 40,000 people live.[3] There were no clinics, missions, schools, government offices, or stores there when the epidemic hit. Physicians were not available to treat patients or explain what was taking place. Vernacular healers attempted to cope with a disease that baffled them. Santiago Rivera was one of the most respected practitioners of *hoarotu* medicine, which incorporates therapeutic touch in addition to chanting and the ingestion of tobacco. Cholera rewarded his unsuccessful efforts to heal a patient by killing him. A colleague who specialized in *wisidatu* medicine also died from cholera in the early days of the epidemic. The Mariusan community could only speculate that some sort of sorcery was to blame for these sudden, violent, and inexplicable events.

Many Venezuelans died in a cholera epidemic in 1854–57, which reportedly began in the delta.[4] But no cholera cases had appeared since that time, and Mariusans had never even heard of the disease. Medina and José Rivera described the moment at which the unknown disease thrust them into a nightmarish world of terror and dislocation. "We don't know what that disease is. We don't know—it appeared so quickly," said Medina. "Look, we were eating well." "We were just fine," affirmed Rivera. Medina continued the story.

Salomón Medina, Tucupita, November 1992[5]

We were eating well, eating well, eating well, and then all of a sudden we started shitting all the time. . . . We were living as we always had, we were just fine—look, we were happy. And even though we were just fine, he [Santiago Rivera] started shitting in the middle of the night. He shitted, shitted, he shitted four times. He was getting really sick, he was getting really sick. "I'm getting really weak, I'm getting really weak"—[he] spoke his very last words. When he grew silent after saying these words, he died.

   Since we didn't know what was going on, we didn't know why he died. Because we didn't know what was going on, the people, they said, "Damn! That Warao who knows *criollo* sorcery has put a spell on him with a cross, he died from a spell." We didn't know what was going on then, we thought the guy had killed him. We thought that he had killed him with witchcraft. Since we didn't know anything about the illness, that's why, that's how [we thought] he died. Then the next day another person started shitting just the same. We started shitting early in the morning, and the other guy died a little later.

   We were shitting, the guy was shitting, shitting, shitting, shitting, and when he shitted again he passed out. "I'm going"—those were his last words. Look, then horrible cramps would shake our bodies, and people would die right away, people would die right away, that's how they died. Another, another, and another died, and when dawn came another died, another was shitting, another was shitting just the same way, shitting, shitting, shitting, vomiting. And when people started vomiting, they'd say, "I'm going"—those would be their last words.

When this unknown disease killed two of their most respected leaders and seven others within a few days, the Mariusans became even more frightened, believing that all would die. They boarded their canoes in search of the medicine practiced by *criollos*. Many headed for Tucupita and Barrancas (see map 1). It was only the beginning of a series of horrible experiences that revealed the true nature and meaning of social inequality.

   Cholera had been absent from Latin America for nearly a century. It returned to Latin America nine years before the date targeted in the "Health for All by the Year 2000" campaign that was thrust into prominence by the World Health Organization (WHO). Just as a new revolution was supposedly bringing CNN, Coca-Cola, and democracy (or at least the democratic right to consume) to all parts of the globe, the presence of one of the world's most extensive cholera epidemics suggested that "progress" and "modernity" had left many people behind. The growing gap between the haves and the have-nots was, and is, fostered by economic globalization and the trade and labor policies imposed by the World Bank, the International Monetary Fund, the governments of wealthy countries, and transnational corporations, factors that promote competition and free markets and discourage the social "safety nets" designed to help poor populations. The cholera stories that we heard and have recorded here offer sobering testimony about the fate of poor populations, especially people of color, in today's world.

Racism was a crucial factor that placed people in Delta Amacuro state "at risk" from cholera. Venezuelans who live in the delta region are classified as either *indígenas* or *criollos*—as either indigenous or nonindigenous persons. Most of those who died from the disease in the region were *indígenas,* classified as members of the "Warao ethnic group," which numbers about 24,000.[6] Both *indígenas* and *criollos* are Venezuelan citizens, but a person's racial classification shapes nearly every aspect of day-to-day life in the region. These people died, by and large, because racism affected the distribution of vital government services such as health care and water and waste treatment facilities, as well as economic and other resources, and affected how individuals who received them were treated. When germs and race mix, however inadvertently, the result is often fatal.

The devastating effects of the epidemic continued to be felt long after it was officially declared to have ended in mid-1993. Faith in vernacular healing was undermined, and institutional physicians and their medicines, particularly antibiotics, came to be seen by many delta residents as possessing magical powers. After the cholera scandal had passed and the reporters had returned to Caracas, the impressive infusion of physicians, medicines, boats, and gasoline disappeared. The cholera epidemic and the subsequent exodus of Mariusans and their neighbors to major cities had discomfited the state government, threatened its legitimacy, and further stigmatized Delta Amacuro as being a bastion of backwardness and ignorance, a premodern cancer on a modernizing country. "The Warao" were seen not simply as an embarrassment and an obstacle to exploitation of the delta's resources, but as a political liability. Therefore, the few clinics established in this vast area were often without even aspirin on their shelves. When patients were turned away by disillusioned physicians and nurses, institutional medicine was also delegitimated. "When they wanted to save our lives, they did," noted one delta resident. "Now they want us to die."

This scene may seem far removed from the experience of residents of Europe and North America. Cholera is, after all, not a major concern in wealthy countries of "the North." Or is it? Government officials worry that epidemics of Third World diseases, whether spread accidentally or disseminated deliberately by terrorists, could produce widespread death. Agencies such as the U.S. Department of Defense and the Centers for Disease Control have created units to plan for the threat of bioterrorism, which security analysts in the United States commonly cite as the new clear and present national danger. Films such as *Contagious* and *Outbreak* and books such as Laurie Garrett's bestseller *The Coming Plague: Newly Emerging Diseases in a World out of Balance* have contributed to the public's growing fear of killer "bugs." As anthrax circulated through the U.S. Postal Service and killed five persons in the fall of 2001, these fears came to life as people opened the daily mail and watched the evening news. Emerging and "re-emerging" diseases are tied to anxieties that deadly germs are passing from Asian, African, and Latin American bodies and environments into white bodies, anxieties that are exacerbated by talk of immigration and population increase. Race and class clearly lie at the core of these fears.

THE IMPORTANCE OF NARRATIVE

The story of the cholera epidemic in Delta Amacuro is not a simple tale of Machiavellian conspiracies or evil power mongers who gleefully marked others for death. It is, rather, a story of well-trained professionals who, in general, took their obligation to protect the health of the public quite seriously. It is not a tale of a backward Third World country where callous officials were ignorant of or unconcerned with modernizing health care. The citizens of oil-rich Venezuela have long prided themselves on being a shining example of democracy and modernity in Latin America. Moreover, the denigrating images and timeworn stereotypes attached to the *indígenas* and the poor in the epidemic were not invented in Venezuela alone. Medicines, techniques of diagnosis and treatment, technologies, manuals, statistics, reports, and interpretations are transnational, moving rapidly among public health institutions around the world.

Images of Latin American cholera patients began to circle the globe in reports issued by WHO and the Pan American Health Organization (PAHO) as soon as the first cases were reported in Peru in January 1991, and they found their way into government agencies and newspaper articles and television reports. Descriptions of cholera patients were circulating in Venezuela ten months before *Vibrio cholerae* crossed the border, affecting how Venezuelans perceived the disease and the people it infected. Ideologies and practices of social inequality—particularly ways of perceiving and relating to persons in terms of their ability to internalize modern hygiene and bio-medical conceptions of health and disease—were disseminated at the same time.

Each cholera story created a dramatis personae, a series of events, and a set of causal inferences, casting some parties as heroes who acted wisely and courageously, others as villains who promoted death for gain or glory, and still others as pathetic bystanders not smart enough to get out of the way. Employees in the public health sector, from the state director to physicians and nurses in small rural clinics, people who survived the illness and relatives and neighbors of those who did not, vernacular healers, politicians, government officials, political activists, entrepreneurs, soldiers, journalists, and the people in the street all told cholera narratives. Stories circulated throughout the region with incredible rapidity. Governors, public health officials, taxi drivers, and patients frequently told the same narratives, albeit in different ways.

It is, of course, not simply the content of cholera narratives that rendered them potent. Until stories are retold, they have little impact. It is crucial to ask how stories circulate. Which stories became part of official statements by regional, national, and international public health authorities? Which accounts of cholera made it into the regional and national press? How were explanations of cholera morbidity and mortality—who gets infected and who dies—retold in policy statements? And how were stories that provide alternative explanations kept from circulating or denied legitimacy? In examining the mechanisms through which stories were produced, transmitted, imbued with legitimacy, and challenged, we see that narratives had very real effects on how people lived and died.[7]

Does it matter what sort of stories were told? Wasn't it more important to figure out why people were dying and what could be done to prevent additional deaths? The problem is that stories are just as real as germs and bottles of rehydration solution. Stories reported by the media were particularly powerful. Accounts in Caracas newspapers included what reporters saw and heard on the streets of Tucupita. Their stories put public health institutions on the line. They forced officials to act. Nevertheless, by constantly quoting public health officials and using their statements, journalists shaped the language that came to characterize the epidemic and inadvertently confirmed these officials' status as the sole authoritative source of information regarding the epidemic. Alternative stories, including those told by people living in the most deeply affected communities, became nearly invisible.

Cholera historian Charles Rosenberg suggests that epidemics follow a routine dramatic structure, in that they "start at a moment in time, proceed on a stage limited in space and duration, following a plot line of increasing and revelatory tension, move to a crisis of individual and collective character, then drift toward closure." At the same time, epidemics are "mirrors held up to society," revealing differences of ideology and power as well as the special terrors that haunt different populations. Thus, while illness narratives told during and after epidemics may help people cope with the search for order that takes place when sickness shatters our commonsense perspectives on daily life,[8] much as the exchange of stories helps people deal collectively with disasters,[9] competing narratives characterize the same events in quite different ways and invite highly contrastive sorts of remedial action. For many public health officials, stories that explained "why *they* are dying," directed to politicians, colleagues, journalists, and the public, involved survival of a different sort: institutional survival. When pictures of dying *indígenas* appeared in national newspapers and television programs, officials in Caracas and politicians in Tucupita started looking for scapegoats. Stories that attributed the epidemic to the geography of the delta and particularly to the culture of the *indígena* population transferred the blame onto the communities in which deaths abounded.

To be sure, cholera stories varied widely. Nevertheless, narrators tended to view the epidemic either in terms of its broad social, political, and historical factors or as a medical and epidemiological phenomenon. For those who adopted the first strategy, the epidemic thus took its place among stories of racism, labor exploitation, land expropriation, human rights violations, transnational commerce, environmental degradation, and international conflict. What people knew or learned about the Persian Gulf War, international commerce, and the environmental problems produced by transnational corporations deeply affected how they perceived and reacted to the disease. Cholera was cast in some of these narratives as the unintentional by-product of broad economic and social forces; in others it was a weapon of mass destruction used intentionally to finish a job begun five hundred years earlier: the extermination of *indígenas*. According to this perspective, the sharp increases in social inequality produced by the Venezuelan economic crisis of the 1980s had created expendable populations without access to health, economic well-being, or justice. And according to this perspective, the fact that cholera was killing poor people of color should have surprised no one. These stories would suggest that *cholera is a disease of modernity, globalization, and social inequality.*

Other narratives treated cholera as a biomedical phenomenon that could be explained by the introduction and spread of *Vibrio cholerae*. These stories isolated the epidemic not only from the economic crisis but also from the way that racialization—a process of imbuing a broad range of phenomena (for example, bacteria) with racial meanings—structured access to health care, jobs, education, and other services.[10] The disease became an "indigenous problem," closely aligned with an entire population, at the same time that it was individualized—that is, tied to the attitudes and behaviors of the specific people it infected. These narratives were created largely by public health officials and disseminated widely by the media. They came to play a key role in shaping the ideologies that guided institutional practices. At the heart of these narratives and their ideological effects lay the anthropological language of culture. Having identified *indígenas* or, more specifically, "the Warao," as responsible for transmission of the disease, the stories detailed how cultural beliefs and practices transformed individual bodies into natural bearers of disease. One of the major concerns of this book is the institutional use of cultural reasoning to blame poor populations for the devastating effects of racism and economic globalization, which is evident far beyond the rain forests of Delta Amacuro.

Cholera created a charged, high-stakes debate about the lives of the people it infected, and competing stories bore quite different policy implications. Some of these narratives cast people who suffered from the disease as modern subjects who demanded the political, economic, legal, and health rights they deserved. If you accept these stories, the solution would seem to lie in ending institutional racism and making fundamental changes in how power and resources are distributed. If you believe the individualizing, cultural narratives, then there is little that *can* be done, since culture cannot be changed through legislation or institutional policies. Cholera stories thus illustrate the dual significance of images of social inequality, serving both as representations of how poor people of color are placed within modernity and as a means of regulating access to jobs, education, legal protection, medical treatment, and capital. In other words, in purporting to describe the lives of the poor, such discourses play a key role in shaping them. Given the role in fostering social inequality played by globalization, its moral and political legitimacy hangs in the balance.

Because public health officials, reporters, and politicians believed that the blame ultimately lay in cultural difference, it was easier to adopt short-term policies aimed at ending the scandal than to move toward medical and social justice. Once the dust had settled, health conditions were worse in the delta, and persons classified as *indígenas* became the targets of more virulent racism. Pinned with the responsibility for branding Delta Amacuro as a backward, cholera-ridden region, they became even less welcome in the land they have occupied for centuries. Those who moved to the small cities near the fluvial area did so because they believed that they would never escape death in the delta. In these cities they lived in the most inhumane conditions. To this day, *indígenas* travel to Caracas to beg on the streets. Their lives are certainly no less "at risk" than they were during the epidemic—the nature of the risk has simply changed.

The epidemic and the stories told about it point to the crucial importance of people's relationship to medicine, public health, and hygiene in determining the way they are treated by nation-states—in other words, in determining their status as citizens. Although the language of citizenship has been connected frequently with questions of inclusion and equality, scholars have recently argued that it has often provided a framework for excluding or subordinating particular communities; accordingly, "citizenship has entailed a discussion [of], and a struggle over, the meaning and the scope of membership of the community in which one lives."[11] Scholars have suggested that citizenship involves civil and social as well as political elements.[12] Arguing for a notion of cultural citizenship, a number of Latino researchers have suggested that the notion of a dominant culture can serve to exclude individuals and communities who are believed to embody a distinct culture.[13]

Sanitary citizenship is one of the key mechanisms for deciding who is accorded substantive access to the civil and social rights of citizenship. Public health officials, physicians, politicians, and the press depict some individuals and communities as possessing modern medical understandings of the body, health, and illness, practicing hygiene, and depending on doctors and nurses when they are sick. These people become *sanitary citizens*. People who are judged to be incapable of adopting this modern medical relationship to the body, hygiene, illness, and healing—or who refuse to do so—become *unsanitary subjects*. I explore how becoming infected with cholera became a key means of characterizing *indígenas* and other poor Venezuelans as unsanitary subjects.

Once a population was cast into the realm of the unsanitary subject, the characteristics of race, class, and gender that seem to exclude them from the ranks of sanitary citizens often led to differential treatment of individuals who bore such characteristics by clinicians and public health professionals. In analogy with the way drivers of color are often singled out in the United States for traffic stops and searches ("racial profiling"), we refer to differences in the distribution of medical services and the way individuals are treated based on their race, class, gender, or sexuality as *medical profiling*. Thus, assumptions made about "the Warao," delta residents classified as *indígenas*, affected who was warned about the possibility of an epidemic, how communities in which cholera cases were reported got treated by doctors, politicians, and the military, how they were characterized in the press, and what decisions were taken once the epidemic had ended. The implications of being relegated to the status of unsanitary subjects were profound, affecting people's access to the political, social, and civil dimensions of citizenship—and, ironically, to health care itself.

AUTHOR AS NARRATOR

A reader's perception that a story "tells itself" is a powerful illusion created by the author, who extracts a story from the words of its narrator and the setting in which the story emerges. Retelling cholera narratives plays a crucial part in shaping their social and political impact. By resituating so many stories in these pages, we too become part of the politics of the epidemic and of social inequality. So it seems only fair to tell my own story of how I became a part of this narrative process.

Trained as an anthropologist, I conducted research in my home state of New Mexico for fourteen years, as both an activist and a scholar. There I concentrated principally on documenting ways that Spanish speakers, who often call themselves *mexicanos,* talk about the past. I attempted to discern the role that such talk plays in communities that are fighting for cultural and political-economic survival.

I first went to Delta Amacuro state in 1985, drawn by the advice of Venezuelan colleagues who suggested that research on social dimensions of the predominant language used in the delta, Warao, and how it interacts with Spanish might be useful in bolstering programs in bilingual education and health care. I lived in Delta Amacuro from August 1986 to July 1987, working primarily in two areas, Mariusa and Murako (see map 1). The people who live in Mariusa had not previously welcomed a researcher into their midst. Since very little Spanish was spoken there at the time, Mariusa proved to be an excellent place to improve my linguistic skills. In both areas I documented how social relations and power were shaped by the different ways that people used language in telling stories and in gossiping, giving speeches, mediating conflicts, teaching, asking for jobs and government services, and defending themselves against land expropriation, exploitation, and assaults on dignity and human rights. A key focus was the role of speech, song, and therapeutic touch in vernacular medical practices. I left in August 1987, but I have returned to these communities nearly every summer.

In 1992 a letter from a bilingual schoolteacher reached me in New York, bearing the forbidden word *cholera.* Newspapers published in Caracas ran stories on the outbreak, and subsequently other friends conveyed the news to me in letters, the occasional telephone call, and even an e-mail message or two. Conversations with anthropologists and others who had worked with Warao communities for decades countered this information. First I was told, "It's not cholera, it's just the normal diarrhea that kills Warao this time of year." Given the high rate of death due to diarrheal disease, this was hardly good news. Later the story changed to "isolated cases of cholera." Having spent a week in the midst of a cholera epidemic in Ecuador in 1991, I was skeptical. Except in areas where cholera has become endemic or where chlorinated water and sewage treatment are widely available, the chances of there being only "isolated cases" are few. My response was typically gringo: "Can't we *do* something? I can raise money to help with treatment and relief efforts. Can't IVIC [the Instituto Venezolano de Investigaciones Científicas, the leading scientific university] send a medical team?" My colleagues repeated that there were only a few cases, that the situation was under control. I wasn't reassured. When María Eugenia Villalón, a fine Ph.D. student of mine, defended her dissertation at IVIC, I went to Caracas for the examination. I decided to go to Tucupita for a couple of days to see for myself just what "isolated cases of cholera" might entail.

What I found horrified me. I listened to story after story of cholera, how it had come, whom it had infected, how their bodies had been afflicted. And I decided that if I ever wanted to make what I had learned during my stay in the delta of any real value, now was the time to act. I made plans to return the following summer. In June and July 1993 I worked with leaders of the Mariusan community and government officials to enhance the community's ability to prevent cholera and other illnesses and to increase access to health care. I also recorded a wide range of accounts of the epidemic.

In June 1993 I met Dr. Clara Mantini, then director of the Rural and Indigenous Health Program for the Dirección Regional de Salud (Regional Health Office). Clara began her career working with a team of left-leaning activist physicians in Amazonas state (map 2). Amazonas, which lies on Venezuela's southern border, is also recognized as an "*indígena* state." It and neighboring states in Brazil are home to *indígenas* called Yanomami. Massacres by Brazilian gold miners and recent accusations that anthropologists promoted warfare and epidemics to enhance their own reputations have thrust these communities into the global media.[14] Clara was the director and resident physician of a small clinic that served a population classified as belonging to the Piaroa and Guahibo *étnias*. (*Étnias* are defined as communities of *indígenas* living within a particular territory.)

Clara then accepted a post in Delta Amacuro. Although she expected to

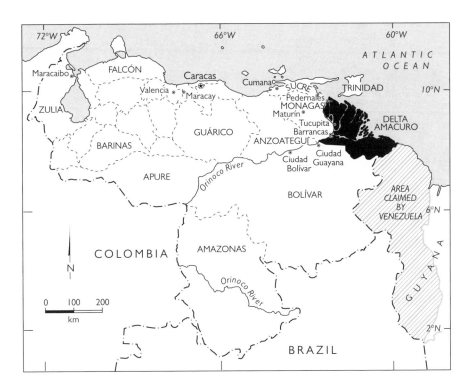

Map 2. Venezuela, showing states and cities mentioned in the text. Darkly shaded states are those with substantial indigenous populations.

do extensive work with *indígenas* in the fluvial region, she was initially denied permission to travel into the delta. Budgetary limitations were cited. The ban ensured that she could not have much direct impact on health conditions there. When the first cholera cases were reported in Pedernales (map 1), however, administrators were only too happy to accept her offer to lead efforts to treat patients and to stop transmission of the disease. She accordingly gained a great deal of firsthand experience with the epidemic, both in communities in the fluvial region and in public health offices in Tucupita, where she worked as the assistant to the regional epidemiologist.

After meeting in 1993, Clara and I began to work together. We inaugurated a pilot project in Mariusa designed to demonstrate that it is possible to deliver community health services and to create a health education program that can change health outcomes even in an area where lack of access to health care is acute and health conditions are among the worst. We worked to establish collegial relations between vernacular healers and representatives of the public health sector. At the same time, since future cholera epidemics in the delta were extremely likely, we decided to collaborate in an intensive, systematic study that would be tied to a health education program aimed at preventing cholera and other infectious diseases. After undertaking preliminary work in 1993, we began fifteen months of intensive work in June 1994.

Clara and I visited every area of the delta. We were accompanied by Tirso Gómez, an intelligent, knowledgeable, and energetic resident of a community near Nabasanuka. We conducted interviews in most of the larger communities and a multitude of smaller settlements. We assessed the impact of the cholera epidemic on each community and probed the range of social, cultural, and political responses it engendered. Our goal was to document (1) how many individuals had been infected by cholera and how many had died, (2) how residents used vernacular and institutional medical systems, (3) how various actors conceived of cholera and its etiology, and (4) how the epidemic had affected the community in both the short and the long run. In the delta we interviewed fifty-three people in Warao, thirty-three in Spanish, three in English, and seven bilingually in Spanish and Warao.[15] In the course of one encounter near the Guyanese border I interviewed three people simultaneously, one in English, one in Spanish, and one in Warao; I will never forget either the exchange or the roar of the waterfall in the background.

We selected interviewees in such a way as to obtain maximum geographic coverage, since experiences even in neighboring communities were often quite different, and a cross-section in terms of age, gender, social position, occupation, and degree of bilingualism. We attempted to speak with all medical personnel who had had close contact with cholera patients. Although we did not use written protocols, we tried to get the same baseline information for each area while leaving plenty of room for people to tell their stories with as few interruptions as possible. We interviewed a wide range of persons, including patients, relatives of individuals who had died from cholera, lay and institutional medical practitioners, community leaders and government officials, missionaries, entrepreneurs, fishermen, and other residents. With the help of community leaders and vernacular healers, we conducted nineteen focus groups aimed at sparking collective discussions of the epidemic and its aftermath.

In addition, Clara assessed health conditions in the communities we visited. Equipped with supplies provided by the Dirección Regional de Salud, she provided free medical attention. In communities with very limited access to health care she sometimes treated fifty patients a day. When a nurse was not available I assumed that role, even though I doubt that I was a credit to the profession. In each area we inaugurated a health education program that centered on preventing future outbreaks of cholera and diminishing the incidence of other diseases.

The recordings made in the delta were supplemented by extensive interviews in Tucupita and surrounding cities. We spoke with physicians, nurses, and other medical workers who had treated cholera patients, as well as with politicians, missionaries, merchants, taxi drivers, journalists, and officials in a wide range of government agencies. In addition to documenting the epidemic, we studied political, economic, and legal dimensions of contemporaneous events. In Caracas and other cities we interviewed officials in the Ministerio de Sanidad y Asistencia Social (MSAS, the Ministry of Health and Public Assistance) and other institutions, members of Congress, officials in the U.S. embassy, and representatives of other agencies. In Tucupita, Caracas, and other parts of Venezuela (excluding the fluvial area), we interviewed fifty-three people in Spanish, twenty-six people in Warao, one person in Spanish and Warao, and one person in English. We also participated in three focus groups each in Warao and Spanish. At the same time that we attempted to maintain a good cross-section in terms of age, gender, social position, and occupation, we focused on eliciting as broad a range of types of experience as possible and on interviewing important players in the epidemic, including the governor, the directors of the regional health service and the regional epidemiologist, the director of the regional office of indigenous affairs, *indígena* activists, opposition politicians, journalists, and others.

Visits to New York (UNICEF and other agencies), Atlanta (the Centers for Disease Control, or CDC), Washington (PAHO), Geneva (WHO), and Bangladesh (International Centre for Diarrhoeal Disease Research, Bangladesh) provided us with firsthand information on how cholera research is conducted and how clinical and policy-oriented formulations are generated at the international level. We conducted eleven interviews in Spanish and eleven in English in these sites, and we also attended meetings and conferences at which cholera was discussed. Whenever possible, interview materials were supplemented by documentary evidence, including regional and national newspapers, official reports and publications, manuals, flyers, correspondence, and photographs.

Nearly all of the interviews were tape-recorded; the only exceptions were in places (such as the U.S. embassy in Caracas) where recording was not allowed. Recordings in Warao were transcribed and translated into Spanish by Rosalino Fernández of San Francisco de Guayo, who was assisted for several months by Elizabeth Gómez. Estrella Mantini transcribed all the recordings in Spanish. Several individuals, including the author, transcribed the interviews in English. Given this tremendous volume of material, I had to be very selective in deciding which interviews to use in this book. I tried to include a variety of experiences while highlighting narrators who particularly illuminated what took place. Since respondents often commented on a number of aspects of the epidemic, it was often necessary to draw material from different parts of the interview. Ellipses indicate where these breaks occur or where shorter segments have been edited out to eliminate repetitions, asides, and the like. The transcriptions are verbatim, except when I edited out my own exclamations or other responses that did not seem to significantly shape what was said.

Many narratives retold here poignantly portray a situation of profound human suffering. The way that people talked about cholera exerted very real effects on who lived and who died in Delta Amacuro. Although the racialization of cholera centered its fatal effects on people classified as *indígenas*, we are all affected by the larger process of globalization and the invocation of a logic based on strategies that attempt to rationalize social inequality in order to justify institutional shortcomings. Failing to take adequate measures aimed at preventing cholera epidemics among the poor and then asserting that their deaths provide evidence of their inferiority were crucial by-products of attempts by individuals, populations, and nations to claim the mantle of the modern. Cholera narratives suggest just how powerful these imaginings of modernity continue to be and, at the same time, reveal the magical sleight of hand that sustains them. Preventing such unconscionable and unnecessary deaths demands a concerted and collective effort to challenge denigrating imaginings of modernity, race, and inequality and the practices they justify. In the case of infectious diseases, this project must cross lines of race, class, and nation. Once undertaken, it will enhance the chances of survival and the level of well-being for all of us.

Witnessing this human catastrophe in Delta Amacuro and being involved in attempts to prevent more needless suffering and death left me with a deep sense of responsibility. I feel it is particularly important to convey this information to as wide an audience as possible because much of it has been actively suppressed, thereby precluding more visible and substantive responses on the part of national and international audiences and organizations. At a time when "emerging" and "re-emerging" infectious diseases threaten populations in both the so-called Third and First Worlds, reflecting on the outbreak of cholera in Venezuela and on the regional, national, and transnational forces that made it so deadly raises crucial questions about globalization's nature and effects. We need to recognize why these diseases are creating critical social and political as well as medical problems worldwide as we begin the twenty-first century. I hope to increase awareness of the fact that people in industrialized countries play active roles in *creating* these problems, not simply in extending acts of charity aimed at lessening their brutal impact. This book attempts to disrupt the circulation of stories and practices that kill, foster critical awareness of the politics of health and inequality, and support global cooperation and justice.

1 Preparing for a Bacterial Invasion

Cholera and Inequality in Venezuela

Peruvian public health officials formally notified their Venezuelan counterparts of the cholera epidemic in January 1991. The announcement generated immediate anxiety within the Ministerio de Sanidad y Asistencia Social (MSAS), the national agency responsible for Venezuela's public health infrastructure. Although cholera was not officially reported in Venezuela for ten months, the disease became the primary focus of attention. MSAS became, to borrow Michael Taussig's pun, a nervous system.[1]

The national offices of MSAS are in the South Tower of Plaza Caracas (photograph 1), a complex that houses the bureaucracies responsible for national policies on immigration, culture, employment, justice, and taxation, as well as public health. Venezuelan citizens and foreign residents stand for hours or days on sidewalks and in waiting rooms, hallways, and staircases, hoping to obtain the magical pieces of paper that are believed to hold the power to link individual interests to state power. MSAS occupies hundreds of offices on all eight floors and in the basement of the South Tower, but no patients are seen here. It is a publicly inaccessible zone.

Regional MSAS offices throughout the country are closely attuned to the words and numbers produced within the South Tower's walls. Long before MSAS announced the first cases of cholera, its efforts to promote a flow of information were coupled with a deep concern about its regulation. Using cholera guidelines and materials developed by the World Health Organization (WHO) and sent to MSAS by an equally nervous Pan American Health Organization (PAHO), MSAS began to produce its own materials for officials and physicians. In May 1991 MSAS published a booklet oriented toward public health professionals, the *Manual de normas y procedimientos para la prevención y manejo de enfermedades diarréicas y cólera* (Manual of norms and procedures for the prevention and management of diarrheal

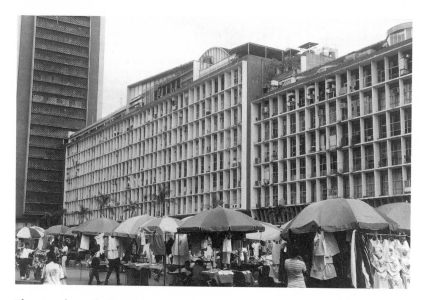

Photograph 1. The headquarters of the Ministry of Health and Public Assistance, in Caracas, is located in the building on the right, overlooking a plaza often occupied by street vendors. Photograph by Charles L. Briggs.

diseases and cholera). Besides promoting "coordinated activities of prevention and control," it sought to "extend through all of the areas of Public Health the unification of basic, current knowledge and strategies to pursue in the fight against cholera and all diarrheal diseases."[2]

Cholera also began to dominate the relationship between MSAS and the press. The publication of stories about cholera involved a daily dance between officials and reporters. Starting in early February 1991, articles appeared almost daily in the benchmark newspapers *El Nacional* and *El Universal,* and they appeared frequently in national tabloids, the regional press, and television and radio news reports. International news services, including Agencia EFE, the Associated Press, the New York Times News Service, Reuters, and United Press International, carried stories on the Latin American cholera epidemic. In addition to using these sources, Venezuela's larger papers soon began assigning their own reporters to develop articles that drew upon press briefings, meetings, and on-the-street observations in exploring the possibility of an epidemic in the country. Venezuelans were largely dependent for their knowledge of the epidemic on this intense interaction between public health officials—particularly the minister of health, Pedro Páez Camargo—and reporters.

From the start, the language used to describe cholera was spatial. Defining the epidemic in terms of its location within and capacity to "spread" beyond national borders provided a narrative structure that appeared over and over. Just as cholera was characterized as having been "born in India,"[3] Peru became the point of origin for the disease and its permanent home in the Americas. A standard line in articles began, "The epidemic, which first appeared in Peru...."[4] The focus of cholera stories progressed through a number of stages: a neighboring country was "threatened" by cholera; the beginning of the "invasion" was signaled by the first few cases, which were usually portrayed as "imported" from another nation-state; a rising morbidity and mortality count was adumbrated; and then cholera moved toward a new national border. Thus, through a slow cyclical process, cholera, like the unseen specter in a ghost story that comes closer and closer to the protagonists, remained newsworthy for months, generating new events that demanded the attention of reporters and readers.

In these stories Venezuela was depicted metaphorically as a corporeal or social body that was about to be invaded by the disease. *El Nacional* characterized the nation as a house that was being secured against the threat of an intruder: "Cholera has two doors by which to enter Venezuela: Zulia, where it is already looking in, and Bolívar state, due to the riverine port and the movement of Brazilian miners and *indígenas* who are closely associated with Colombia."[5] Here cholera was anthropomorphized—granted the capacity to create plans of action and to use them in reshaping social and natural worlds—by being likened to a criminal staring in through the window, waiting for an opportunity to break into the house. In *El Mundo* cholera was cast as a wolf waiting to attack.[6] One article, "The Assassin at the Door," stated that "like one of the horsemen of the Apocalypse, the infectious agent *Vibrio cholerae* gained speed as it rode toward the borders of Latin American countries."[7] Cholera became a threat to the health of not just individuals but also the nation-state.

Such metaphors created a sense of impending doom while generating the reassuring feeling that public health authorities were protecting the body politic by securing the country's borders. Military metaphors were used in regard to neighboring Colombia—"declaration of war on the Colombian-Venezuelan border"—a rhetoric that was, ironically, often juxtaposed with statements about binational cooperation.[8] Since Colombia acknowledged cholera cases in mid-March 1991 and the first official cases were not reported in Venezuela until early December, this militaristic lexicon had a long time to coalesce. The metaphor of a Colombian invasion fit a familiar national rhetoric: Venezuela regularly blamed its neighbor for a host of economic and political problems. The power of spatial and nationalistic language was remarkable. Cholera was clearly an international phenomenon, in terms of its "pandemic" reach across continents and the effects that economic globalization had on public health infrastructures and health care systems and the rapid circulation of capital, people, goods, information, and germs. Nevertheless, these reports seemed to make the nation-state and its geopolitical boundaries more real, confirming them as the natural units for understanding something as important as the threat of widespread death and disruption.[9]

Another dimension of the metaphorical construal of cholera had to do with its agency—the capacity to act in accordance with a concrete plan. *Vibrio cholerae* cannot get very far under their own steam. Human beings and the machines they build, along with ocean and riverine currents and the like, move these bacteria from place to place. Nevertheless, newspaper accounts, like many reports by leading scientists and public health officials, imbued *Vibrio cholerae* with quasimilitary agency by implying that cholera was a force that could conquer new terrain and push across national borders. Other metaphorical constructions granted cholera the capacity to move but denied it intentionality, equating it with other processes of diffusion. Adopting a metaphor that was particularly appropriate for a major oil-producing country, Pedro Páez Camargo asserted in August 1991, cholera "spreads slowly like an oil stain *[mancha de aceite]*, and there are no methods that enable us to know when it will arrive."[10]

Great pressure was placed on MSAS "to intensify epidemiological surveillance in order to prevent the consequences of a possible entrance of the cholera epidemic in our country."[11] Cholera, a bacterial disease, was often characterized as a virus, perhaps owing to concern over HIV, Ebola, Hanta, and other "killer" viruses or over the persistent presence of dengue. In mid-February MSAS reported that it had established a "cordon sanitaire" on its border with Colombia. This measure apparently consisted of subjecting persons arriving from countries where cholera cases had been reported to rigorous inspection and, in some cases, continuing to keep track of these individuals for several days. In February it was reported that closing the border was being considered among various "emergency measures."[12] "Cholera controls" greeted airplanes and ships arriving in Venezuela from "affected countries."[13] When cholera cases were reported in Colombia, public health and other government institutions in Venezuela were placed on "maximum alert."[14] All these measures involved close collaboration between military and public health personnel.

That this nationalistic discourse had at least some effect on popular perceptions of the disease is evident in polls taken on the streets of Caracas in late April. *El Nacional* reported that 91 percent of Venezuelans believed that their country's borders should be closed to prevent a cholera epidemic.[15] To be sure, talk of defending Venezuela's borders against Peruvians, Ecuadorians, and Colombians and the image of foreign carriers of cholera entering the country, perhaps illegally, linked cholera to anti-immigrant discourses that blamed citizens of these countries for economic and social problems.[16]

STATISTICAL IMAGININGS AND OFFICIAL AUTHORITY

Weaving the nation-state into the fabric of cholera stories augmented the authority of public health authorities not only over preventative measures but also over who would control information about an epidemic. Venezuelan law grants the director of the Oficina Nacional de Epidemiología (National Office of Epidemiology) the authority to provide information about "controlled diseases," such as cholera, to other institutions and the public. Article 20 of the "Rules Governing Obligatorily Reported Diseases," which became law in 1939, states that "all data that officials of the [ministry of] Health obtain regarding obligatorily reported disease are by their nature private, [and] officials who reveal them are subject to" fines, imprisonment, or removal from their positions.[17] The legislation pertains only to epidemics, however, and the statements issued between February and November 1991 all preceded the first reported case of cholera in Venezuela. The primary spokespeople on cholera were Pedro Páez Camargo and Luís Echezuría, head of the Oficina Nacional de Epidemiología.[18] Their authority was enhanced by newspaper articles that treated press briefings by these and other national officials as newsworthy events.[19]

How could Venezuelan authorities be so sure that their information was correct? Figure 1, which depicts the structure of the offices of epidemiology, is taken from the MSAS *Boletín Epidemiológico Semanal,* an official means of conveying national health policy and information to regional offices.[20] The head of the División de Enfermedades Transmisibles (Division of Communicable Diseases) has access to information provided by other countries and by international health authorities such as PAHO and WHO. This division head, in turn, consults with the minister of health and other officials. At the bottom of the chain of command, district epidemiologists pass along policies and procedures to local hospitals, clinics, and other offices. These agencies are required to report statistics on the cases they encounter to the district epidemiologist, who sends them back up the chain to the national office. Parallel to this chain of command is a hierarchy of laboratories that extends from local to national facilities. The national laboratory, in turn, forwards some

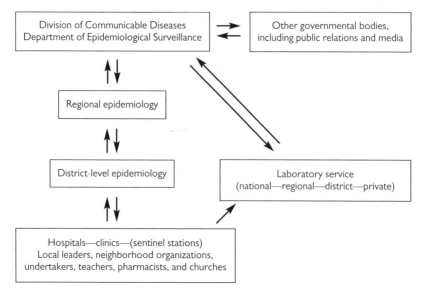

Figure 1. Flow chart of schema of epidemiological surveillance for cholera, MSAS, adapted from the *Boletín Epidemiológico Semanal* 46 (1991): 71. Courtesy of the Ministry of Health and Social Development.

samples to international reference laboratories such as the one at CDC in Atlanta. The lines that connect epidemiological and laboratory departments are crucial. Epidemiologists determine which samples are to be processed by their corresponding laboratory, and they have official access to the results.

Because the microbiological knowledge produced in national MSAS facilities was privileged, MSAS could declare competing information to be false. The laboratory facilities of the Instituto Nacional de Higiene (INH, the National Institute of Hygiene) in Caracas were refurbished to enable MSAS to analyze samples of feces, water, and food for the presence of *Vibrio cholerae.* The press, which covered the renovation, assured the public that INH personnel were working seven days a week to maintain their vigilance over the disease.[21] The institute's director declared in May 1991, "It is up to the INH, with the support of its investigations, to say: 'cholera has begun.'"[22] The INH laboratory provided MSAS with a scientific monopoly over the technologies that control the production of truth and falsity in statements about cholera,[23] thus Páez Camargo, Echezuría, and the national reference laboratory of the Instituto Nacional de Higiene became distinct obligatory passage points in controlling the flow of information about the disease.[24] Cholera could not officially arrive in Venezuela without passing through the INH laboratory, and information on the disease could not reach the press or the public without passing through the mouths or pens of the two designated MSAS officials.

At the same time, public health authorities went to great pains to point out that cholera is *trans*national, that it "does not recognize borders."[25] On the same day that the first cases in Colombia were reported, an article in *El Nacional* asserted, "The experience gained since the appearance of cholera has demonstrated that outbreaks cannot be prevented in any country, but its dissemination can be contained through control measures."[26] It was similarly stated that "no Latin American country is immune to the cholera epidemic" and that the disease "is now invading the continent without respecting its borders."[27] WHO and PAHO had long stressed that quarantines, cordons sanitaires, and import and export embargoes are ineffective because too many carriers are asymptomatic and too much illegal immigration and trade occurs. They also emphasized that focusing on such measures diverts energy and resources away from much more effective steps, such as improving sanitary infrastructures, creating cholera prevention committees, and training health professionals and the public. Although this transnational rhetoric seemed to contradict the nationalistic language that appeared so frequently, using both enabled MSAS to enhance its institutional power—which is generally much less than that of the military or the interior ministry, for example—*and* to try to avoid being blamed once the "inevitable" occurred and cholera "invaded" Venezuela.

One of the major modes of telling the story of the cholera epidemic was through statistics. Totals for the number of cases and deaths in particular countries and in the Americas as a whole were often the main focus of stories. The release of new cholera statistics by PAHO or WHO officials was covered by international news services. Just as societies have come to be imagined in statistical terms,[28] questions of health and disease are projected statistically in public health discourse; in turn, the mass media have come to see the use of numbers as being just as central to public health as to demographics and economics.

A common focus in such accounts was on numbers that were explicitly imaginary—projections of the future course of an epidemic. Thus, 270,000 cholera cases were projected for Guatemala in July 1991, and 3 million cases, with 30,000 deaths, for Brazil in December 1991. Estimates of between 90 million and 120 million cases were projected for the Americas in July 1991, and in June 1991 *El Nacional* reported WHO's estimate that 25 percent of Latin America's population was "in danger" of contracting cholera.[29]

Cholera was similarly imagined in Venezuela before cases were reported.

One estimate suggested that 83 percent of Venezuelans were "vulnerable" to cholera.[30] Just as statistical constructions of what is "normal," "marginal," and "deviant" can influence perception of a population, statistics shaped how Venezuelan readers placed themselves in relationship to cholera. If 83 percent of the population was "vulnerable," then relatively few persons could afford the luxury of positioning themselves as neutral observers. If they believed the numbers, most people had to imagine that the scenario was one from which they could not easily escape. Nevertheless, race, class, and gender shaped how people placed themselves with respect to these projections.

TYING CHOLERA TO POVERTY

Discussions of cholera in other countries and the possibility of an epidemic in Venezuela created a prominent public space for debating questions of social inequality, as Páez Camargo implied in 1991: "Cholera is an undemocratic disease because it affects a very specific part of the population in which hygienic variables are extremely marked."[31] A crucial focus, both before and after the first case of cholera was reported in Venezuela, was denoting exactly which part of the population was most "susceptible" to the disease—and why.

In the popular imagination cholera is widely associated with Asia, specifically India. An article that appeared in *El Nacional* in April 1991 cast cholera as a disease whose "date of birth coincides with the development of ancient Oriental civilizations." The newspaper tied the illness to India's poverty in cultural terms: "Because of religious beliefs the cows are worshipped while the population dies of hunger." Poverty, filth, and superstition were all set in opposition to modern medical science: "The Hindus considered the Ganges as a sacred river, but just the same they threw their excrement there, just as they drank and bathed. Thinking that it was a punishment by the gods, they let themselves die without knowing that it was the work of a simple bacillus that leveled entire populations in a matter of days."[32]

Even when transposed into the final years of the twentieth century and onto the American continent, cholera continued to be characterized as the disease of poverty, the Third World, and underdevelopment. Cholera had become a leading means of sustaining Orientalism, the notion that peoples from North Africa, the Middle East, and Asia occupy a social realm that is forever alien, premodern, superstitious, and undemocratic.[33] In fact, epidemiological historians have suggested that cholera is a modern disease, one that dates from the demographic and economic transformations of the early nineteenth century, notwithstanding the possibility that similar microbes with less epidemic potential may have existed previously.[34]

Two distinct if overlapping discourses linked poverty and cholera to Latin America and the present.[35] One characterized both as *hemispheric* problems, as dimensions of a broad economic crisis; the other treated them as national problems tied to a particular segment of society. PAHO director Caryle Guerra de Macedo took the first view, stating that cholera "could cause 6 million cases and leave 40,000 dead, because it is fed by the poverty and marginality that is punishing the region."[36] A number of writers suggested that the depth and breadth of poverty was the result of economic crises that had led to cutbacks in public services and to the deterioration of water and sewage infrastructures. In Peru radical voices blamed structural adjustment programs imposed by international lending organizations, thereby characterizing the problem as a result of globalization and deeply implicating the industrialized nations of North America and Europe. This discourse of cholera and poverty pointed to the powerful as bearing substantial responsibility for a possible epidemic. Because the debate on social inequality was related to a significant threat to human life, it was charged with a sense of danger and urgency. Peruvian critics developed this critique much more forcefully into a broad attack on neoliberalism.[37] They placed poverty within a larger political-economic frame, resisting the discourse of poverty that stigmatizes the poor as producing their own misery.

In Venezuela, even though globalization was partly responsible for a rapid slide into poverty and structural adjustment programs were a prime target of the 1989 popular insurrection, these issues seldom emerged explicitly in public discourse about the epidemic. Since running water and sewage facilities had become central indicators of modernity during the nineteenth and twentieth centuries, some critics pointed to the growing inaccessibility of these services for vast segments of the Venezuelan population. For opposition politicians, particularly members of the Partido Movimiento al Socialismo (Movement toward Socialism Party), talking about cholera and poverty was an accessible means of attacking the Partido Acción Democrática (Democratic Action Party), which was in power at the time. It seems plausible to suggest that this debate helped create the critical discourse on power and poverty that Lieutenant Colonel Hugo Chávez Frías attempted to transform into a political base through the coup attempt that he directed on 4 February 1992, two months after the Venezuelan epidemic began.

Statistical constructions of poverty provided a highly visible arena for political debate. Public health authorities, nongovernmental organizations, opposition politicians, and journalists all generated their own superimpositions of these discourses. *El Nacional* reporter Ludmila Vinogradoff suggested that the newspaper's staff relied on figures taken from the second national inventory of barrios in Venezuela to project that "seventy-two Caracas barrios would be prey to cholera."[38] When a parastatal agency, Fundacresa, announced that 35.63 percent of the population fell below the "relative poverty line" and that 43.56 percent lived in "a state of critical poverty," *El Nacional* reporter Marlene Rizk declared that these figures indicated that 83 percent of Venezuelans were vulnerable to cholera.[39] Although Rizk did not indicate who made this extrapolation from demographic to public health projections, cholera and poverty were so deeply connected in the minds of everyone that such implications seemed to follow automatically.

The debate on social inequality, like so many others, rested on an unstable base. Demographic projections were taken as reliable scientific windows on the social world, crystal balls that could be used to read the choleric—and perhaps political—future. Even when these figures were used to attack government actions and institutions or neoliberal policies, they confirmed the authority of statistics for imagining the public, foreseeing the future, and planning the nation. Statistical constructions are generated by institutions.[40] Although some institutions are "nongovernmental," they are generally staffed by professionals, and they derive their funding from either the state or the bourgeoisie—individuals who enjoy the material advantages of the middle class and assume their social superiority to the working class. Thus, even spokespeople who criticized the government and neoliberal policies on behalf of the people confirmed that professional discourses—and the people and agencies that produced them—were more powerful than the forms of knowledge produced by the people whose possible suffering and death were foretold.

A second and quite pervasive way of imagining poverty and cholera looked precisely in the opposite direction, to persons who had *less* access to power and resources, in characterizing the way the two phenomena were linked. Given the nationalistic frame of the discussion, this "geography of blame," as scholar, physician, and activist Paul Farmer has trenchantly called it, often took the form of stories about why other countries were reporting cholera cases.[41] Constantly referred to as the place where the epidemic began, Peru became cholera's hemispheric point of origin, its natural American home. The epidemic in Peru was attributed to that country's status as "one of the poorest nations in South America," its economic collapse "caused by civil war and a growing external debt." The crisis that deprived residents of clean water and sewage facilities was blamed on "years of neglect" by Peruvian governments that "ignored sanitary measures."[42]

Nevertheless, the sources that created a space for nationalistic comparisons between Venezuela and its seemingly poorer and more backward neighbors were *trans*national. In an article on Peru that was published in *The New York Times* and reprinted in *El Nacional*, poverty was described as being not simply economic but *cultural*: "In Pampas San Juan, a fly-infested barrio that is typical of the barrios that surround the city of Lima, clean water is a prohibitive luxury. An open-air hut is the communal bathroom, and you have to walk a long way to find a sanitary installation." In such descriptions "sanitation" and "hygiene" became questions not just of infrastructure but of the population's lack of "hygienic practices." Echoing the stereotypes that link India and cholera, the article asserted that "in some places, poverty also engenders fatal superstitions." The poor thus became at least partly responsible for their own status as patients because they believed that the cholera outbreak was caused by the evil eye and because they obtained help from "a primitive curandero." These superstitions reportedly prevented them from believing that cholera can be transmitted by water—even though the article also described a single mother of three who spent the majority of her income "trying to obtain clean water."[43] Here the power attached to the circulation of cholera narratives becomes apparent: a reporter took images of poverty, filth, and premodernity and imbued them with an eyewitness's sense of immediacy and authenticity; the result was a story that naturalized North American imaginings of South Americans and then recirculated them in South American newspapers.

The "origin" of this account within the U.S. press is particularly ironic. The story nationalized cholera as Peru's problem, thereby leaving out the role of the United States, other rich nations, and international organizations in fostering the policies and practices that played a key role in creating the situation. The title of the story suggests that the article is about South America, not just Peru. I want to underline this point. By reprinting it, the Venezuelan press pointed a finger at Peru, Ecuador, Colombia, and other neighbors and helped circulate and add legitimacy to stigmatizing stories that ultimately denigrated Venezuela as well. The images of social inequality used in attempts to deflect blame ultimately disempower everyone.

The geography of blame that linked cholera and poverty remapped Venezuela itself. In an address delivered at a conference, "Cholera Is Everyone's Problem," and reported in *El Mundo*, Dr. Francisco Aráez asserted, "Cholera is an infection that typically and almost exclusively affects very poor people."[44] The term Aráez used, *gente miserable*, is also commonly used to designate individuals who are villainous. Discussions of poverty and cholera in the press focused on the *cerros* ("hills," referring to hillside communities) or *barrios marginales* of Caracas and other urban centers. In this context "marginal" conveyed a sense of people who stand outside democratic politics, the formal economy, the law, and morality. In the bourgeois imagination, *barrios marginales* are places where promiscuity, violence, criminality, and psychopathology are pervasive and natural.[45] Discourses of poverty decontextualize and depoliticize images.[46] The link between hillside barrios, the poor, and cholera helped to reimagine popular protest as a timeless product of poverty rather than a strategy for dealing with the differentially distributed effects of a particular political-economic crisis.

The residents of these communities figured prominently in the popular protests in 1989 over President Carlos Andrés Pérez's attempt to impose neoliberal economic policies at the beginning of his term. This sector continued to be the focus of resistance, middle-class anxiety, and political repression in the early 1990s.[47] The bourgeoisie referred to the 1989 action as *cuando bajaron los cerros*, "when they came down from the hills." Reporter Asdrubal Barrios's reference to "the daily descent of tons of fecal material from the hills" that was converting Caracas into a cholera "time bomb" merged powerful images of people and sewage, thereby juxtaposing fears of cholera and those associated with popular insurrection.[48]

Reporters and public health authorities often refined the notion that cholera is the disease of poverty by linking the disease explicitly to filth, thereby helping to exclude the first way of connecting cholera and poverty. Vinogradoff suggested that "filth [*suciedad*] is this character's [cholera's] favorite habitat for multiplying its fatal action. And the best place it has found for propagating is the marginal areas."[49] Suggesting that the streets of Caracas "smell of cholera," Barrios referred to *suciedad* as the parent of cholera and "its best ally."[50] Milagros Polanco, chief of the División de Control de Alimentos (Food Control Division) of INH, stated that "in the places where poverty reigns, people are often not educated to be able to perceive cleanliness as a healthy way to live."[51] The phrase she used, *falta la educación*, can refer either to a lack of education or, more idiomatically, to a lack of sophistication and manners. Whichever way you read the statement, it reflects the common conviction that barrio residents were ignorant of and failed to practice hygienic norms. By creating filthy environments "they" marked themselves as the likely targets of cholera. The equation became firmly established: barrio = poor = dirty = cholera.

Poverty was not the only characteristic that accorded communities the dubious honor of being "at high risk" for cholera—*indígenas* took their place alongside the poor and "residents of hillside barrios" as potential bearers of the disease. Zulia state (see map 2, page 13) contains the largest population of persons in Venezuela who are classified as *indígenas*. They are generally referred to as "the Waayú" (also spelled "Guayú") or "the Guajíro."[52] Even before the first cases were reported in Venezuela, Senator Lolita Aniyar de Castro linked "the Waayú" to cholera:

> With the entrance of cholera in Zulia state, there is a serious risk of an epidemic of considerable proportions among the members of the Waayú *étnia*, since the great majority of those who live in Sinamaica and Paraguaipo don't have the most elementary sanitary services in the region, in addition to which they drink water from springs *[jagueyes]*, where the animals drink, they don't have latrines, and their hygienic habits are primitive.[53]

The two rhetorics of poverty intersect here, drawing attention simultaneously to the paucity of public services in the Sinamaica and Paraguaipo areas and to the "hygienic habits" of the Waayú, which, according to the senator's statement, seem to predestine them to become bearers of cholera. The image of the *jaguey* evokes an old stereotype that equates *indígenas* with animals.

When he was pressured to close the border with Colombia, Páez Camargo stated that the action "makes no sense because the Guayú indigenous ethnic group, which is the one that has been affected by the disease, is geographically and culturally a single entity, which feels the same in Colombia as in Venezuela and has no concept of physical border."[54] Any resident who did not recognize the importance of the Venezuela-Colombia border was not a participant in the political life of the nation and could make only weak claims to substantive citizenship. Páez Camargo made the statement during an epoch in which *indígenas* were pressing for recognition of their political, territorial, and human rights. This statement could have been interpreted as supporting the view that political parties and government institutions need not respond to the *indígenas'* demands for political representation because they had excluded *themselves* from the political process.

Reporters played a key role in turning official statements into public opinion. Given their professional concern with separating "fact" from "opinion" or "rumor" and relying on objective and authoritative sources, journalists often depended heavily on institutions, which could be counted on to generate news on a regular basis. Knowledge of the disease was medicalized—as such knowledge usually is—meaning that biomedical professionals were the primary sources of authoritative information.[55] Because the cholera story involved epidemiological information, and because the government employed most epidemiologists and controlled the production of health statistics, the symbiosis between reporters and institutions was especially pronounced as both sought to imagine a possible epidemic. Venezuelan newspapers often incorporate the perspectives of interest groups or opposition parties that differ with official stances, but since lay and public health perspectives were accorded such different weights, reporters found it unnecessary, even impossible, to look for the opposing points of view that would give their stories a "balanced" or "objective" perspective. Páez Camargo and Echezuría thus became the primary definers of the cholera story. They evoked the discourses of nationalism, poverty, and race that were used in telling it; they proposed the metaphors that would shape perceptions of the disease, its "victims," and persons and institutions responsible for prevention and control efforts; and they decided who could become characters in the story and what sorts of roles they would play.[56]

This is not to say that journalists simply repeated what these individuals said. They exercised selectivity, deciding which statements were newsworthy and how to make them interesting to readers. This problem was acute in that reporters had to hold their audience's attention as they continued to tell essentially the same story day after day. To be sure, playing on people's growing fear as cholera cases were reported closer and closer to Venezuela was crucial, but the spatial element proved to be insufficient from mid-March until early December, when cases were reported in Colombia but not, as expected, in Venezuela. One technique was to link cholera to ongoing journalistic themes such as poverty, popular unrest, crime, drug trafficking, urban decay, and, to some extent, *indígenas.* Another was to bring in bizarre elements or to add humorous and/or grotesque touches, as with Barrios's reference to "the daily descent of tons of fecal material from the hills."

The active role of reporters is perhaps most evident in the way they translated clinical, microbiological, epidemiological, and other types of technical information into lay terms. The result was a heteroglossic language containing enough technical jargon to impart the authority and prestige of science into paraphrases of public health information and statements cast as the words of the proverbial person on the street. Journalists represented the public by incorporating public reactions through quotes and polls and summarizing public reactions to official statements (that is, to stories they had already published). The cycle of cholera reporting that emerged from January through November of 1991 thus achieved closure, setting the limits as to what sorts of information were deemed relevant to the cholera story, who the players were, and what roles they were assigned—and making it difficult to get other types of accounts into the press. Even if MSAS was sometimes judged to be playing its part badly, its officials could count on reporters to naturalize the rules they sought to establish for representing cholera in the public sphere; this cycle was established before any cases were reported in the country and MSAS could be held accountable. Claiming to speak for those who presumably could not speak for themselves—the poor and the *indígenas*—disguised the complex process through which journalists helped create a hegemonic discourse. Only a cold and heartless person could question the politics of their expressions of concern for the downtrodden.

Representing the public also helped draw attention away from the process through which cholera stories portrayed Venezuelans. Those whose habits and mental dispositions seemed to place them beyond cholera's grasp were construed as *sanitary citizens*. They became complex subjects who possessed a full set of normative economic, cultural, familial, legal, educational, sexual, and medical characteristics. Sanitary citizens were identified by their status as Venezuelans rather than being marked specifically in terms of a single dimension, such as social class. The state assumed the obligation of protecting them from *Vibrio cholerae* after suggesting that they were in any case unlikely to be infected. Persons whose ignorance, place of residence, occupation, poverty, race, and unhygienic habits placed them at risk for cholera became *unsanitary subjects*. They were identified primarily by means of one feature of their social identities, either class (often coded in terms of place of residence, occupation, or speech) or race, thereby becoming simple or one-sided subjects. Unsanitary subjects lacked the broader set of characteristics that would have enabled them to adequately fit the model of the modern citizen, and thus they could be denied access to jobs, legal protections, and human dignity. They seemed to be intrinsically linked to a particular package of premodern or "marginal" characteristics—poverty, criminality, ignorance, illiteracy, promiscuity, filth, and a lack of the relations and feelings that define the nuclear family. Because the bodies and minds of unsanitary subjects seemed to be inseparable from their despicable environments, the state had to protect them from their own natures and desires—in short, from themselves. At the same time, the state isolated its unsanitary subjects because its sanitary citizens had to be protected.

THE HEALTH EDUCATION CAMPAIGN

Television, radio, and print media carried statements by public health authorities that stressed the need to take cholera prevention measures. In addition to weaving recommendations into articles on the epidemic, newspapers frequently printed guidelines as a separate section, intended to be cut out and posted, such as this one entitled "Measures for Avoiding Cholera":

- Wash vegetables with water and vinegar for half an hour.
- Cook fish and seafood well.

· Avoid foods purchased from street vendors [comidas ambulantes].
· Wash fruit before eating.
· Boil drinking water ten minutes or freeze filtered or bottled water.
· Also wash kitchen utensils with boiled water.
· Wash hands with soap and water before preparing food, serving children, [and] after going to the bathroom, taking care of someone who is ill, or cleaning up after children.
· Combat flies; since they come to rest on feces and contaminated water, [they] become vehicles of transmission. Use insecticides, and deposit trash in plastic bags and keep them shut.
· Use bathrooms and latrines.
· Prepare powdered milk with boiled water or drink pasteurized milk.[57]

Institutions often formulated their own sets of rules or guidelines, thereby getting advice on cholera prevention—and their agency's names—into the press.

The health education program adopted what Cindy Patton refers to as a classic hypodermic model—that is, the idea that problems can be solved by a direct injection of information.[58] MSAS created an authoritarian discourse that projected the sense that only one proper response was available to viewers: receiving the information exactly as it was intended by state authorities and using it to produce the desired behaviors.[59] Venezuelan public health authorities constantly underlined the centrality of "individual responsibility."[60] A top public health official of Táchira state declared, "It won't help at all if we health authorities make the effort to fight against the disease if the community doesn't support us by paying attention to the recommendations."[61] Politicians articulated the importance of health education through the language of citizenship and civic participation. A Caracas high official attempted to mobilize "the community" by setting up "anti-cholera commandos" consisting of a local official, a physician, and five neighborhood leaders for each parish. Rather than waiting with crossed arms for the government to act, he stressed the importance of "making each citizen into an ally."[62] A member of the Cámara de Diputados (Chamber of Deputies) similarly suggested that "each citizen must transform himself into a guardian [fiscal, literally, "prosecutor"] of his own home, place of study or employment, and community, to demand compliance with the rules that have been issued; and when we can make sure that our neighbor protects himself adequately, we are protecting ourselves as well."[63] This is not to say, however, that everyone accepted this attempted transfer of responsibility. One reporter noted that in response to efforts to organize "anti-cholera commandos" and health education messages, "the neighbors complain that the anti-cholera campaign has focused in such a way that it seems as if the only one who is responsible is the ordinary citizen. 'Doesn't the government also have to assume some responsibilities, such as provisioning the hospitals, cleaning up the streams, providing the population with potable water?'"[64]

To whom was the health education "campaign" directed? This question seems silly at first glance. The use of the mass media and the placement of posters in such public spaces as bus terminals and government offices would seem to target all Venezuelans. Nevertheless, televised messages showed well-dressed women demonstrating hygienic measures in well-equipped, middle-class kitchens. The media campaign seemed oblivious to the economic constraints that rendered the implementation of such procedures difficult or impossible for the majority of Venezuelans. Polanco and the PAHO representative for Venezuela commented that, in contrast, Colombian authorities directed their cholera education campaign at working-class audiences.[65] The health education program was thus burdened with a fatal contradiction. Although public health authorities produced statistics that placed the majority of Venezuelans in poverty and constantly asserted that the poor were at the greatest risk from cholera, the thrust of health education efforts was toward a minority of Venezuelans, precisely the population that was characterized as being much less at risk.

The use of an information deficit model that located threats to public health in the ignorance of individuals effectively divided Venezuelans, once again, into sanitary citizens and unsanitary subjects. Being rational and modern, the former were deemed to possess the knowledge of science and hygiene and the educational foundation needed to assimilate information regarding the prevention and treatment of cholera. Such widely used models of health education assume a linear relationship between knowledge, attitude, behavior, and practices; thus, sanitary citizens would acquire the proffered knowledge, display the appropriate attitudes, adopt the desired behaviors, and incorporate them into their routine practices, thereby confirming their rationality and normalcy.[66] Unsanitary subjects purportedly departed from this model at all points, failing to acquire the proper knowledge, being resistant or uncooperative, not adopting the appropriate behaviors, and failing to change their routine practices. The breakdown of health education programs confirmed their lack of rationality, modernity, and civility, the factors required for full citizenship, sanitary or otherwise. The importance of this perceived failure to master cholera prevention measures for defining sanitary citizenship was heightened by the tendency to look for people to blame during epidemics of infectious diseases, especially ones that spread rapidly and are associated with premodernity and poverty.[67]

The state could then construct its responsibility to unsanitary subjects as twofold: the highly visible health education efforts theoretically provided people relegated to this class with the means of converting themselves into sanitary citizens. If the "campaign" failed, an outcome that was foretold from the beginning, then medical profiling—conducting surveillance and control efforts aimed at particular populations—seemed to be the only option. The possibility of confronting health—and thus economic and social—inequities thereby disappeared from official and media discourses.

The government's role could be defined as providing information and conducting surveillance of unsanitary subjects, not overcoming health inequalities. By being asked to regulate the conduct of family members, neighbors, and co-workers, sanitary citizens were invited to help the state to police the border that separated them from unsanitary subjects. The state succeeded in deflecting the blame for a cholera epidemic—in advance—onto its unsanitary subjects and rationalizing their lack of access to health care, highquality education, sanitary infrastructures, housing, political representation, and justice.

Even if health education programs were misdirected from an epidemiological point of view, they seem to have been well designed to cope with institutional and political fallout. The prospect of a cholera epidemic must have seemed to officials like a powder keg ready to ignite popular discontent with an increasingly unpopular president and to provide fuel for opposition politicians. By focusing on health education, officials could partially deflect criticism from the nation-state and onto individuals who failed to embody modern citizenship. The discourses of risk and transmission placed responsibility particularly on the backs of the poor; the *indígenas*, who had long defined the limits of "the national society" by virtue of their exclusion from it; and the residents of the barrios, who were the standard scapegoats for the social evils associated with the economic and political crisis. The photographs of poor communities that often accompanied these articles helped to make this shift in responsibility seem real and natural. At the same time, health education efforts individualized cholera—the disease was linked to the beliefs and behavior of individuals and households. In televised images and the wording of articles and guidelines, cholera was also gendered: women were portrayed as bearing the primary responsibility for protecting their families against cholera through good hygiene.

Addressing the health education "campaign" primarily to the middle class made sense from another angle. The two parties that dominated Venezuelan politics from the time that democracy was reestablished in 1958 until the 1990s, the Partido Acción Democrática and the Comité de Organización Política Electoral Independiente (COPEI), had excluded peasants, *indígenas*, and the urban working class from real political power.[68] Facing the possibility of a political crisis if cholera claimed many lives in Venezuela, officials followed the same strategy by presenting an educational program that targeted the middle class as the embodiment of sanitary citizenship—that is, as individuals who were capable of preventing cholera. In the event of a catastrophe the politically potent bourgeoisie would be convinced that the government had done everything possible to prevent cholera. At the same time, the distribution of cholera cases would mark those communities that had apparently failed to embrace health education and hygiene—in short, that had caused the epidemic through myriad individual acts of failure to follow guidelines. The bourgeoisie could once again blame the poor, rural and urban, for the persistence of the premodern world in Venezuela.[69]

The most strident and consistent criticism was directed toward street vendors who sold hot dogs and hamburgers, homemade candy, drinks, fruit, and other items. Public health authorities warned the public not to purchase food or drinks on the street, and the press focused on health risks associated with itinerant food vendors. Even though some articles acknowledged that many customers were middle class, the sale of food on the street was cast as one of the "cultural effects" of poverty and was described as "Third Worldish" *(tercermundista)*.[70] Journalists created vivid images of filthy food stalls replete with swarming flies, cockroaches, and "microbes and bacteria that make fun of cleanliness and dance to the cholera beat *[el son del cólera]*."[71] Cholera had become so thoroughly identified with street vendors by late October 1991 that the reporter who fashioned this poetic image, Barrios, could describe these sites as exhibiting "a proclivity for all kinds of disease, principally cholera," even though no cases had been reported in Venezuela. Barrios also linked dirt and disease to other vices:

> From the corners of Puente Nuevo to those of Puerto Escondido, this reality beats plainly *[pulsa crudamente]* in dark alleyways where [people] play with the health of citizens in the domain of foodstuffs and also in the domain of pleasures, converting one of these corners into a pimping strip where ladies of the night catch the innocent.
> This picture is rounded out by the sale of cigarettes in the new method, one by one—twenty-five of these enterprises could be counted in the narrow space of these central capital district streets, not to mention the bars,

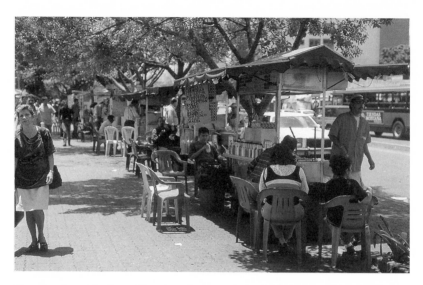

Photograph 2. Vendors of hot dogs, homemade foods, desserts, and beverages line up near Plaza Venezuela in Caracas. Photograph by Charles L. Briggs.

lottery ticket sales, terminals and other gaming devices, forming a daily flirtation with vice and corruption.[72]

Poetic pretensions aside, Barrios's story provides a striking example of the use of strong negative imagery in suggesting that street vendors were breaking not only sanitary but also moral codes, linking them to a sexist image of predatory sex workers. This article, like so many others, was accompanied by photographs of street vendors, tying these often extravagant descriptions to everyday scenes from the sidewalks of Caracas (photograph 2). Even researchers, journalists, and opposition politicians who used the epidemic to criticize the government generated images of street vendors as unscrupulous purveyors of cholera.

It would appear, however, that this attempt to transfer blame onto a politically and economically marginal sector backfired to some degree. Journalists, opposition politicians, representatives of nongovernmental organizations, and others began to criticize MSAS and local governments for failing to undertake their responsibilities in inspecting and regulating the vendors. As a result, MSAS joined municipal health authorities, groups representing the itinerant merchants, the police, and the military in an effort to increase the regulation of street food, prohibiting items (such as cabbage and homemade sauces) deemed most likely to spread cholera, inspecting sanitary conditions, issuing permits, offering courses in hygiene, and confiscating the carts of noncompliant vendors. These well-publicized efforts affected only a tiny fraction of the fifty thousand persons estimated by Páez Camargo to make their living in this manner.[73] Admitting in advance the failure of this program, officials disseminated guidelines to the public that effectively asked potential customers to take on the role of inspectors, transferring the government's responsibility to "the consumer himself."[74]

There is a larger lesson here. The sale and consumption of food and drink on the street grew markedly in the 1980s and 1990s. In the face of massive underemployment, unemployment, and prices that were increasing much more rapidly than wages, some workers had been driven out of the formal economy and into the ranks of vendors, while others used these sales to supplement wages.[75] Many of their customers faced longer work schedules, longer commutes, and/or the need to work more than one job. For them, cheap food purchased on the street helped meet both temporal and economic constraints. The press placed these enterprises in the informal economy, and it depicted officials in a tragic role: intent on wiping out this threat to public health, they were unable to do so in the face of popular demand. This "vicious cycle" of cholera transmission was squarely rooted in interactions between people on the street. The focus on street vendors implied that government institutions and "formal" capitalism were out of the picture, except as critics, which helped to shield them from blame.

By presenting themselves as neutral observers of urban disorder and by relaying public health officials' characterizations of urban residents, neighborhoods, and street vendors, reporters helped to maintain the illusion that the people themselves—rather than economic globalization or government policies and practices—were responsible. By fetishizing the vendors' transactions, the health education program transformed a pervasive social and political-economic *effect* of globalization into the *cause* of increased incidences of infectious diseases. Rather than a predilection on the part of individual vendors and consumers, these conditions are part of a process that has engulfed many Latin American cities in a structural chaos so deep that the state can no longer effectively claim the ability to maintain order.[76] This inversion of cause and effect—and the adoption of medical profiling procedures—was accomplished by cholera discourses even before *Vibrio cholerae* appeared in Venezuela.

REPRESENTING AN EPIDEMIC

It happened in early December 1991: the first case of cholera was reported in Venezuela. A truck driver from Colombia apparently ate food contaminated with *Vibrio cholerae* before crossing the border en route to Caracas. After entering Zulia state, he became ill and checked into a Maracaibo hospital on the morning of 3 December. Páez Camargo did not learn of this event until eleven o'clock on the morning of 4 December, an hour after having testified in Congress that there was no cholera in Venezuela. Although clearly embarrassed, he told the press that he was not alarmed. The country was not in a state of emergency because the incident involved "an imported case."[77]

On 14 December *El Nacional* reported that another crucial chapter in the cholera story was being written. The first cholera death had occurred in Venezuela. The sixty-year-old victim was identified as "an itinerant ice cream vendor, of the indigenous ethnic group wayú," who lived near the Colombian border. The first "fatal victim" of the disease thus seemed to belong simultaneously to *all* the at-risk populations that epidemiologists had identified, being poor, *indígena*, an ambulatory food vendor, and a border crosser.[78] The epidemiological projections that had emerged during the previous eleven months were thus confirmed. Páez Camargo later asserted that the man had in fact died from a rotavirus rather than from cholera.[79]

The rhetoric of the "imported case" lost a great deal of credibility with the death of a five-year-old in Maracaibo on 14 December. The girl had been infected in Venezuela, and tests confirmed that *Vibrio cholerae* was present.[80] This case was so clear that health authorities felt it necessary to declare Zulia in a state of emergency. Despite this, Páez Camargo quickly distanced himself and his country from the death. The girl's father, according to the minister, had commercial contacts in the Colombian city of Maicao, where cholera cases had been reported, and he had probably infected the child. Páez Camargo blamed the girl's death on "the negligence of her relatives, because they didn't take her to a hospital."[81] The collaboration between reporters and officials that thrust this family—rather than Venezuela as a whole— into the geography of blame did not stop there. The family, which was characterized as being "Guajira"—that is, *indígena*—was accused of hiding the cause of death: when the corpse was taken to a cemetery for burial, employees reported a "suspicious death" to health authorities.[82] Public health authorities imposed a cordon sanitaire of two blocks around the child's house and ordered residents of the community to bury their vomit and excrement. This stipulation revealed the poverty of the health infrastructures in the area, a form of "negligence" that could not be assigned to the family.

From this point on Venezuelan papers carried almost daily articles presenting the national body count—the number of cholera cases and fatalities reported by MSAS. The narrative structure that had traced the spread of the disease from country to country was transposed into stories that mapped cholera from state to state. The appearance of the first cases in Táchira (December 1991), the Federal District (January 1992), Miranda (February 1992), Carabobo (February 1992), Mérida (April 1992), and Sucre (June 1992) became newsworthy in turn. Indeed, the stories repeated the nation-to-nation pattern: first came the possibility of an epidemic in a new region, then denials that cholera was present, then claims that the first cases were imported from Colombia or other states, and, finally, a declaration of a public health emergency.

This is not to say that nationalism disappeared from the cholera picture. For example, one headline, "Four Cholera Cases a Day in Venezuela," was followed with the statement "Peru reports 600 a day."[83] Public health officials frequently stressed that Venezuela's epidemic would not be as bad as Peru's because Venezuela was "privileged" in that it had "more sewer facilities than many countries."[84] One of the most important measures of the success of public health systems during a cholera epidemic is the case fatality rate (i.e., the percentage of cases that result in death), and Venezuelan officials congratulated themselves on their success in this regard. The governor of Zulia state proclaimed that mortality had dropped to "zero" in recent months, "thanks to the primary care system that we have been developing since last year."[85]

The transmission of cholera was a central concern of public health authorities. The attack on itinerant food and beverage vendors intensified, and sellers of raw oysters and other shellfish were characterized as the main culprits. These products were prohibited, and criminal action was threatened. Public health authorities were particularly concerned about population movements in connection with Christmas, Carnival, and Holy Week. Since the latter two are popular times for going to the beach, officials worried that bathers would become infected with cholera by swimming in contaminated water or by eating raw clams and oysters sold on beaches. The infected would then return to their homes, spreading cholera throughout Venezuela. Health authorities also blamed the public for failing to follow their guidelines. Finally, *indígenas* received a good deal of attention as cholera epicenters. The ministry's focus was on "the Waayú" of Lake Sinamaica in Zulia and other parts of the border area. Although reporters mentioned the inadequacy of health infrastructures in this area, attention was directed toward questions of hygiene. One MSAS epidemiologist suggested that individuals had infected their own family members, an assertion that was gendered as well as racialized, since *indígena* women were considered to be responsible for family hygiene.[86] The old theme of the Waayú's propensity for frequently moving back and forth across the Colombia-Venezuela border also re-emerged.

Questions of race were often transformed into issues of culture. Epidemiologist Miriam Morales declared some three weeks into the Zulian epidemic that it was "very difficult to work with this population because it is nomadic *[errante]*, and their distinct culture makes them afraid of the steps taken by our physicians."[87] When Páez Camargo was fired as a result of the epidemic, his replacement, Rafael Orihuela, similarly asserted in late January that *indígena* culture was to blame because it led its bearers to actively reject biomedicine: "The problem with the Guajiros is that they don't permit preventive treatment. Their customs, their culture, makes the work very difficult."[88] Echezuría added reliance on alternative medical practices to the list of cultural factors that promoted resistance: "They delay seeking treatment because they prefer their own medical rituals. These deaths in some way follow from sociocultural factors."[89] To counter accusations regarding the government's failure to provide adequate sanitary infrastructures, residents were accused of refusing to use latrines provided by MSAS.

A strong sense of verisimilitude was infused into these accounts through institutional and journalistic ventriloquism. When MSAS built more than a hundred latrines in Zulia, a reporter suggested that *indígena* fishermen rejected them: "'The smell closes in on you, and it bothers us,' some say, trying to justify themselves. Others speak more clearly. 'I don't like them, I prefer the lake.'"[90] The positions of the institutional primary definers of the cholera narrative were thus translated into popular, as well as journalistic, voices. Echoing the long-standing transformation of state violence against *indígenas* into acts of violence perpetrated by *indígenas,* Echezuría asserted that in "Guajiro" neighborhoods residents "arm themselves and confront health commissions."[91] These powerful images created the sense that the situation was so hopeless that cholera would become endemic in this area; accordingly, *indígenas* would be fixed inside a geography of blame and outside the nation-state and modernity. State institutions were cast in the role of generous benefactors who were doing everything possible to provide a surplus of health-related resources to people. *Indígenas,* who are often stereotyped as ungrateful beggars, were depicted as actively rejecting MSAS's gifts, thereby threatening not only their health but also that of all Venezuelans.

Blaming the poor, including *indígenas,* for the epidemic was far more than a means of protecting public health institutions and their officials. Politicians, including President Pérez, were quite concerned that a large epidemic would crush tourism (which it did in 1992) and curtail exports (which it apparently did not). Just as important, Venezuelan leaders of the twentieth century, democratic and authoritarian alike, had worked assiduously to cultivate an image of the country as a bastion of progress and modernity in Latin America.[92] Cholera, with its strong associations with poverty, backwardness, filth, ignorance, and the premodern world, threatened to place Venezuela alongside Ecuador and Peru in the court of world opinion despite its decades of effort to distinguish itself from its "poor neighbors." President Pérez reportedly said before the first cases were announced that Venezuela would never broadcast news of a cholera epidemic should one occur.[93] In anticipating the epidemic, public health discourse sought to isolate cholera in precisely the social sectors that supposedly had rejected the national project of modernity. Once the nightmare was converted into everyday reality, this strategy allowed the Venezuelan government to continue to claim that the modernist core of the nation remained intact.

METAPHORS AND INSTITUTIONAL INSECURITY

Official control over the circulation of information about cholera helped deflect criticism of the Venezuelan government and its agencies. This is not to say that public health officials cunningly used the threat of death to create a sanitary dictatorship. Such a characterization would be false for a number of reasons. First, public health officials' authority to act as the sole source of information regarding cholera did not go unchallenged. Starting in May, the Venezuelan press would commonly report that a cholera case had appeared in Venezuela, only to publish an official denial of the statement's accuracy the following day.[94] Interestingly, public health authorities sometimes challenged the statistics offered by other countries. Richard Huntington, head of PAHO's Cholera Working Group, stated with respect to Latin America as a whole that "the reported cases probably represent barely a small part of the real figures that have emerged in marginal barrios or areas of extreme poverty."[95] It would stand to reason that such statements might lead to popular skepticism regarding the statistical projections of all public health officials.

Second, people sometimes doubted the words of officials and reporters. Many believed that officials were hiding the presence of the disease in Venezuela. An *El Nacional* poll taken in July 1991 reported that 50 percent of the 168 respondents believed that cholera "had indeed come to Venezuela," but that MSAS was "hiding the cases." Only 36 percent of those polled believed that MSAS was telling the truth, while 14 percent said they didn't know.[96] A newspaper poll conducted in February 1991 suggested that 65 percent of Venezuelans "said that they do NOT believe that the authorities will do everything necessary for prevention of the disease." The data revealed a striking gender gap: among the 65 percent of respondents who expressed a lack of confidence in public health officials, women outnumbered men by more than two to one, while nearly eight times as many men believed that MSAS efforts were sufficient.[97]

Some Venezuelans asserted that the "threat" of cholera was entirely illusory. Just as the state was using cholera to shape an image of the poor, popular sectors used the disease to shape the public's opinion of the state. Stepped-up repression after the 27 February 1989 popular insurrection augmented the uncertainty of life in poor neighborhoods. The coup attempt organized by Chávez on 4 February 1992 may have failed, but it created a more visible space for debating the role of the government and evaluating its policies. Popular mistrust contributed to the tendency to regard cholera stories as a smokescreen (cortina de humo) conjured up to keep people from thinking about the crisis and criticizing the government. The degree of closure achieved by public health officials and reporters in limiting the narrative conventions of cholera stories augmented the sense that cholera was a circus act meant to entertain the people while power operated behind the stage, generally to the detriment of those not part of the middle class. Press statements that transferred blame to "marginal barrios" undoubtedly exacerbated such reactions. Similarly subversive readings also emerged in television comedy programs that presented parodies of official statements.

Finally, the word cholera represented perhaps the greatest threat to date to the viability of MSAS. As institutions go, health ministries or administrations have relatively little power. When they compete with military, police, immigration, foreign affairs, and other institutions for influence and resources, health officials seldom bargain from a position of strength. Cholera placed MSAS under intense scrutiny and opened the door to widespread criticism. Before the epidemic began many Venezuelans believed that MSAS had not prepared the country for cholera. An El Nacional poll conducted in late April found that only 1 percent of respondents thought that hospitals were "well prepared" for a possible epidemic, 27 percent believed that hospitals were "somewhat prepared," and a full 72 percent thought that they were "not prepared at all."[98]

From the time that the first cases were reported, people in the street often accused MSAS of a heartless disregard for public health, and this attitude was sometimes echoed by reporters. El Nuevo País captioned a photograph of a broadly smiling MSAS minister as follows: "[Rafael Orihuela] leaves the [presidential] Palace wearing his best smile, in spite of the resurgence of infectious diseases, such as dengue, malaria, and cholera, generated by the complete lack of attention on the part of the government of President

Pérez to health issues (the IMF is only interested in payment of the debt and handing over state industries)." The richly parodic article accompanying the photograph countered Orihuela's contention that "Venezuela can relax" because the government had controlled the outbreak of cholera, asserting that "the risk of new outbreaks of malaria and dengue, newly reborn Third World diseases [*enfermedades tercermundistas*], along with cholera" presented clear and immediate dangers.[99] At the same time that reporters and opposition politicians largely accepted MSAS's biomedical view of the epidemic, they sometimes used cholera as a means of portraying the institution as deceitful, unconcerned with the health of citizens, and responsible for stripping Venezuela of its claims to modernity and thrusting it back into the Third World.

INSTITUTIONALIZING INEQUALITY

Official statements and press reports fundamentally shaped cholera narratives in Venezuela, helping to determine what could be said about cholera and who could say it in public debate. Blaming the poor and *indígenas* for cholera accorded MSAS a key role in reproducing social inequality and legitimating the many sorts of violence that were directed at the people MSAS was attempting to help. Along with nationalist rhetoric, this language of blame encouraged sanitary citizens to place themselves outside of the picture, to think that cholera affected only Peruvians, Colombians, barrio residents, and *indígenas*. It helped to maintain the nineteenth-century idea that contracting cholera is a mark, a stigma, a confirmation of one's status as premodern, unhygienic, ignorant, poor, and Other. It thus helped to undermine the very health education program that MSAS was promoting, since people were not likely to heed advice that did not directly relate to their own situation and that placed them in a stigmatized position. While these statements and reports did not stop people from criticizing inadequacies in health care and health infrastructures, they created a dominant narrative that focused on cultural difference and individual behavior and blamed the epidemic on foreign countries, immigrants, and street vendors. MSAS was portrayed as a benign, if not necessarily powerful, force seeking to penetrate pathological social spheres that it had no hand in making.

I believe that MSAS officials told the story in this way not to consolidate power but to defend their institutions against a tremendous threat to their legitimacy. I think that they were fundamentally guided by the belief that these measures constituted the best available means of preventing a cholera epidemic or at least limiting its extent. I am not talking about vil-

lains or power mongers but about people under political fire. It is crucial to
remember that the way public health officials and others prepared for and
responded to the cholera epidemic does not reflect some sort of Venezuelan
or Latin American cultural pattern. A variety of different perspectives were
evident in official debates and an even wider range emerged on the streets
and within homes. Official statements about cholera were tremendously il-
luminating, revealing the collusion of the leading political parties to adopt
policies that exacerbated social inequality and rhetorics that made it seem
natural and normal. Nevertheless, many Venezuelans began to identify social inequality as the major problem that confronted their society, and they
began to criticize national and international institutions and transnational
corporations for their role in fostering it. Ideologies that justified social inequality and blamed the poor were coming under increasing attack. This was,
of course, precisely the focus of Chávez's coup attempt and subsequent electoral campaign.

This story is not about Venezuela alone. Many of these cholera stories—
and, particularly, the narrative patterns that generated them—were produced
in other countries and by journalists for international press agencies and
officials of international public health organizations. Official reports by
PAHO and WHO, the most influential public health institutions in the
world, also contained echoes of these rhetorics. At the same time, however,
PAHO officials urged their counterparts in Latin America to use cholera as
a context for pressing their governments to make the infrastructural investments in potable water, sewage disposal, and waste treatment that would
help prevent communicable diseases in the long term. One important limitation that hampered such efforts in Venezuela was international in origin:
austerity conditions imposed by international lenders, the World Bank, and
the International Monetary Fund left little room for new investments in
public works.

All the talk about cholera and poverty obscured the factors that fostered
a cholera epidemic in Venezuela. Public health scholars Vicente Navarro and
Richard Wilkinson argue that poverty, in and of itself, does not correlate as
closely with health outcomes as social inequality does.[100] They suggest that
even countries with similar levels of per capita gross domestic product have
very different rates of life expectancy, infant mortality, and other measures
when different degrees of social inequality are present. Although the United
States and Bangladesh lie at opposite ends of the income spectrum, the age-
specific mortality rate for some age groups in the Harlem area of New York
City is higher than it is in Bangladesh.[101] Moreover, it is misleading to limit
poverty to measures of income level, which displaces other factors that re-

late to well-being and the political processes that shape it.[102] In Venezuela, identifying cholera with poverty thus drew attention away from broader questions of social inequality that shaped the likelihood of an epidemic, its potential severity, and effective forms of prevention and treatment. Medical profiling exacerbates social inequality, both by decreasing access to health services for people classified as unsanitary subjects and the quality of care that they receive, further limiting their enjoyment of other citizenship rights, and by creating a social and political climate that is more hostile to them. If social inequality affects health outcomes, then medical profiling is sure to worsen conditions for populations in which life is already precarious.

These assertions served to blame the most powerless members of society for creating the conditions in which they were forced to live. In the end, connecting the disease with "marginal" sectors of society, including *indígenas*, eroded the very conceptual and political foundations of public health. An effective health policy regards health and disease as conditions and concerns that are shared by everyone, not just model sanitary citizens. MSAS and the press attempted to place this sense of a shared mission at the core of the cholera "campaign." As an editorial in the newspaper *2001* put it, "Such a situation calls forth a country to come together [*confluir*] at all levels in a frontal attack on cholera, a task for all Venezuelans, even if it belongs primarily" to MSAS.[103] Citizens were exhorted to assume personal responsibility for cholera control at the same time that they were expected to recognize that they were participating in a collective effort—and to recognize the authority of MSAS to direct it. An outbreak of cholera should bring people together, not give rise to partisan politics and attacks on the government and its institutions. Equating cholera with poverty, immigration, and *indígenas* shattered this conception of *public* health and invited many Venezuelans to excuse themselves from participation. An image of dirty, defective, defecating bodies contradicted nationalistic rhetorics that presented a larger vision of the body politic. This dialectic was particularly fatal when it emerged in Delta Amacuro.

2 Epidemic at the Door
Cholera Prevention in the Bureaucratic Imaginary of Delta Amacuro

As soon as authorities in Caracas learned of the cholera outbreak in Peru, they warned regional public health officials that a cholera epidemic was quite likely to emerge in Venezuela. In accordance with WHO and PAHO directives, MSAS required each state to set up an anti-cholera committee, which was charged with organizing health education campaigns and ensuring that medical institutions were prepared. National officials deemed cholera important enough to merit a week-long course on prevention and control of the disease, held in Caracas in mid-June 1991. Delta Amacuro was represented by its highest institutional officials: Dr. Magdalena Benavides, regional director of MSAS for Delta Amacuro state, and Dr. Daniel Rodríguez, chief of the Oficina Epidemiólogica Regional (Office of the Regional Epidemiologist).

Caracas officials warned Benavides and Rodríguez pointedly that if cholera reached Venezuela it was certain to create an epidemic of cataclysmic proportions in the Orinoco delta. They based their alert on two premises: first, the delta is one of the poorest regions in the country, and the incidence of malnutrition and infant mortality from diarrheal diseases is among the highest in the country; second, the state is deeply associated with "the Warao," who stand alongside "the Yanomami" as quintessential *indígenas* in the national imagination. The death of hundreds or thousands of *indígenas* would cause a national and, perhaps, an international scandal. The implication was clear: Benavides's and Rodríguez's jobs were on the line.

The message did not fall on deaf ears in the case of the regional epidemiologist. Rodríguez is originally from Maracaibo, on the opposite side of the country. He is tall and thin, with short, straight black hair and a long, serious countenance. He exudes the sense that potential chaos and catastrophe are being held in abeyance at every moment through his dogged de-

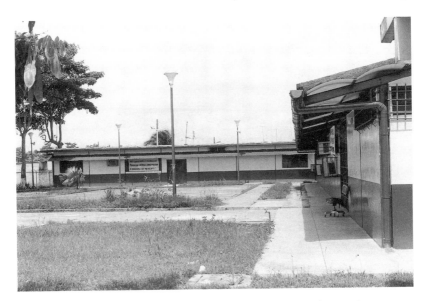

Photograph 3. Office of the Regional Epidemiologist and an adjacent clinic in suburban Tucupita. Photograph by Charles L. Briggs.

termination. Rodríguez regards the mountains of statistics and the manuals of procedures that surround him as objects of devotion, contrasting sharply with most officials in Delta Amacuro, to whom power and money and friendship and connections are at least as important in advancing personal and institutional agendas as statistics, reports, or projects.

After the meeting Rodríguez traveled directly to Tucupita, leaving early in the evening and arriving the following morning at dawn. The bus always passes the outdoor market, which is packed with fish, meat, fruit, and vegetable vendors and customers at this hour, even though the stores, bars, billiard halls, bakeries, cafes, and curio shops of the main plaza are still closed. Rodríguez's office is not located in the MSAS complex in Tucupita proper, but in an unpretentious cinderblock building in Hacienda del Medio, a cross between a middle-class suburb and a poor barrio (photograph 3). The office is the nerve center for epidemiological statistics in Delta Amacuro. Lives, deaths, and illnesses, converted into numbers, are summarized, compared, explained, and sent to Caracas. As one enters the building the heat and relative quiet of the surrounding neighborhood give way to the roar of air conditioners. The regional epidemiologist's office, with its stark furnishings, bare walls, and serene atmosphere, mirrors the occupant's controlled, earnest demeanor.

Fighting off the fatigue from his journey, Rodríguez thrust himself head-long into mounting an effective cholera prevention campaign. If MSAS's goals were met, the citizens of Delta Amacuro would be aware of the disease, would understand how to prevent it, and would know what to do if suspicious symptoms were observed. Medical personnel would be trained in the prevention and treatment of cholera, medical facilities would have stockpiles of supplies, including chlorine for water purification, antibiotics, and rehydration solutions, and an adequate number of hospital beds would be available for cholera patients on an emergency basis.

Rodríguez was determined to pull together a nonpartisan group of top officials within each of the agencies whose support would be needed to meet these goals. Benavides helped decide which institutions and officials to include. The list of members of the anti-cholera committee—the Comité Regional de Prevención y Control del Cólera (Regional Committee for the Prevention and Control of Cholera)—read like a *Who's Who* of institutional power in the state. In addition to public health officials, members included the governor of Delta Amacuro, the mayor of Tucupita, and representatives from the Guardia Nacional (the main unit of the armed forces), the ministries of education, environment, public works, and transportation and communications, and the Corporación Venezolana de Guayana (a powerful government agency that regulates public works and mining for the eastern part of the country), as well as firemen, presidents of neighborhood associations, and representatives of the Defensa Civil, the Capuchin Franciscan mission, and the press.

In an interview conducted in January 1994 Rodríguez described his efforts to carry out the orders he had received in Caracas:

Daniel Rodríguez, Tucupita, 14 January 1994

We formed the Committee for the Prevention and Control of Cholera, in '91. Yes, okay, they were formed in the different states of Venezuela on instructions of the office—the Division of Communicable Diseases—and at the same time on instructions generated by the ministry. . . . Yes, well, it's true that many people from the different agencies didn't come. They didn't come. When a problem arose, that's when they developed a momentary, transitory interest, and everybody met. And when, of course, the representatives from the ministry [in Caracas] came, then they did come, they were present. But the support wasn't what we could call serious. . . . The other agencies, I don't know, weren't sufficiently cognizant, even though there was a very large informational campaign [*campaña de humanización*] here. We even had informational programs long before cholera appeared, where we expressed our concern, those of us who came. I was thinking, what we have been saying here is that, most of all, the most heavily impacted population was going to be the *indígenas,* the *indígenas* and the part of the population that is least served from a sanitary point of view—it's logical, in that there's no hope [for them]. But at no time did the people who could have helped pay attention. They were all, they made some gesture for a few moments. And when we said, "We need this," then there was a series of obstacles.

As he uttered these words, Rodríguez's voice swelled with a mixture of anger and pride, albeit carefully muted. He was quite clearly the only public health official in the state who took cholera seriously, at least in more than a fleeting sense, in 1991. Nevertheless, by characterizing cholera as a potential threat to *indígenas*—and, secondarily, to the poor—he and other public health officials placed the disease within the pervasive system of racialization. Since the *indígenas* were virtually excluded from "the national society," a serious threat to them was of little social, political, or institutional significance. Once the photo opportunity presented by the initial meeting had passed and the write-up had appeared in *Notidiario,* Tucupita's local newspaper, the officials and their agencies had little to gain from investing time or resources in the anti-cholera committee. Accordingly, between February 1991 and July 1992 the committee was born, allowed to become moribund, and then briefly resuscitated several times.

INSTITUTIONAL INDIFFERENCE

Official indifference was strikingly apparent during meetings of the committee. I (Clara Mantini-Briggs) participated in three or four of these gatherings, which took place on a weekly basis. I was bursting with enthusiasm, eager to participate in the decision making that would shape policies for cholera prevention. My sense of urgency had been fueled by having seen cholera cases in Apure and Zulia states. In Amazonas, I was involved in a campaign that targeted a multilingual and multicultural population located in areas accessible only by motorboat and airplane. We trained that population to purify household water supplies by adding drops of chlorine. I thought that Delta Amacuro officials might be interested in the strategies that we used, given that no cholera cases had been reported in Amazonas even when the disease had been reported in neighboring states.

The first meeting I attended in Tucupita, in April 1992, was held in the firehouse. As Rodríguez guided me into the building through a back door, I was greeted by the young firemen. Impressed by the immaculate condition of the firehouse, the modern and shiny fire engine, and the proud, confident, and professional look of the firemen, I asked how many times each year they were confronted with emergencies. Someone responded, "There haven't been any fires in four or five years, but we participate in the vaccination campaign." Someone else added, "And, well, with electoral campaigns as well." Representatives arrived from the governor's office, a number of state ministries, the Malariología (Malarial Institute), the Oficina Regional de Asuntos Indígenas (ORAI, Regional Office of Indigenous Affairs), the office of the Defensa Civil, and the press, but we could not begin the meeting without Benavides.

Benavides, who spent much of her childhood in Pedernales, was trained in social medicine in Mexico. She is short and solidly built and has straight, shoulder-length black hair. Her penetrating eyes convey seriousness and authority. She speaks with a conviction and self-assurance born of having served for years as Delta Amacuro's highest public health official, a leading figure in the Democratic Action Party (AD), and a confidant of political boss and ex-governor José García Gómez. She once surprised high officials from Caracas during a dinner that she was hosting by serenading her guests in full mariachi dress, backed up by a local ensemble. An engaging and often poetic narrator, she can draw her listeners deeply into her accounts. Benavides arrived at the meeting some two hours after the scheduled time. With her entrance the lively exchange of small talk and gossip suddenly gave way to a tense, somber atmosphere. The participants put on timid smiles and began to watch, waiting to see who would score the first point and at whose expense. The meeting abruptly commenced.

Rodríguez took the lead, passing around a list of attendees that he asked each of us to sign. He began the meeting by attempting to convey the preoccupation that had been expressed by national officials during his most recent visit to Caracas, noting that he had been questioned regarding what advances had been made toward preparing for an epidemic now that cholera was spreading to more Venezuelan states. He attempted to dramatize the importance of taking concrete action, but he could not refrain from adding that he would be unable to attend more of these important meetings in Caracas if he was forced to continue paying for travel expenses from his own pocket.

This complaint proved to be a strategic misstep. Benavides saw her opportunity to steal the show. She interrupted, in a maternal voice, "That's true, my boy [mi hijo]. The problem is that allocations by the governor's office for the Regional Health Service's budget have been," she paused momentarily, "suspended." When the governor's representative tried to respond, Benavides cut him short and, pointing to me, announced, "Today we have the pleasure of welcoming a new doctor to the delta, Dr. Clara Mantini, who worked in Amazonas and will be directing the Program in Peasant and Indigenous Health. As you well know, this is the program that I personally created, and if we are graced with the financial support of the governor's office it will enable us to make sure that cholera doesn't come here." Silently the participants, except for the official from the governor's office, smiled in my direction. Rodríguez then pointed out that having a prevention strategy in hand was crucial, which gave me the opportunity to outline procedures for home chlorination of drinking water. Benavides confronted the governor's representative, asking flatly whether his office would be able to donate the eyedroppers and small plastic bottles that would be needed for the program. His reply consisted of a detailed explanation of government procurement procedures that I found impossible to follow, but which Rodríguez succinctly translated as "yes."

Isabel Romero, second-in-command of the Dirección Regional de Salud, interjected that the national MSAS office had offered to donate concentrated chlorine solution and containers for storing water safely in rural communities. As if the lever of a Rube Goldberg device had been tripped, setting off a long series of complexly interconnected events that serve no purpose, the various officials each began offering excuses as to why they could not commit their institutions to providing the gasoline, truck, driver, or whatever part of the operation had been assigned to them. Suddenly Benavides leapt up from the table, declaring that she had to leave for another meeting.

This level of drama and intrigue was absent in the majority of meetings. On some occasions the regional epidemiologist and the fire chief appeared to be deeply absorbed in watching the blades of the fan, the sole source of movement in the room, since no other participants appeared. The frustrating and painful silence at these meetings was interrupted only by the incomprehensible but seemingly mocking commentary offered by the red macaw that was the station's mascot and by Rodríguez's declaration that the meeting was adjourned for lack of a quorum.

This institutional indifference, further expressed by the absence of any institutional commitments, dominated anti-cholera committee meetings until *Vibrio cholerae* appeared in Delta Amacuro in August 1992. As a result, the efforts that were made to prepare Delta Amacuro for a possible cholera epidemic were limited in the extreme. The articles that appeared in *Notidiario* and Caracas newspapers and the news clips broadcast by Caracas television stations gave many residents of Tucupita basic information regarding the disease and guidelines for treatment and prevention. Rodríguez and his staff helped keep the media interested in the subject, and they targeted some health education information at Tucupita's 44,000 residents. In early 1992, for example, the sale of such items as ice, raw seafood, and *tetas* (homemade frozen sweets), as well as the use of raw vegetables in hot dogs and other foods, was officially prohibited, in keeping with national MSAS guidelines.[1]

Probably the most significant step that was taken was to train MSAS physicians and nurses in cholera prevention and treatment. Primary health care was available to the population of the fluvial area largely through type-I clinics, which were staffed by nurses, and the five type-II clinics, which boasted a resident physician. From west to east, these sites were in Pedernales, La Horqueta, Nabasanuka, Guayo, and Curiapo (see map 1, page 2). Patients also visited hospitals and clinics in Tucupita and Barrancas. Doctors in the rural clinics were generally *médicos rurales,* newly graduated physicians who were completing their required year of service with an underserved population. In May 1991 all of the *médicos rurales* were called to Tucupita for a one-day course on cholera prevention and treatment.[2] They subsequently conveyed this information to the nursing staffs in their clinics. This step probably saved many lives when patients with cholera symptoms began to show up en masse in August 1992. It would have been more effective, however, if it had been repeated. By the time cholera appeared, many of the *médicos rurales* who had participated in the training session had been replaced by new physicians.

Unfortunately, this single training session was virtually the only substantive action that was undertaken in the fluvial area to minimize the impact of cholera. Apart from meetings of the anti-cholera committee, the most publicized MSAS activities were occasional *operativos*—intensive efforts over one or a few days aimed at particular communities. *Operativos* were effective in institutional terms because they involved little sustained effort and minimal stays in the fluvial area for town-dwelling personnel yet created an illusion of concern and generated impressive articles in *Notidiario.* Treating a hundred patients in one day does little to transform overall health conditions.

No systematic effort was undertaken to teach the residents of the vast fluvial area cholera prevention and treatment, even though regional health authorities accepted the claim by national officials that the *indígenas* were particularly "at risk." Television and newspapers were seldom available in the fluvial area. Some bilinguals, usually residents who had been schooled in the missions, did learn about cholera before August 1992 from Radio Tucupita. Nevertheless, Radio Tucupita seldom reached many communities because reception was poor and residents lacked the funds to buy radios and batteries. Moreover, the information that was transmitted generally assumed that listeners shared a biomedical model—the belief that infectious diseases are caused by viral, bacterial, and other agents that can be identified by scientists. Many delta residents were more familiar with other theories of disease, including those focusing on sorcery and nonmaterial forces ("spirits"). When people began to have diarrhea and to vomit in August 1992, few residents in the fluvial area had ever heard of cholera. They didn't know that their lives depended on obtaining treatment in a matter of hours.

It could be argued that it would be impossible to inaugurate an effective cholera prevention program for a multilingual and multicultural population in rural areas dominated by rainforest and to expect positive results within a year or so. To be sure, neoliberal economic policies, restraints on social spending imposed by international lending agencies, and an economic crisis certainly made it more difficult to obtain the resources needed to accomplish this goal. Nevertheless, the Federal Territory of Amazonas, in southern Venezuela, did just that. There, Gilberto Rodríguez Ochoa directed a regional health service that served 38,208 *indígenas* identified with nineteen *étnias*,[3] a situation that was certainly no less complex than that in Delta Amacuro.

When González was given the message by national MSAS officials that Amazonas was in the line of fire for cholera—a message that was later reinforced by the nearby presence of cases in Colombia—he held a workshop for all medical personnel, including nurses. Teams consisting of nurses, teachers, and sometimes physicians traveled from community to community, teaching about cholera and how to prevent and treat it. All rural households were given small bottles of chlorine, eyedroppers, and instructions on how to prevent diarrhea by treating drinking water. One community representative was chosen to make sure that water was chlorinated and stored properly and to ensure that household chlorine supplies were replaced when exhausted. In addition, an oral rehydration center was established in each locale. Finally, radios were placed in all clinics, and a team was dispatched from the capital, Puerto Ayacucho, when an outbreak of any type of diarrheal disease was reported. No cholera cases were reported in Amazonas from 1991 through 1993.

BEYOND MODERNITY'S REACH

The failure to make adequate preparations for an outbreak of cholera in Delta Amacuro was exacerbated by discourses that circulated in Caracas and in the delta regarding the separation of the region from the nation-state. The presence of cholera was quite visible in Caracas and other parts of Venezuela, and it provided a means of exposing, representing, and controlling social inequality and attacking President Pérez and the AD party. Cholera stories here were often clothed in the language of nationalism. The situation in Delta Amacuro was quite different. Before August 1992 cholera was not so evident in public discourse in the region. This difference was linked to the way the region positioned itself and was positioned vis-à-vis the nation.

Delta Amacuro state is often described as *el fin de Venezuela* (the end of Venezuela). Another expression heard from time to time in other parts of the country likens the nation to a human body and Delta Amacuro to its anus. As a cab driver in Caracas recently put it, "Delta Amacuro is the end of the world. There is nothing there but wilderness and Indians *[monte e indios].*" Within the region the "non-*indígena*" residents view *indígenas*—not the region as a whole—as constituting the border that fixes the limits of Venezuelan modernity. The hierarchical relationship formed by relations of inclusion and exclusion places the *indígena* population of Delta Amacuro—and, when viewed from Caracas, the state as a whole—beyond the limits of the nation-state and modernity.

This is not to say that the residents of Tucupita and other areas of Delta Amacuro do not consider themselves to be Venezuelans, do not identify with the nation in many contexts, or do not make claims on the resources of the nation-state. Nevertheless, nationalist discourses and issues that take center stage in the political life of Caracas and many other (but certainly not all) parts of the country often fail to dominate political discourse and action in Delta Amacuro. The popular insurrection of February 1989, for example, never caused a stir in Tucupita. In February and November 1992, people often joked that any number of coup attempts could be launched in Caracas and elsewhere without their effects ever reaching the delta. The political struggle between García Gómez and rival Bernardo Alonzo for political control of Delta Amacuro, on the other hand, led to frequent street demonstrations that blocked the main arteries into Tucupita and were the constant foci of rumor, attention by the local media, and political maneuverings. These events seemed real and immediate. Those that rocked the nation-state seemed far away and illusory.

The "threat" of a cholera epidemic was read in different ways in the region, providing a range of competing discourses of citizenship, the nation-state, and modernity. Since Delta Amacuro is one of the poorest states in Venezuela and has one of the highest rates of malnutrition and infant mortality, this discourse could have influenced how cholera was perceived and represented and what steps were taken to anticipate its possible arrival. But it didn't. This disjuncture seems to have resulted from the widespread perception that modernity had never really arrived in Delta Amacuro.

In the delta any discourse on poverty just seemed naturally to apply to "the Warao." Articles that projected the disappearance of the Warao appeared periodically in *Notidiario* and occasionally in Caracas newspapers. A prominent five-part article published on consecutive days in early August 1991 in *El Nacional* declared that the Warao "will disappear due to hunger."[4] The article quoted anthropologist Dieter Heinen in suggesting that the Warao had formerly maintained "a delicate equilibrium between man, nature, and supernatural beings." According to public health and other authorities, in the wake of acculturation the Warao had been affected by "malnutrition, promiscuity, marginality, and extreme poverty."[5]

Whereas anthropological, public health, and other experts were often cited to claim that modernity had left the *indígenas* behind, these articles sometimes employed a romantic discourse that pictured modernity as having corrupted the delta's premodern Others and as threatening their existence. The possibility of a cholera epidemic breathed new life into these narratives of extinction, and the cholera connection became a rhetorical strategy used by leaders of delta communities and government agencies, including the Dirección Regional de Salud, in requesting more resources. Nevertheless, because many *criollos* thought that "their" disappearance would be no great loss, linking cholera and extinction did not produce much in the way of genuine concern or concerted action. Although exclusion of the *indígenas* from the ranks of sanitary citizens made them seem like natural targets for cholera, this status deprived them of the right to have access to substantive prevention programs. Unsanitary subjects would, in any case, be considered incapable of taking advantage of efforts aimed at sanitary citizens.

The popular perception that all the talk about cholera was simply a "smokescreen" concocted by the government to hide the real motives of decisionmakers was another discourse tailor-made for Delta Amacuro. The real motives were advancing individual and party goals, strengthening personal networks, weakening enemies, and misappropriating public funds. Since the content of exhortations by politicians and institutional officials was thought by many to be a much less effective guide to action than assessments of hidden interests and political relations, it was only logical that the presence of *Vibrio cholerae* was interpreted by many as a fictional construct. In the delta this view did not necessarily regard official talk about cholera in negative terms. Some party stalwarts and agency officials concluded that the Dirección Regional de Salud and other agencies were intelligently seizing the fiction to attract funds to the region and to line their own pockets.[6]

The effect of these discourses was greatly enhanced by the sense that cholera would never find its way to the region. If cholera was a concern of the nation-state and formed part of its struggle to achieve and preserve modernity, then it, like the anti-neoliberal insurrection of 1989 and the coup attempts of 1992, had little relevance in the delta. Even when cholera cases were reported in neighboring Sucre state, which lies just across the Gulf of Paria from the delta, most Delta Amacuro residents honestly believed that they were inoculated, as it were, against the disease: "How could cholera reach the delta if it's so far away? Nothing reaches us here in Tucupita, right?" A related attitude combined the sense that cholera was remote with the racialization of the disease. Professionals in Tucupita stated that "this cholera couldn't come here to Tucupita, because the only ones who could get that disease are the Indians [indios]—and they are so cursed with diarrheas, tuberculosis, and malaria that nothing else could strike them!"

The privileges of race and class led criollo residents of Tucupita to believe that they had nothing to fear from cholera. Paradoxically, even as "marginality"—the exclusion from substantive participation in the nation-state and modernity—was identified in Caracas as the short road to cholera, this relationship between cholera and citizenship—that is, who was considered to be a member of the nation-state and in what way—was inverted in Delta Amacuro. Bilingual teachers and other professionals in the delta with access to the Spanish-language media imagined an impassable spatial gulf between the delta and the disease. The social construction of citizenship crucially shaped how people perceived the disease and what they were willing to do in preparation for a possible epidemic. The epidemic, in turn, reshaped categories of citizenship and how social and political exclusion affected people's lives.

3 Stories of an Epidemic Foretold

Cholera Reaches Mariusa

From the perspective of the residents of Tucupita, Mariusa is just plain off the map. Not only is it "inaccessible," it is the home of the most "isolated" and "uncivilized" of "the Warao." Getting to Mariusa from Tucupita requires following the Mariusa River beyond Tortuga Island along a lengthy uninhabited stretch to the coastline (see map 1, page 2). The better-traveled route goes to Nabasanuka and Winikina and then through the Caribbean, which can be rough, dangerous, even impassable. Few government officials would even consider making the trip. Persistent requests by Mariusans over decades for a clinic, a school, a water tank, and polling places have fallen on deaf ears.[1]

In 1992 the population of Mariusa moved in somewhat regular cycles between the moriche palm groves near the coast and communities built above the river at its mouth. In the forest Mariusans depend almost entirely on extracting the starch from moriche palms and collecting swamp fish, fruit, and other forest products (photographs 4 and 5). The moriche palm provides the floor and thatched roof of Mariusan dwellings as well as hammocks, the only furniture, and stronger woods contribute the posts and beams. Baskets are fashioned from the bark of *sehoro* bushes. Getting from place to place requires trudging through the mud—there is almost no dry land—or balancing on small tree trunks laid out to make a slimy, precarious path that often rises six or more feet above the ground. Although others maintained a sense of balance that rivaled that of professional equilibrists, I (Charles Briggs) often fell into the mud.

Although some families have continued to live in the forests most of the time, in part to minimize contact with exploitative *criollos*, others return when modernity fails them—when, that is, they cannot sell crabs or earn wages working for fishermen. The profound economic downfall that gripped

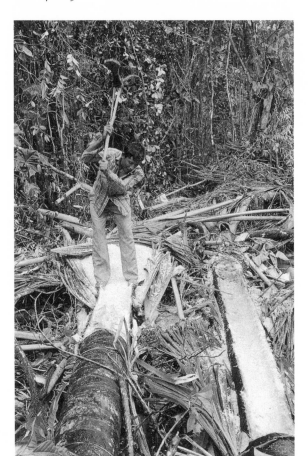

Photograph 4. Man hoeing the starchy pulp from
a moriche palm log in Nabaribuhu. Photograph by
Charles L. Briggs.

the country starting in the 1980s forced many people back into the forest.
Ironically, it is modernity that induced many Mariusans to return to a way
of life that has been seen as the quintessence of the premodern world. Others generally return only once a year, when all Mariusans gather in the forest for the *nahanamu* festival. The ritual high point of the year, the *nahanamu* is given for the *hebu* spirits that bring disease upon a community.
The "father," or "owner," of the spirits, the *wisidatu,* learns through a dream
that the *hebu* are "hungry" for starch extracted from the moriche palm, and
then he announces to the community when the *nahanamu* will take place.

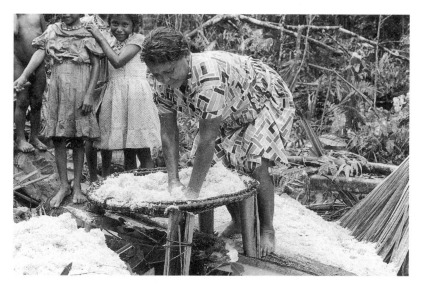

Photograph 5. Young girls watch as a woman kneads moriche palm pulp to extract the starch in Nabaribuhu. Photograph by Charles L. Briggs.

Participants dance through the night, leaving the days for the laborious preparations (photograph 6). My first visit to Mariusa was occasioned by a chance invitation from friends to attend the festival. When *kobenahoro* Santiago Rivera saw that I had learned the appropriate dance steps and could speak English, he ordered me to return, promising to teach me Warao in return for English lessons.

The size of the population that lives in the forest is often rivaled by the number of people who live above the Mariusa River at the point where it reaches the Caribbean (photograph 7). Posts, sunk into the river bottom, support houses that consist of log floors and thatched roofs. The open sides provide excellent ventilation in the subtropical climate. Houses are furnished much as they are in the moriche groves—with sewing machines, occasional boom boxes and a mélange of items fashioned from palm fiber and *sehoro* bark—except that fishing nets are crucial on the coast.

Mariusans are hardly isolated. Commercial fishermen have exploited Mariusans for decades, thereby creating a "contact zone,"[2] a place where people from very different places have access to very different types of power and can exchange goods, labor, languages, and ideas. Promising employment and food, *criollo* fisherman, who are generally from Barrancas, Tucupita, or Sucre state, make a deal with the *kobenahoro* and move into one of the houses, often forcing a local family to move out. Most fishermen then hire

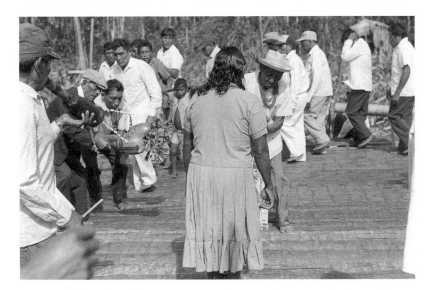

Photograph 6. A *wisidatu* healer dances opposite a prominent woman in Nabari-buhu, with *wisidatu*, sacred rattles, and *isimoi* clarinet visible on left. Photograph by Charles L. Briggs.

a "secretary"—a young woman often barely past puberty—from whom they obtain sexual and domestic services in exchange for food and gifts. I have known fishermen who live with as many as three women at one time. When a fisherman moves on, in a matter of months or years, his "secretary" and any children are generally abandoned. The fishermen do little more than sit around. The Mariusan men sink posts into the sandy bottom of the river or coastal waters, fasten nets to them, and bring in the catch, filling the large iceboxes used for transporting the fish to Barrancas or Tucupita. The fishermen bring flour and cornmeal, sugar, tobacco, batteries, plantains, mangos, and other articles from town. These are sold to the workers by crediting the purchases against their wages. Prices are often three times as much as those in Tucupita or Barrancas. Mariusans cannot read, write, or keep numerical accounts because they have never had a school.[3] Therefore they cannot check their employers' records. The fishermen pay Mariusans little, often claiming that they purchased more goods than their wages were worth.

Indígena laborers have no redress against *criollo* operators if they take their claims to town. The fishermen joke that Mariusans don't know that they are getting cheated and are happy with whatever comes their way. Not likely. Carlos Romero, who had gained a position of responsibility with An-

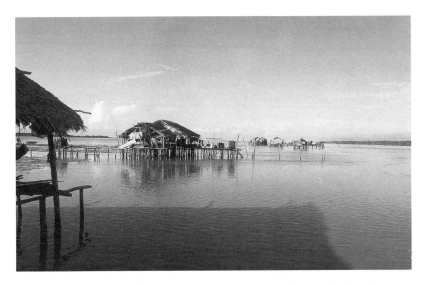

Photograph 7. Clusters of houses on stilts stretch along the mouth of the Mariusa River. Photograph by Charles L. Briggs.

tonio Bustamante, one of the fishermen, noted wryly that "when the *criollo* workers get to Barrancas, [their boss] gives them 20,000 *Bolívares,* but he only gives us 2,000, 2,500, maybe 2,800 *Bolívares.*"[4] The workers know how labor gets racialized—especially on payday. That was, in part, why Santiago Rivera was so keen on learning Spanish and English and on having a school in his community. Some fishermen also bring cases and cases of cheap liquor. When they leave the community they take the major source of protein in the local diet—fish—and leave provisions for what in some households can become a twenty-four-hour drinking binge. Their contribution to the malnutrition that fosters some of the most appalling health conditions on the planet is painfully evident.

Mariusa is also a decidedly transnational zone. Trinidadians and Venezuelans run contraband goods between their two countries on a regular basis. A substantial quantity of Colombian cocaine reportedly also travels this route, although explicit signs of this trade are seldom apparent. For generations, probably for centuries, Mariusans have traveled about seven miles across the Caribbean to trade with persons living on the southern coast of Trinidad.[5] Until cholera arrived, Trinidadians came on a weekly basis to buy crabs that had been gathered by Mariusans in nearby swamps. To harvest crabs the Mariusans lie in the mud, hoping to avoid stingrays and poisonous snakes, and pull the crabs from their holes. In the early 1990s eighty-pound sacks of medium-sized red and blue crabs brought from two to five dollars each in cash.[6] Rivera wanted to learn English so that he could bargain for fairer prices. Rivera was a good student, and he mastered enough English to carry on simple conversations with the Trinidadians. But he never got much more money for his crabs.

THE *CRIOLLO* FISHERMAN'S STRANGE DISEASE

When Salomón Medina and José Rivera described the death of Santiago Rivera, they mentioned a crucial detail: they did not think that Santiago Rivera was the first person in the region to be infected by the strange disease. They and others reported that a commercial fisherman from San Félix, a major industrial area southwest of the delta, had become ill as he was passing through Mariusa. A skilled healer, Rivera attempted a cure. After smoking a ritual cigar to muster his healing powers and to focus his concentration on the task at hand, he began to chant. He ran through a long series of segments of curing texts, hoping to intone the name of the *hebu* that was afflicting his patient. Curers such as Rivera use tobacco smoke and song to open a pathway between the visible world of the patient and the invisible world occupied by the disease, which has both spiritual and physical dimensions. Massage is used to locate the source of the illness and feel its tactile characteristics. When the secret name of the disease appears in the song, the pathogen "stands up" and begins to lose its hold on the patient's body and spirit. The causal agent can then be extracted through massage and sent back to its invisible, distant home.

Rivera called upon spirits that dwell in a wide range of regions of the delta and spaces that reach from the surface of the water and the land up to the highest reaches of the sky, hoping to find the culprit. None responded. Touching the man's diarrhea-soaked body exposed Rivera to cholera. Mariusans eat with their hands. Thus, Rivera could easily have contracted cholera in this manner. This is where social inequality comes into the picture. The fisherman had a motorboat, and he immediately left the region in search of medical attention. If there had been a clinic in Mariusa or if Rivera had owned a working motorboat, he, too, would have sought help from medical personnel, and he would have lived.

Rivera's death had a devastating psychological impact on his community, not only because the Mariusans had lost a strong leader to a frightful disease but also because all attempts to save his life failed. When their *kobenahoro* became ill the Mariusans assumed that the virulent diarrhea was caused by *hebu* spirits. They turned to the only healers in their area, the lay practitioners.[7] They went to the chief *wisidatu* specialist, the "owner" of ancestral *hebu* spirits, Claudio Martín. The keeper of the most important ritual objects in the community and the ritual director of the *nahanamu* cycle, Martín was charged with curing individual patients and protecting the entire community from disease and death. (Two *wisidatu* practitioners, rattles in hand, are visible on the left in photograph 6, earlier in this chapter.)

Moved by the fear of Rivera's relatives and their sense of urgency, Martín climbed into Rivera's canoe and made the short journey downriver, arriving at the *kobenahoro*'s house after midnight. After smoking a huge cigar of tobacco wrapped in palm leaves, Martín worked until dawn, massaging Rivera's abdomen vigorously. Martín was unable to make out the shape and feel of a *hebu* within his body. He similarly evoked the names of every *hebu* he had ever heard of that had been known to cause diarrhea and vomiting. As dawn arrived and Rivera's condition worsened, Martín declared that he was unable to find the pathogen. He had no explanation for what seemed to be a case of *hebu* sickness. He slept in the early morning hours, hoping to be visited in his dreams by the *hebu* spirits responsible for the disease, but this powerful source of diagnostic information also failed him.

Like institutional medicine, the forms of healing practices in delta communities are divided into a host of specialties. When the *wisidatu* failed, Rivera was visited by a *hoarotu*, a healer who cures *hoa* sickness. The *hoarotu* sang, massaged Rivera's abdomen, and then gave up, declaring that the problem was not caused by *hoa*. He could hide neither his ignorance of the illness nor his impotence to cure it. Other specialists were similarly baffled. When the Mariusans lost Santiago Rivera their tremendous faith in vernacular curing was compromised and they became engulfed in terror and confusion.

WHY DID SO MANY DIE?

Fishermen tell a different story. One of the key protagonists in this early part of the story was Antonio Bustamante. His ties to the Mariusan community are deep. Bustamante, who was in his late forties at the time of the epidemic, had been raised primarily in the delta, where his mother was a schoolteacher. He is of average height, relatively thin, and has brown hair. Years of sun and wind have darkened and toughened his complexion. His gait is uncertain on land, as if his feet were still negotiating a rocking boat. Unlike many delta fishermen, he is not easy to engage in conversation. When he chose to speak his words emerged in machine-gun bursts of narrative fragments, offering summaries of stories rather than full performances. He had run a fishing operation in Mariusa for about fifteen years, and he employed more than a dozen men. A few helped him in the large house that also served as dock, warehouse, and store. Most placed the nets and then returned to haul in the catch, receiving their pay per kilogram of fish. He bragged that he had had seven wives in Mariusa, and in 1992 he was living with two women from the community.

When we saw Bustamante in June 1993 he was extremely reticent to talk about cholera, and he claimed that he had been in Barrancas when the epidemic began. His son Jacobo, he said, had been in Mariusa at the time. When we interviewed Jacobo in 1994, he claimed that all of the Bustamantes were in Barrancas and that only an employee had remained in the fishing camp. We interviewed Antonio Bustamante again in August 2000 about oil exploration in Mariusa. Cholera was no longer of concern to him, and he seemed to have forgotten that it was of interest to us. He brought up the question of the epidemic: "Yes, those poor people [pobrecitos], they are hungry here, life is hard for them, so cholera gets them and kills them right away. . . . I came here about six or seven years ago, and it made me sad. When we arrived we saw about three corpses that had been killed by cholera."[8]

Why were both father and son so anxious to distance themselves from these deaths in the years following the epidemic? The viability of their business was very much on the line. The death of many Mariusans and the exodus from Mariusa could have led to the scrutiny of fishermen's operations that Santiago Rivera had sought for so long. Moreover, the association of cholera with the coastal waters of the delta—specifically the fish caught in its waters—could potentially destroy the family's livelihood. Indeed, sales in the fish markets in Tucupita were down by about 90 percent during the epidemic, particularly after MSAS officials temporarily banned the sale of crabs and fish from the region (photograph 8).[9] Fishermen were so intent on controlling the spin on this information that they sought to popularize the theory that the epidemic was not produced by cholera at all. Jacobo Bustamante stated, "I imagined that, well, [the Mariusans] would never return here," pointing to concern with the possible loss of the Bustamantes' labor supply.[10] Since commercial fishermen do relatively little of the hard work of setting nets and retrieving fish, they would be forced to scale back their operations—as they did from August through October 1992—permanently.

The father's and son's stories of the epidemic—including their efforts to distance themselves from the role of narrator—converged in one important regard: they offered the same explanation for the high number of deaths in Mariusa. "So when there was cholera," Jacobo stated, "all of them got scared, and they didn't know where this disease came from. And it's pow-

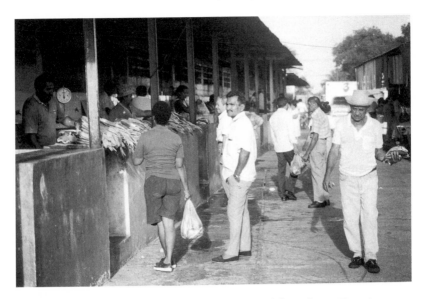

Photograph 8. Stalls lined up along a mostly empty fish market in Tucupita. Photograph by Charles L. Briggs.

erful! Perhaps because so many of them died, because they are a kind of people who don't know anything, they got scared."[11] The problem was ignorance, he asserted, and a passivity that resulted from fear and a superstitious response to a medical emergency. The Mariusans, according to the Bustamantes, froze—they could not think of any way to remove themselves from harm's way.

Salomón Medina's explanation of the Mariusans' immobility was quite different. "We were very aware of the extent of the danger—well, we were all facing death," he said. "Even though there was an outboard motor and a boat, we couldn't use them to take patients to the doctor because [Bustamante] was too stingy to loan us the motorboat, too stingy to loan us the gasoline. He was stingy, and that's why so many of us died."[12]

The question that lurks here is not of "merely historical" interest. Persons who considered themselves to be *criollos* generally argued that the failure of people classified as *indígenas* to get timely medical help resulted from ignorance, resistance, and superstition. Mariusans, in other words, *chose* to remain on the coast until the number of deaths induced them to run away like scared cattle. Mariusans point to their lack of access to resources—boats, motors, gasoline, and clinics. Their accounts of how they were denied access to the boats that were available in Mariusa indicate that racialized lives are accorded less value, particularly when saving them might get in the way of institutional or corporate objectives. Although Bustamante was more honest and scrupulous than most fishermen, the terms that guided his operation were strictly economic and individualist: he paid his workers exactly what he thought they had coming, and he recognized no obligations to the community as a whole. Except for selling small packets of Alka-Seltzer, he brought no medications to Mariusa other than those for himself, his sons, and his employees. In an area in which some 36 percent of children die in their first year of life,[13] questions of life and death were deemed to be the private concern of Mariusan families, and generating a profit was his. If we read the opening days of the epidemic through the lens of Bustamante's story, loaning gasoline and a motorboat to transport a gravely ill patient to a clinic or hospital was too costly and disruptive. The death of Mariusans was too common an occurrence to warrant any deviation from business as usual.

THE EXODUS FROM MARIUSA

In Mariusa the death of a loved one is not received with pathos or passivity. All available therapeutic resources are exhausted, including the full range of spirit-based techniques that are primarily used by men, the herbal therapies practiced mainly by women, and the therapies available at the clinics and hospitals, when they are accessible.[14] If the patient dies, the women who have been caring for him or her crowd around the body and begin to wail. They are joined by other relatives, and the torrent of powerful poetry, intense emotion, and musical polyphony continues until the mourners return from the burial ground. Women take turns composing *sana*, texted funerary laments that women sing collectively. These verses transform notable features of the person's life into collective memories and excoriate anyone who they believe contributed to the death. Powerful healers and political leaders are often the objects of scathing, ironic, and often salacious criticism.[15] The wailing generally lasts all night, although the singers stop to rest their voices from time to time. Although women are seldom able to directly challenge men's voices in the meetings and mediation sessions in which power is visible or to participate in curing rituals, wailing women x-ray the state of social and political relations in their community. Men can only listen in silence.[16] This display of intense emotion and collective introspection greets every death in most communities, including the altogether too frequent deaths of infants.

Life was rapidly becoming impossible in Mariusa. Eight people had died within the space of about four days. The *wisidatu, hoarotu, bahanarotu,* and other healers had all failed. The fishermen had denied them a motorboat and gasoline to transport patients to the clinic in Nabasanuka or to the hospital in Barrancas. People were hungry and exhausted. Since most of the deaths occurred in the early morning, the lamentation and other ritual activities continued all day and night, ending late the following morning—just in time to begin mourning someone else. Unlike many Latin American communities, where wakes and funerals are punctuated with communal meals, Mariusans feel unable to eat or prepare food until the person has been placed in his or her hammock, then placed in a special wooden canoe, wrapped in palms and vines, and hung in an above-ground grave, often in the forks of a tree. With one death on top of another in a community where most folks are related in some way, few Mariusans slept or ate much in the days following the *kobenahoro*'s death.

The final straw came when the *kanobo arima*, the *wisidatu* who guards the ancestral spirits and is charged with defending the community against illness, got sick. I had worked extensively with the *kanobo arima*, Claudio Martín, one summer, trying to make sense of the way that *wisidatus* treat individual patients and seek to control *hebu* in the course of the *nahanamu* ritual cycles.[17] Very thin, he seemed to ingest more tobacco smoke—which helped increase his power over *hebu*—than food. He seemed wholly disinterested in day-to-day affairs. As we listened to recordings of *hebu* songs and exhortations, however, his eyes and face came alive, and he spoke rapidly, often almost feverishly, when discussing the invisible and philosophically complex world of *hebu*.

Martín spoke for hours about the home of the ancestral spirits on Bubu, a mountain located on the southeast coast of Trinidad, relating the attributes of the individual spirits, how they lived, their hierarchical social relations, and their origins.[18] Although he had never been there physically, he visited this and other realms in the dreams that gave him entrée into the world of *hebu*. He shared the philosopher's penchant for dissecting language, exploring the full range of the meanings and uses of individual words from the healer's lexicon. His ability to ward off illness within the community and to cure patients with acute respiratory and other diseases depended on his skill in calling *hebu*, engaging them in dialogue, and commanding them to return to their home. A patient's life is believed to hang just as much on the power of Martín's dreams as on his vast repertoire of songs for controlling spirits and his ability to extract *hebu* through massage. When he raised his rattle, garnished with parrot feathers, Martín waged hand-to-hand combat with the *hebu*—meaning both spirits and physical pathogens—that attack individuals and entire communities.

When Martín confessed that he was incapable of naming the *hebu* afflicting the Mariusa, people became even more frightened. When the "owner" of the *hebu* spirits himself died in the same rapid, horrible way, people lost faith entirely in their ability to stay alive in Mariusa. Several Mariusans emphasized that this powerful healer had become impotent by stressing that his last words were just like everyone else's—he had no special knowledge of or power over the disease. Many people reported that their faith in vernacular healing in general was shaken.

At this point the Mariusans did not seek a boat to take just the sick to the clinic in Nabasanuka—they used every means available to get everyone out of Mariusa. A fisherman from Cumaná helped some leave. Perhaps he accepted the gravity of the situation since he was from Sucre state, which had already reported cholera cases. He worked in Mariusa only occasionally, so he also had less to lose than Bustamante did. Carlos Romero, Bustamante's right-hand man, said that Bustamante loaned gasoline and a boat. Other Mariusans dispute this point. Many families had no access to an outboard motor, and they painfully recalled paddling their way to safety.

Some went to Yakariyene, a rudimentary shelter established on the outskirts of Tucupita for persons classified as *indígenas* (see photograph 9). Perched on a narrow strip of land between the Manamo River and the main highway into Tucupita, Yakariyene consists of two cement floors with pitched metal roofs overhead. It is a government architect's vision in metal and concrete of an authentic *indígena* house. Although the structure was made for 150 to 200 persons, 400 or 500 often hung their hammocks there, filling every available inch. The communal toilets, sinks, and showers were so inadequate that residents depended on the river and the open ground beyond the shelters for bathing and other necessities. People would stay at Yakariyene for periods ranging from a few days to several years. It symbolized the way that the municipal government and the residents of Tucupita tried to segregate *indígenas* from *criollos*. By housing *indígenas* in this squalid, overcrowded, and unsafe mini-ghetto, they made sure that the *indígenas* were kept out of town. The living conditions at Yakariyene were widely regarded as proof that *indígenas* are ignorant, backward, filthy, and lazy.

Yakariyene was a living nightmare in the second half of 1992, packed beyond belief with hungry, frightened people. Since no space remained in the sheltered areas, Medina and José Rivera lived with about a hundred others in dwellings fashioned from ragged pieces of plastic held in place by sticks that had been torn from nearby trees. Since it was the rainy season, water poured through gaps in the plastic, prompting people to migrate frequently within these tiny spaces in search of dry spots. Handouts and odd jobs hardly

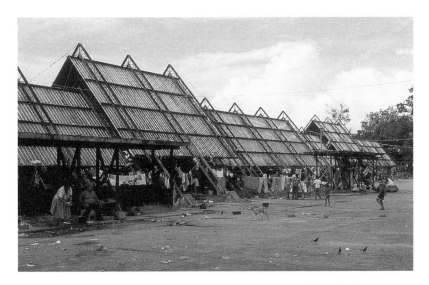

Photograph 9. Yakariyene, "the *indígena* house." Photograph by Charles L. Briggs.

provided an adequate economic base, and hunger was acute. The high-pitched laughter and the flurry of activity that usually emanate from Mariusan households gave way to silence, broken only by low murmurs and the creak of slowly rocking hammocks. A few perfunctory efforts were made to keep fires going—a small measure of defense against the pervasive dampness.

Some Mariusans headed for the clinic in Nabasanuka. Another large group got as far out of the delta as they could, heading straight for Barrancas. The amazing thing is that nearly everybody found a way to leave within a single day of Martín's death, and the few remaining people left the day following. Never wealthy, the Mariusans had to leave nearly all of their belongings behind.

IN SEARCH OF A STORY:
MARIUSAN EXPLANATIONS OF THE CHOLERA EPIDEMIC

When Santiago Rivera tried to make sense of his symptoms, he reportedly accused an old rival of killing him through sorcery. The word *cholera* was not available; no one could recognize the disease or treat it, let alone prevent its spread. Rivera used the modes of explanation that he had at his disposal. Mariusans repeated his words over and over, looking for clues that might enable them to sort out what was happening and what they should do.

It might seem less relevant to discuss these initial attempts to explain

Rivera's death than to press on with the action, particularly since these explanations were fairly short-lived: within six months or so, most people had decided that sorcery had not been the killer (although the accusations continued to augment tensions between rival families for years). The situation was not quite so simple. The stories that people told about Santiago's death shaped people's understandings of what was happening, affecting both what took place next and the long-term psychological and social impact of these early days of the epidemic. The stories, in short, are no less a part of the action than *Vibrio cholerae*, unsuccessful treatments, and the comings and goings of *criollo* fishermen.

Narrating the epidemic was a collective process. Family members each contributed details and perspectives to the stories in the course of each successive retelling. Versions were circulated among homes in Mariusa and then, in the course of the diaspora, throughout the delta. But the narratives told by men like Medina and José Rivera were fragmentary and disjointed. They contained few details and failed to portray accurately the events leading to the outbreak. Women, on the other hand, told much richer and more elaborate stories regarding the *kobenahoro*'s death and the early days of the epidemic.

María Rivera recounted the death of Santiago Rivera, who was her brother, in November 1992. Rivera is a remarkable woman. She divides her time between Mariusa and Nabasanuka, spending part of each year in a community with a Catholic mission, a clinic, stores, and a school, and the other in an area in which all of these institutions are absent. About fifty years old, the youth and beauty of her face and her physical strength belie her age. She always wears a long, brightly colored dress with floral patterns, like most Mariusan women, and she boasts a large beaded necklace graced with old silver *fuertes* (coins worth five *Bolívares*) and a small picture of the popular saint and healer José Gregorio Hernández.

Rivera is shrewd and hardworking. A widow with two young children to support (her older children are already married), Rivera had turned down a host of marriage proposals. And with good reason: she defies gender restrictions with relish. Being postmenopausal, taboos on menstrual blood do not disqualify her from learning the healing practices dominated by men. Women are also excluded from the performance of *dehe nobo*, the "ancestral stories" that reveal powerful secrets about how the world came to have its present form. Rivera, however, relishes the chance to tell *dehe nobo*. I have never seen another woman take a leadership role in *monikata nome anaka*—the meetings that community leaders organize to mediate disputes. Rivera sometimes attempts to take charge of these events. Her appropriation of the words and leadership roles that are closely guarded by men is not accepted passively, and attempts are often made to silence or discredit her. She lives with two of her brothers, who also circumvent accepted gender roles by weaving hammocks, cooking, raising children, and doing other sorts of "women's work."

I had stayed in María Rivera's home on many occasions, but the following conversation took place in a dingy hotel room on the plaza of Tucupita. Having taken refuge from the epidemic at Yakariyene, she learned from Medina that I was in town and came to visit. We sat opposite each other on two creaky beds. Her usual composure and self-confidence had vanished, her slightly round figure had been reduced to a thin and frail outline, her rich sense of humor was nowhere in evidence, and her face was drawn and tired, etched with worry and fear. As she spoke, her tone rarely rose above a whisper, producing the sense that she was imparting information that could be dangerous to both of us.

Rivera began by recounting the trip she, the *kobenahoro*, and other Mariusans had taken to a part of the forest where large logs are cut and carved into canoes. They had run out of food, and Santiago Rivera was weaving a basket that they would use as they extracted starch from a moriche palm. Manuel Torres, whom she accuses of murdering her brother, arrived with his family.

María Rivera, Tucupita, 13 November 1992

He arrived, damn! "How are you? How are you, Santiago?" He greeted [Santiago] by name! "I've come here to drink honey, I've come to drink honey."

Santiago answered him, "There's no honey here. Up on the hill, way up there on the hill, that's where there's honey."

Santiago was sitting over here weaving the basket, and he sat over here. [Rivera's] back was to him, and he was upwind of [Rivera]. Then he left, he left alone. His [Torres's] wife stayed in the house. . . . Manuel went alone, he left alone. "I'm going for honey, I'm going to collect honey." He left with the jug he had for bringing the honey.

[Rivera] kept on weaving the colander [used to collect the palm starch], slowly. Having gone there to fell logs for a canoe, he kept on weaving the colander. After [Torres] left, he kept on weaving the colander, weaving.

So then [Torres] came back around the other side of the house, circling around the other side. And having come up from behind, he came right up to him for just a moment, really close to him. [Rivera] was weaving intently, and when he turned around like this—"What could that sickness be?"—he nearly passed out from a horrible pain in his abdomen. "Damn!" . . . he said to his [Rivera's] wife. "Damn! I've been

struck by some kind of illness, it really hurts. I've massaged and massaged and massaged it and it's getting a little better, it's getting a little
better."

Then he grabbed a machete, saying, "Manuel inflicted me with this
sickness. Let's go look for him up there!" He ran off in that direction at
once. He ran off in that direction, he ran off following the tracks, he ran
off following the tracks.

He ran after him until he came to a path. When he hit the path, he
couldn't distinguish the tracks. "If this hadn't happened, look [at what
I would have done with] this machete!" . . . He would have killed him.
[Rivera] was furious when he went after him; but he didn't find him.
Manuel fled to the other side, far away from the house. And when he
came back to the house, he left immediately. "I'm going back now, I'm
in a hurry." [She laughs.]

So he went back without honey, without swamp fish, empty-handed!
Right after he left to look for honey, to bring some swamp fish, he came
back empty-handed! He inflicted a really bad sickness [and] that's why
[Rivera died].

Santiago Rivera had been a powerful ally of Manuel Torres until about
1989.[19] The relationship reportedly went sour when Torres's third wife—
Rivera's daughter—left him, and Torres reportedly blamed Rivera. María
Rivera went on to tell how her brother had planned to kill his daughter when
she rejected her old and reportedly abusive husband. The woman escaped
to Tucupita with a young lover. Rivera and Torres alike believed that the
young woman had been wrong to defy the practice of making political al-
liances by bartering the sexuality of young women; nonetheless, the event
turned the two patriarchs into implacable enemies. From the late 1980s until the beginning of the cholera epidemic their struggle provided a framework that people used in their attempts to explain illnesses and death. I was
a close friend of both men and their families, and their enmity often placed
me in a bind.

The narratives told by José Rivera and Medina in November 1992 cover
the same ground—the trip to cut logs for a new canoe, the return home via
Nabasanuka, Santiago Rivera's death, and the accusation against Torres. As
stories, however, they are worlds apart. Torres is not a character in Medina's version, although he is referred to, but not named, in the quote from
the dying *kobenahoro.* In María Rivera's rendition Torres comes fully to
life as his words, actions, intentions, and deceitfulness are dramatically recre-
ated. In relaying Torres's words, Rivera used a tone that is frequently invoked in *dehe nobo* for the voice that powerful monsters use in attempting
to beguile their prey. Santiago Rivera is not fooled, and he unravels the lie:

"There's no honey here." The listener's suspicions are confirmed when Torres returns to town shortly after having reportedly used sorcery against his adversary and without having made an effort to collect honey or swamp fish. Rivera brings the sorcery accusation to life by suggesting that Torres twice placed himself behind and upwind of his victim so that he could blow the invisible spirit arrow that he had prepared. Torres's cowardly treachery stands in stark contrast to Santiago Rivera's bravery.

María Rivera's narrative and personal stance was clearly embodied in her portrayal of the two characters. She related exactly what her brother ate and drank between the time of the incident and his death. Medina only alluded to Torres's anger, but Rivera replayed a dramatic dialogue between her late brother and his daughter. Rivera embedded in the *kobenahoro*'s words the accusation that Teresa was to blame for turning the two allies against each other. The profound differences between Rivera's account and the depictions that her nephew and Medina gave on the previous day go beyond differences in narrative ability—all three are quite good storytellers.

Both within the delta and far beyond, how people reacted to the epidemic, how they talked about it, and what (if anything) they did about it related closely to their social position. Different social addresses afforded different liabilities, interests, and resources, both discursive and material. In the case of narratives that were told in delta communities, the gender of the narrator was crucial: women generally told much more detailed and evocative stories. Rivera weaves an explanation of why her brother died into the fabric of her story. To make the incomprehensible into a phenomenon that could be apprehended and managed, she looks to a standing social conflict, the medical system most accessible to the Mariusans, and the details of daily life that are known by women. The narrative form provides her with a means not only of bringing these elements together but also of finding causal links between them. The details that bring the scenes to life also add credibility to her story, showing that Torres's actions were precisely calculated to put him in a position to use sorcery. Medina deprived his account of authority by constantly asserting, "We don't know," but Rivera used detail to infuse her story with legitimacy.

In the end, however, the stories told by Medina, José Rivera, María Rivera, and other Mariusans were clearly incapable of encompassing the events that they described. The reality was simply too huge and too terrible to be contained by a single story, particularly one that relied on familiar political struggles and therapeutic schemas. Other people died in Mariusa after Manuel Torres had returned to Barrancas, and the rivalry lost its explanatory power. When their full range of explanatory frameworks failed, Mariusans no longer had a strategy for comprehending the tragedy, and they were unable to gain any sense of closure. The phrase "We don't know" continued to echo through the provisional shelters in which they sought refuge from cholera and terror.

SHAPING CULTURAL MEMORY

When they were most needed, the powers of the Mariusans' vernacular healers failed them. By the same token, the art of the storyteller largely failed them as well. In November, over three months after the death of Rivera and the others, the Mariusans I visited still felt that they could not understand, explain, or adequately cope with what was happening. They had heard cholera stories from physicians, politicians, and many others, and these accounts had been deeply incorporated into the way they viewed the disease. Nevertheless, instead of detailed descriptions of specific episodes laid out in chronological sequence and deftly connected by logical connections (*because . . . , in spite of . . . ,* and the like), Mariusan men could only provide fragmentary and disjointed stories.

The source of the problem certainly did not lie in any lack of narrative virtuosity. Delta residents have achieved international fame as storytellers through a number of publications.[20] Their stories unleash the power of the imagination to make the adventures of culture heroes, battles against cannibals and monsters, the racialized violence of the nation-state, and even the exploits of a rabbit trickster figure seem compelling and real. Santiago Rivera was widely recognized as a virtuosic storyteller, and his stories helped shape the way that Mariusans connected their past and present, thus constructing both in the process.[21] Rivera told "The Origin of the *Criollos*" to me shortly after I arrived in Mariusa. The tale described a primordial giveaway that left *criollos* with nearly all of the goods. In the denouement Rivera connected this mythological event to efforts then being undertaken by delta residents to resist the expropriation of their lands. By categorizing me as one of the greedy *criollo* newcomers, his story subtly warned me not to add myself to the long list of people who exploited the Mariusans. He also seemed to suggest that I could not avoid taking sides in the struggle over land and human rights.[22]

The Mariusans were adept at using the sense-making power of storytelling to reinforce established cognitive and social orders. What happened to these narrative skills when cholera entered their lives? Why were the men in particular capable of telling only stories that they knew were grossly inadequate to depict their experiences and encourage their tenacity? As they related their stories in November 1992, Medina and José Rivera were clearly attempting to make sense of their most baffling and terrifying moments—but terror can make a mockery of sense-making.[23]

Many students of narrative have stressed the importance of sequentiality—the linear structure of stories—suggesting that narratives set up a one-to-one relationship between a series of sentences and a linear sequence of actions.[24] The sequential structure of the text thus imposes a structure on the events that it encodes, helping to shape the way that we perceive and remember them. Some suggest that narrators use linearity and other poetic properties to construct relations of cause and effect in representations of social life,[25] arguing that this "inherent sequentiality" is one of the properties that make narratives such a vital element in cognitive processing and sociocultural interactions of human beings.[26] The relationship between the temporality of human action and the "irreducible temporality" of the narrative is seen as a key to our understandings of time, being, and the world.[27]

The stories told by Mariusan men were not presented in linear fashion. Actions did not unfold, one after another; instead, events were presented in fragments, with very little connection. If we were to accept arguments that stress the importance of linear structure, we could deny these accounts the status of narrative for their incoherence and lack of sequentiality. To do so, however, would simply provide another example of scholarship's Procrustean tendency to throw out phenomena that do not fit received categories. Moreover, it is clear that residents of the Mariusan area of the delta were *trying* to cast ineffable experiences in narrative form, that they were trying to tell stories. It is equally clear that they were cognizant of the inadequacy of their efforts.

Perhaps these stories can teach us a deeper lesson. The sequential unfolding of events in a story is neither intrinsic nor inherent because events do not consist of some readymade reflection of the past. Narratives *make* events by fashioning aspects of social life into discrete, relatively bounded wholes.[28] These tiny social worlds, which portray configurations of characters, settings, and actions, can then be linked through constructions of time, space, and human agency. The early Mariusan accounts are evidence of the importance of this literary and social process and suggest that it can be achieved to quite different degrees. Medina, José Rivera, and the other men felt that if they could relate discrete events, weave them into linear strings, and discern causal relations among them, they would be able to create a story that would allow them to overcome their terror and confusion.

A crucial dimension of the role of narrative is its ability to create cultural memory. Cultural memory can be defined as "a field of contested meanings" that lies between personal memory and history; it is the product of the ongoing struggle to construct—to understand—the identities, relations, and actions of the past. These constructions shape our understanding of the present.[29] Narratives play a crucial role in the production of cultural memory. The poetic properties of stories influence how often they will be retold and whether fragments of them will be inserted into conversations, texts, policy statements, and so forth. Bounded, tightly structured, linearly organized narratives can be easily extracted from the contexts in which they are told (be these written, oral, or electronic) and recontextualized in a wide range of settings. In the process narratives become objectified: they become floating icons of the events they describe, which are inscribed in memory as authentic and authoritative reflections of the world. As a result, the events themselves come to be objectified, as existing apart from individual constructions of them. We can say that the more tightly memory is constructed in narrative features, the more real it seems.[30]

The fragmentary narratives of Mariusan men accorded central stage to ghosts—the people, places, objects, events, and explanations that could not be assimilated in conventional social and epistemological categories.[31] Their stories related the uncertainties, the incomprehensibility, and the terror that people experienced during the epidemic. These emotions opened up a desperate search for new perceptions, strategies, connections, and meanings that had previously been sealed off or unexplored. The initial stories told by Mariusan men during the epidemic did not last. They were progressively erased by accounts that were laid out in linear fashion, in keeping with monolithic explanations of why people had died. The more formal and epistemologically elaborated stories that superseded the Mariusans' initial representations banished some ghosts as they shaped which aspects of the epidemic would be remembered and which nearly forgotten. Despite the power of these screen memories (to borrow a phrase of Freud's), they could not erase the terror of the epidemic.[32] It became a powerful cultural memory, one that continued to inform the present, although in less pervasive and unpredictable ways.

In delta communities the narratives considered the most authoritative purport to reveal the *ahotana*, the "beginning," of the events in question. Therein lies the tremendous interest in *dehe nobo*, particularly ones that depict how human beings, cultural practices, and features of the natural world came into being. Santiago Rivera's "Story of the Origin of *Criollos*" is an example. Similarly, a diagnosis is considered to be definitive when the healer has a dream after treating the patient; if spirits or an ill-intentioned practitioner appear in the dream, the narrative that reports the dream is considered to be the ultimate proof of the cause of the illness. These narratives imagine events—either primordial or contemporaneous—in particular ways. When Rivera got sick, Mariusans immediately turned to these diagnostic practices in an attempt to discern the *ahotana* of the strange virulent disease, but they came up empty-handed. Since the men's claims to knowledge and authority rested on this sort of evidence, their narrative abilities were reduced to shots in the dark that convinced no one, not even themselves.

Because access to the world of *dehe nobo* and diagnostic dreams is primarily limited to men, the construction of cultural memory is highly gendered. Mariusan women tell narratives about daily life and significant contemporary events. Although they generally lack knowledge of *ahotana*, women acquire information through their roles of providing care to children and the sick as well as preparing and distributing food. When they describe illness and death, their narratives richly detail the patient's actions, meals, and words. Ordinarily their stories are deemed by men to be much less significant than tales of spirits and sorcerers, but when someone dies, women's narratives become *sana*. *Sana* open up a broad range of explanations of the death, from emotions, to interpersonal conflict, to relations with the nation-state and economic elites.[33] No *ahotana* exist in *sana;* there is little closing down of imaginative possibilities.

Clara and I witnessed time and time again a reversal of these gender roles when cholera stories were told. On many occasions women stole the floor from men when the latter were attempting to talk about the epidemic. This phenomenon was still occurring two years after cholera first appeared in the delta. This is not to say that patriarchy suddenly disappeared in Mariusa or that the epidemic granted women undisputed control over their communities. Men's voices have many sources of power, and the threat of physical violence remains one of them. Women's narratives, however, provided key tools for coming to terms with one of the most devastating crises that had ever hit the delta.

It took Mariusan men about a year to start imbuing their narratives of the epidemic with coherence and sequentiality. The cholera deaths had shattered a knowledge system that had imbued men with a great deal of power to impose narrative closure, to determine the events, perspectives, and explanations preserved as dominant cultural memory, and to banish ghostly presences. When people were dying from cholera, stories that lacked authority, recounted details of daily life, and juxtaposed multiple orders of epistemology and political action provided the only available means of sorting out what had happened, what was taking place, and what should be done. These narratives would not, of course, ordinarily be repeated or recognized as being of importance. Foreign scholars and senior *indígena* men ordinarily cast these stories into the dustbin. When cholera arrived in the delta, however, men lost their control of cultural memory. The richly detailed stories told by women continue to shape the way that Mariusans remember the epidemic and perceive questions of life and death, health and disease.

None of the stories told by Mariusans got much chance to influence how other people perceived and reacted to the epidemic. The question was not simply one of "access to the press": reporters interviewed Mariusans shortly after they left the coast, and several stories about them appeared in *Notidiario*. Nonetheless, Mariusans and other *indígenas* were not portrayed in newspapers and television stories as persons who were exploring narrative and intellectual models that would help them make sense of either their situation or what was taking place in the region. Instead, they appeared as ignorant and helpless victims whose only choice was to accept or reject the explanations and resources offered by more knowledgeable and powerful public health officials and politicians.

It is easy to dismiss the cholera stories that the Mariusans told as being too poorly formed to count as narratives or as reflecting ignorance of the epidemic's biomedical foundation. To do so, however, is to ignore the pernicious influence of the region's racial economy—the social and political practices that enforced inequality in pervasively racialized terms. The Bustamantes in Mariusa and the reporters, politicians, and officials in Tucupita and Barrancas all ignored these factors, which deprived Mariusans of the chance to prepare for cholera and compromised their attempts to sort things out when people started to get sick.

4 Fighting Death in a Regional Clinic
Cholera Arrives in Pedernales

On 2 August 1992, Daniel Rodríguez, the regional epidemiologist, and I (Clara Mantini-Briggs) were traveling along the Paseo Manamo, one of the larger streets in Tucupita. The river, on our right, was dotted with small boats. Some of the newer vessels were destroying the small-town serenity by traveling at substantial speed, while ancient vessels inched along like water-borne snails. On the other side of the street stretched a line of small mercantile establishments that included at least four liquor stores (photograph 10).

A message on the portable radio in the jeep requested that Rodríguez proceed to the Regional Health Office. Its coda, "cholera in Pedernales," prompted a torrent of angry and frustrated words from Rodríguez. "I knew it! I said so to the doctor [Magdalena Benavides, director of the Regional Health Office], but she never paid any attention to me!"[1] As he spoke, his face grew pale. I couldn't discern whether his fear sprang from his knowledge of the disaster that cholera could produce or from his concern about how people would judge his work. "What can you do with this town? You know what has to be done, and you tell people what has to be done, and yet you lack the power, the authority to make it happen. I have repeatedly told them in Caracas that you just can't get things done here. I have had meetings with the governor, the chief state administrator, the directors of state agencies." He continued by drawing on his prime example. "You saw what happened in the anti-cholera committee. Everybody goes to the meetings, but not a thing happens; everybody makes statements to the press, but they don't do anything. It's a good thing that upstairs [in the national MSAS offices] they know that it's not my fault, that I did everything they told me to do. That's what happens to you."

He then turned to me and asked, "How long have you been here?" Answering his own question, he said, "You have tried to establish your pro-

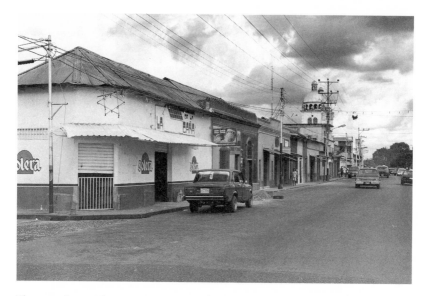

Photograph 10. The Paseo Manamo in front of the river in Tucupita, with one of its liquor stores and the parish church visible. Photograph by Charles L. Briggs.

gram, the Programa de Salud Campesina e Indígena [Peasant and Indigenous Health Program], with tremendous enthusiasm, and the governing party sent [to] you as workers worthless members of the party's faithful, people who were chums of the doctor or ones she had recommended, who do exactly as they please."

Just then we saw Isabel Romero, the director of medical care at the Regional Health Office. She flagged us down and immediately announced, "Cholera broke in on us at Pedernales [*el cólera nos entró por Pedernales*]. The nurses there don't have any medicines, and the doctors are on leave. I just sent them this morning with the medicines that we had on hand. But we already have the first death, an *indígena* girl eleven years old. And on top of everything, the people from Barrancas keep calling the Regional Health Office, the governor's office, and the national offices, saying that they have some of our *indígenas* who are causing health problems there."

"And where's the doctor?" Rodríguez asked.

"You know that she's on leave," replied Romero.

Rodríguez countered, "No, I know she's not around. The doctor is *never* around when anything happens." He turned his head to stare at a group of drunks who were sitting on the sidewalk. They were dangling their feet above the open canal that serves as the town's sewer system (photograph 11). He

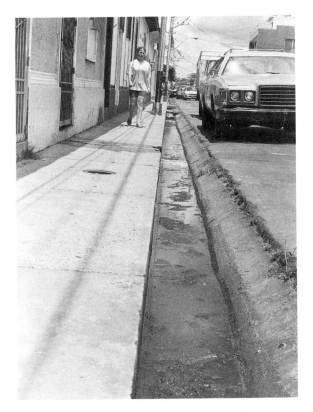

Photograph 11. A main street in the center of Tucupita, with an open sewer. Photograph by Charles L. Briggs.

continued, rage and frustration evident in his voice. "And then they say that I am a troublemaker, as if we could think about disease prevention when you can see that we are in the capital of the state and the sewers are exposed. Sure, the governor's lived here for years, and he doesn't care. I've told them time and time again that they have to invest in health, but that doesn't help them get rich. And in any case, they don't understand. They don't have any foresight or the interests of the people at heart, much less the Indians, who they would rather see disappear. The only thing that would bother them is the ton of votes they would lose."

Romero interrupted. "Oh come on, Daniel, you think that they would be sad about that? If the Indians disappear, they won't have to spend the minuscule sums that they spend every five years to make a few rotten schools, distribute a little food and a few candies to the communities, and, most of all, get all the Indians drunk in order to make them believe that this year their votes will lead to an improvement in their condition. But, Daniel, let's stop talking nonsense—if the doctor isn't around, who is going to be in charge?"

Daniel replied, "Not me!"

"Okay, I'll be," Romero returned. "But remember that the only one who can talk to the press about cholera is you! And the physicians are about to arrive in Pedernales without any idea of what is waiting for them, and the nurses are sending radio messages because patients are arriving by the dozens in canoes. We need to call a meeting of the anti-cholera committee, because now they'll really be afraid. And officials from the national office are coming, and we need to send word to the doctor."

I chose that moment to jump in. "Okay, let me suggest—don't you think it would be better if I went to Pedernales to begin the cholera control procedures?"

The two doctors looked at each other and granted approval with a shrug of their shoulders.

Reconstructing this scene from memory was not difficult, since I have re-lived it many times. These two individuals played essential roles in shaping institutional responses to the cholera epidemic. Their words presaged much of what would be said and done in the coming months. Romero's metaphorical characterization of the beginning of the epidemic—"cholera broke in on us at Pedernales"—is extremely telling. The "us" is an institutional plural that equates the borders of the region and the institutions that administer it with the corporeal space of the human body. It indicates that the most immediate threat was to institutional well-being and to the reputations and jobs of high officials. An important dialectic of power emerges in Rodríguez's response. An infuriating sense of impotence—his inability to take the steps that had been mandated by national officials, public health practices, and rationality because of ignorance and self-interest—is coupled with a desire to avoid making decisions that will be carefully scrutinized.

These remarks also foreshadow the complex way in which public health officials would relate to politicians, the press, the public, and *indígenas* during the course of the epidemic. Rodríguez blames politicians for the acute inadequacy of sanitary infrastructures in Tucupita and the inability to improve public health in general. He had commented earlier that the assignment of unqualified and often undisciplined individuals to the Peasant and Indigenous Health Program that I directed on the basis of their value to the Partido Acción Democrática came at the insistence of Benavides, herself an influential party member. These points of intersection between politics and public health would become particularly crucial during the first election of state and municipal officials in Delta Amacuro, which had become a state in 1991.

Romero's statement to Rodríguez points to her foresight regarding the importance of the role the press was to play in the epidemic. The national epidemiologist—and, by extension, his regional counterparts—had control over the release of information about cholera and the epidemic to other institutions and the press. Regulating the representations of cholera that emerged in the public sphere, particularly in the press, was one of the Regional Health Office's most important jobs during the epidemic. An image of public health officials *versus* the press is too simplistic, however. Institutions often keep a reporter on staff, and for these individuals generating positive images of public health officials was as vital as fending off hostile publicity. Indeed, the press seldom strayed from the parameters set up by public health authorities.

Finally, the epidemic was racialized from the outset. Cholera was closely identified with "Indians." Although the term *indígena* was generally used in public discourse, *indio* ("Indian") was more common in informal conversation, particularly when the implication was pejorative. The question immediately arose as to whether the epidemic would signal the long-expected "extinction" of *la étnia warao*. This question hid a deeper, subversive question: Would the interests of politicians and government officials be best served by the "extinction" or by the "preservation" of this population? In the following months many people classified as *indígenas* asked themselves this question.

Romero's remarks convey the chaos that people experienced during the early days of the epidemic. Almost no preparations had been made, and many clinics lacked physicians and medicine. The response of public health and other institutions to the epidemic was to attempt to move from a situation of emergency, alarm, and crisis to one of order and normalcy. "Control" was the master strategy that guided this effort. The official locus of attempts to control cholera was to contain the disease medically. The "cholera control campaign" brought unprecedented numbers of dedicated individuals, including physicians and other medical personnel, antibiotics, rehydration solutions, and other medical supplies, and boats, gasoline, and food into delta communities.

Officials also sought to control the tremendous threat to their institutions and jobs. An explosion of cases would expose the lack of adequate preparations and the deplorable state of public health in the delta. If this threat

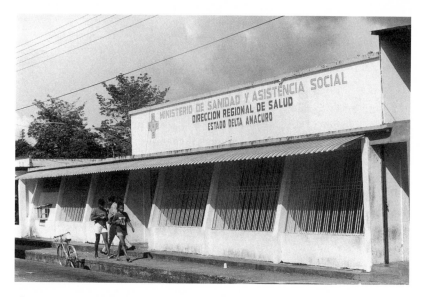

Photograph 12. Headquarters of the Regional Health Service, MSAS, in Tucupita.
Photograph by Charles L. Briggs.

could be adequately controlled, it might even provide opportunities for expanding their agency's power and resources. While officials in Tucupita worried about broad logistical and institutional issues, medical personnel in Nabasanuka and Pedernales did not have the time to stockpile resources or hold endless meetings and press conferences. The problem in these clinics was bodies—lots of them, all emitting diarrhea and vomit, and many of them showing signs of the advanced dehydration that could lead to rapid death.

RACE AND DEATH IN A MEDICAL EMERGENCY

When I arrived at the Tucupita headquarters of the Regional Health Service (photograph 12) on 3 August 1992, one day after the official arrival of cholera, I found Romero shouting instructions to employees who were in the medical supplies storeroom preparing a shipment for Pedernales. I asked about the patients in that area, and Romero replied that seventeen patients had been transported to the Luís Razetti Hospital in Tucupita due to severe dehydration. Only one still needed intravenous rehydration.

On our way from the storeroom to our offices, we stopped at the office of nursing services, where we exchanged greetings with the staff and accepted a hospitable cup of coffee. Anamaría Tejera asked me if it was true that I was going to Pedernales, to which I responded affirmatively. One of the nurses then quipped, "Of course she's going! That's what they're like, traveling around the rivers following those Indians!"

Another nurse interrupted her to add, "That doctor, hmm! She's going to end up married to some Indian over there, you'll see!" Her comment elicited laughter from the rest.

"This business isn't a joke," interrupted Romero, using her usual maternal tone of voice. "The poor doctors there in Pedernales called, saying that they need help, that the clinic is full of Indians, and that things are crazy."

One of the nurses broke in. "Well, this cholera may overrun Tucupita."

Another staff member added, "Once this cholera gets started it won't stop. They say that this disease stays in the population for, minimum, ten years."

Tejera commented, "Okay, it starts over there in the delta. But when it gets here—over where I live we have problems with the water, and this cholera could make things really bad for us."

Trying to calm these fears, Tomasa Gabaldón, chief of the nursing office, said soothingly, "How is cholera going to reach us here? The truth is that it hit the delta because, well, we all know the conditions in which those Indians live—malnourished, tubercular, with mange, malaria. And do you know how they eat? On the floor, with mangy dogs right next to them, eating out of the same plate. They don't even wash the plates when they are going to eat. They're filthy and smelly. And on top of it all, they don't have any supply of clean water, because you know that while they are eating someone is next to them shitting *[cagando]*."

Her statement elicited a chorus of laughter from her staff, who then intoned together, "What did you say, Mrs. Tomasa?"

"S-h-i-t-t-i-n-g," she spelled out with mock seriousness. "Well, I think that the best thing that could happen to them is that they could all die off!"

This remark prompted a general exclamation from several persons and an admonition—"Now really!"—from Romero.

Gabaldón continued, "That just goes to show you—these Indians don't get a break, not from God, not from the Devil, the Adecos, the Copeyanos, or the Masistas.[2] Even the priests exploit them. And now cholera—God must surely have sent it!" With these words ringing in my ears I left the MSAS building and walked down the street to the dock, where a large blue boat was moored, piled high with boxes carefully labeled "Pedernales."

My first trip into the fluvial region began. I watched the vegetation that floats on the river's surface glide past like a green carpet. About four hours later the boat arrived in Pedernales. Located in the northwest corner of the delta, Pedernales is oriented toward the port of Güiria (which lies across the

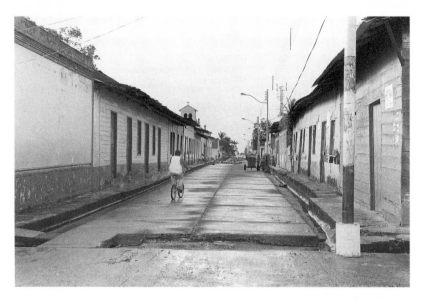

Photograph 13. A street in Pedernales, with its usual vehicular traffic. Photograph by Charles L. Briggs.

Gulf of Paria), Trinidad (for which it serves as the major route into the delta), and Tucupita (see map 1, page 2). Pedernales was discovered by the modern world in 1890, when four oil wells were opened on Capure, an adjacent island. Standard Oil of New Jersey and its Venezuelan affiliates began their oil activities in the area soon after, and operations continued through the mid-1960s. The company was joined at various points by Richmond Exploration Company of Venezuela, Barco, Texas Petroleum Company, and Texaco.[3]

Pedernales is now a major administrative center. It became a municipality with its own administration and budget when Delta Amacuro, formerly a federal territory, became a state in 1991. According to the 1990 census, Pedernales's population of 737 is primarily *"criollo."* If it weren't for the absence of cars, it would be hard to believe that Pedernales is an outpost in the middle of a small island in the delta rather than a town on the mainland. The main part of the town consists of well-constructed houses, featuring tall doors and windows and indoor plumbing, that are lined up along paved streets (photograph 13). The *indígena* population is segregated, living on the southern and eastern fringes of town, beyond the paved streets. Their ramshackle houses are constructed of old pieces of metal roofing and have thatched roofs and walls. Warao residents are not unwelcome in Pedernales, as they are in Tucupita and Barrancas, and many find decent jobs in the fishing industry. Nevertheless, they are second-class citizens, their status marked not only by their poverty but also by the jibes and jokes told by *criollo* residents and the assumption that *criollos* can dupe the *indígenas* with ease, especially adolescent girls.

The clinic is about a block from the "Warao sector" and about four blocks from the municipal dock. As my boat arrived I saw a number of familiar faces, particularly those of the nurses who went each month to Tucupita in search of medicines and paychecks. Other residents waited alongside with a wheelbarrow. After these volunteers helped unload the cargo, the pilot of the boat introduced me: "This is Dr. Clara, the assistant regional epidemiologist." "How long will you be here?" asked the man handling the wheelbarrow. Before I could answer he declared, "Things are bad here! You see this wheelbarrow? This is the local transport. It's how we pick up those Indians when they arrive half-dead." By this time the wheelbarrow was full of boxes. Simulating the sound of an ambulance, the man took off, pushing his vehicle along the streets.

When I arrived at the clinic I greeted the two resident physicians, Marina Parra and Lilibeth Morillo, and was immediately struck by the vast human sea that filled the clinic. One of the larger clinics in the fluvial area, it is a square structure some thirty-five meters on each side, with wards distributed around an interior courtyard. Approximately five hundred persons filled the entrance, hallways, waiting and examining rooms, and courtyard. Their faces reflected exhaustion, confusion, and a strong sense of terror and uncertainty born of the knowledge that they might die from a disease that none of them had heard of the previous week. Clinic director Parra studied my reaction to the scene while remaining thoroughly professional and led me through the tumult of crying children and adults who were hoping for a sign that they would not die. The clamor was so loud that Parra was practically shouting.

The first room we came to held the seven or eight patients in the most critical condition; all were suffering from serious dehydration. In the next room patients in less serious condition lay not in standard metal hospital beds but on blue canvas cots, each with a large hole in the center. Each cot had a trash bag fitted into this opening; the bag hung down into a bucket containing chlorine to kill the *Vibrio cholerae* in the diarrhea that cascaded through the hole. These humble beds were a direct response to guidelines generated in Geneva by WHO and passed via PAHO to MSAS and then to the Regional Health Service in Tucupita.

At times I found it difficult to concentrate on what Parra was saying. My nostrils and lungs were assaulted by the penetrating stench produced by the mixture of feces and chlorine. The nurses and cleaning staff fought valiantly to maintain a semblance of hygiene in that environment. In the middle of the patio a woman wearing gloves, a surgical mask, and an apron was hand-washing all of the linen used in the clinic. Medical gowns, sheets, and other items had been placed in a large tub containing a generous quantity of chlorine and chocolate-colored water drawn from the river by an electric pump.

All the critically ill patients had been brought back from their respective levels of dehydration and were now stabilized. Their bodies were shrunken and sweaty, and their voices, as they tried to respond to Parra's questions, were practically inaudible. She explained to me that although the process of rehydration was remarkably rapid, it was necessary to watch patients carefully since some inexplicably took a sudden downturn. In the main examining room Morillo was examining the less severely dehydrated patients, extracting capsules of antibiotics from large containers, and filling cups with oral rehydration solution from a large plastic cooler. She was accompanied by a nurse who was providing a sputtering translation of the exchanges between doctor and patient. The nurse brought patients forward according to a list of patients.

At that moment a wheelbarrow-ambulance made a dramatic entrance through the main door of the clinic and into the examining room. As the driver simulated the sound of a siren, "*uuuuuu*," his cries temporarily silenced the tumult. The driver tilted his vehicle first to the left, then to the right, avoiding physicians, nurses, and the throng of patients. The wheelbarrow contained the semi-naked body of a man, his arms and legs dangling loosely toward the floor. He resembled a rag doll or, perhaps, an anthropomorphic figure of death. As patients recoiled, giving the driver more room, Parra ordered, "Put him in with the other patients in intensive care." The driver was about to say something, but the nurse interrupted him. "Follow me," he instructed. "I'll help you put him on the bed." The wheelbarrow started down the hallway, and Parra and I began to follow.

As we left the examining room the tumult reached an even greater level. New patients from the boat had entered the clinic. Morillo shouted, "Will the ones who have just arrived stay here!" Children cried and the anxiety of all the patients rose. A woman grabbed Morillo's sleeve and implored disconsolately, "*Maukwatida, maukwatida!*" (My daughter, my daughter!). Women who had arrived the day before took her by the hand and led her to a corner in the hallway. They began to converse with her in Warao while passing her cups of oral rehydration solution. Morillo and two nurses began to add new names to the list of patients and to quickly provide antibiotics and oral rehydration solution for each new person with diarrhea. He also provided asymptomatic family members with doses of antibiotics.

When Parra and I entered intensive care, the man who had been in the wheelbarrow was stretched out on one of the cots, and the ambulance driver was exiting rapidly. He murmured in passing, "I'll be right back with some patients who are too weak to walk." The nurse was already cleaning the patient. Since no verbal information can be elicited from semiconscious patients, we physicians have to rely on what we can observe. The state of the eyes, the turgidity and color of the skin, and blood pressure and heart rate provide good indicators of the degree of dehydration. This patient had experienced a dangerous drop in blood pressure, and we determined that four IVs, one in each arm and ankle, would be necessary to rehydrate him sufficiently to avoid permanent damage to his kidneys or other organs. His bed was a spider's web of bottles and tubes.

When we left the intensive care unit we found that, remarkably, Morillo and the nurses had provided treatment for the patients and their close relatives—who are termed "contacts"—and restored calm. The crowd was sipping cups of rehydration solution and chatting as if they were attending a cocktail party. The physicians slipped away to the relative privacy of the doctors' quarters. As we prepared and ate our dinner we mapped shifts, flipping a coin to decide the order. I then assumed my responsibilities as assistant regional epidemiologist, shifting my focus from treating individual patients to bringing cholera under control in the lower western delta. After Morillo and Parra had provided me with information regarding the location and approximate population of area communities, we designed strategies for ending local outbreaks and preventing new cases. By the time we had finished eating and Parra had left to take the first shift, we had a plan of action and felt ready to put it into place.

Early the next morning I met with community leaders. These included the judge, the police chief, the commander of the local Guardia Nacional, the friar in charge of the Capuchin mission, teachers, owners of the fishing enterprises, presidents of neighborhood organizations, and medical personnel. After taking an inventory of the boats, gasoline, chlorine, medicines, and other supplies that we could use, we decided to launch a door-to-door informational program and to inaugurate a clean-up effort aimed at the public dump and the river shore. The level of fear in the community was such that support was forthcoming from every sector. I then turned to my next task: exhuming the body of the first person to die from cholera and placing lime and chlorine in all of the corpse's orifices, as dictated by MSAS guidelines.

Rodríguez, the regional epidemiologist, arrived later that day. He helped decide which communities to visit first and helped launch the health education program in Pedernales. The arrival of public health physician Roberto Guzmán and nurse Ricardo Simón provided us with much-needed help for the cholera control efforts. Guzmán is tall and relatively thin, with a roundish face that frequently bears a friendly smile. He is a conscientious physician who was quite concerned with the well-being of communities in the fluvial area. Simón was the only person classified as *indígena* and one of only a handful of nurses in the delta who had received a university degree in nursing (rather than the regional standard, the course in simplified medicine, which combines limited coursework and practical experience). The institutional racism that deems *indígenas* incapable of adequately mastering modern epistemologies and practices—and that guards against the possibility that "a Warao" might supervise the work of *criollos*—had denied Simón a position of responsibility, keeping him at the level of a "nursing assistant" *(enfermero auxiliar)*. A member of a politically important family of the Macareo River area, Simón is short, stocky, and strong. He possesses a good sense of humor. He has an extensive knowledge of delta communities and a desire to improve the lot of its residents. Guzmán and Simón assumed responsibility for the Manamo River area.

My team included Alfredo Guacara, a nurse from Tucupita assigned to the regional epidemiologist's office. Guacara had learned a great deal about public health by working with Rodríguez and his staff and through participation in vaccination campaigns. Tall, dark, and athletic, Guacara was reluctant to make concessions to racial hierarchies and had a strong desire to improve health conditions in the fluvial region. These qualities, combined with his great enthusiasm and seemingly inexhaustible energy, were invaluable in the days to come. Neither Guacara nor I spoke Warao, but the driver of our boat had a rudimentary knowledge of the language. He was a strong fellow of about thirty-five with deep black, expressive eyes, a boyish grin, a calming manner, and an impeccable knowledge of the area's rivers and communities. Our team assumed responsibility for the Pedernales River sector.

Each team followed the same routine in each community. Each boat was stocked with a large amount of medicines, chlorine solution, and other supplies, sufficient to treat patients, reequip small clinics, use in health education presentations, and supply local oral rehydration centers. Persons with cholera symptoms were treated where they lay. In each household we trained

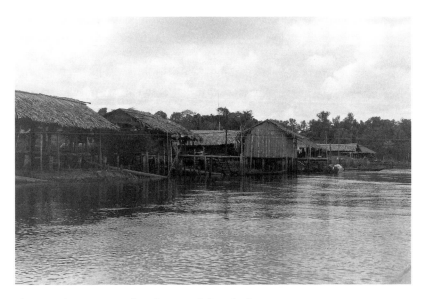

Photograph 14. Waranoko. Photograph by Charles L. Briggs.

one individual to prepare the oral rehydration solution that was used to treat all cases of diarrhea. We also observed the preparation and consumption of food. All present received instruction regarding cholera symptoms and how to prevent and treat the disease. We worked nonstop until nightfall, then we returned to the Pedernales clinic, where we helped until we were overcome by exhaustion.

On one rainy August morning our route took us to Waranoko (see map 1 on page 2 and photograph 14), where we found about three hundred people crowded into the houses of this small community. We soon learned that this sudden population increase was due to an influx of residents from nearby communities who had grabbed their belongings and fled their homes when people began to die. The community's clinic (type I) was located in the home of Casimíro Silva, who received a small salary from MSAS for this service. As we approached the site Silva called to us and appealed for help. Fatigue had transformed the soft features of his young face into a mask. He related that for days his house had been full of patients, that he had run out of medicine, that he was in despair because "the canoes keep coming in all the time with more and more people." As he motioned us inside his house we could see ten of the more seriously dehydrated patients and bottles of rehydration solution dangling from the beams of the thatched roof above their hammocks.

The two nurses and I worked all morning, checking the condition of patients, providing antibiotics to those who had been exposed to the disease and who might be asymptomatic carriers, and showing a member of each household how to prepare oral rehydration solution. We enlisted the assistance of the principal local healer to teach residents about cholera, the benefits of oral rehydration solution, and the importance of using it to treat any type of diarrhea and to impress upon everyone the importance of hygiene. The *comisario*—the local governmental representative—helped the vernacular healer, reporting new cases and keeping track of groups seeking treatment that arrived from other communities.

Just as we were finally wrapping up our work, a profound silence suddenly descended upon the community. Mute children, women, and men stared fixedly at a canoe that was moving painfully slowly along the river toward Silva's house-clinic. As the boat came to shore, men jumped out into the water and dragged it up to the dock. People on the bank, I among them, moved every which way to get a good view of the occupants of the craft. We saw about fifteen people packed into the boat's small quarters. They stared fixedly at the horizon, soaked by rain and undone by terror and dehydration. No one on shore seemed capable of uttering a single word, perhaps holding their breath to see if these emaciated bodies would emit any sign of life. The face of a woman who sat at the far end of the canoe was the most arresting. The sadness and desolation it expressed were striking. Her skin seemed desiccated despite having been moistened by the rain, her eyes had sunk into their sockets, and her body was so thin that her bones were visible beneath the skin on her face. Her head bowed, she stared at an infant who was wrapped in the fold of her bright floral skirt.

The minutes of silence that elapsed as the canoe was pulled to the dock and secured finally ended as our pilot asked the passengers where they lived. He received no reply, but his initiative spurred the onlookers to help the people climb out of the canoe. The order in which the passengers were brought into the clinic-house was determined by their location in the canoe rather than the apparent severity of their condition. I had gone with the nurse to find a new site within the residence that could be claimed for medical care when I heard the pilot shout above the clamor, "Call the doctor— there are four dead bodies here!" I shouted back from the other side of the house, "Leave the dead in the canoe for now. Let's treat the living first!" The fires were stoked with wood in order to boil water and prepare more rehydration solution. We began to distribute what was left from the morning's brew among the newcomers. I hooked up IVs to the more seriously ill and tried to keep these new patients, many of whom were soaked in diarrhea, from reinfecting the people who were being treated. Our efforts to check the condition of patients were impeded by the maze of hammock ropes, the IVs, and the relatives who were seated nearby. We strained to see through clouds of smoke generated by burning green or wet logs. Silva, fully bilingual, communicated with patients and relatives alike, instructing the latter on how to wash their hands with soap after going to the bathroom and before eating. The latter instruction was unintentionally ironic, given that there was already very little to eat in the community and that there were now many additional people to feed.

I was working with the healer and *comisario* when Guacara called me over to the dock. I felt resentful that I had been interrupted until I saw that he and several men were attempt to move the woman in the back of the canoe, who was desperately embracing her child. "Bring her to me," I cried. When someone nearby advised me quietly, "It's that she doesn't want to let go of the child," I added, "Bring them both at the same time." But the men simply looked at me.

The pilot came over and whispered, "Look, doctor, what has happened is that one of the corpses in the canoe is her husband, and the child she has in her arms is dead, too." I tried to repress my own fear and anguish, inspired not so much by the thought that this woman had lost her child and husband as by the sight of her surrounded by corpses and, most of all, by the expression on her face.

To provide the woman with a semblance of privacy and dignity, people turned away as several men gently helped her, still clutching her ghostly child, ascend onto the dock. Women grasped their own children, instinctively trying to protect them, and a profound silence fell once again over the entire community. Everyone had stopped what they were doing and seemed to be reflecting on what this shattered woman must be feeling. Supported by two men, she took several painful steps in the direction of the hammock that had been prepared for her. As she sat down, her hair still shrouding her child, I could barely hear a murmur emanating from her lips. In a voice weakened by dehydration, she repeated over and over, like a secret, constant prayer, "*Maukwatida, maukwatida,*" attempting to intone a *sana*. She lay down in the hammock, holding the child's body to her chest with wrinkled hands. Her eyes seemed focused on another world, and she repeated her prayerful words. She could barely hold on to her infant. She was seriously dehydrated. Diarrhea poured into the bucket beneath the hammock, and her pulse was barely audible. She was nearly unconscious. We gently removed the child, and the two nurses and I hooked up the IVs and gave her antibiotics.

Guacara and I then returned to the canoe to deal with the corpses. He left with several men to fell trees that would be carved into the small canoes that often serve as coffins. Meanwhile, a nurse assisted me in impregnating all orifices of each corpse with chlorine. When the canoe-coffins were ready we dusted the interiors with lime, then laid out the corpses and dusted them with more lime. A funeral procession carried the five canoes into a distant and swampy part of the forest. Each was covered with mud and huge palm leaves and suspended in forks formed above the ground by felling two trees and lashing them together to form an X.

Before departing, we directed the implementation of a prevention program, leaving bottles of chlorine, eyedroppers, and all the medicine and envelopes of oral rehydration salts we could spare. We then checked the patients one more time, promised to return as soon as possible, and left for Pedernales. During the return trip we encountered two large canoes trying to reach the clinic before a number of severely dehydrated passengers died. Bringing the most seriously ill of these passengers with us, we reached Pedernales and helped Morillo prepare for the arrival of some forty more patients before we collapsed. It had been one of the most physically and emotionally trying days of my stay in Pedernales.

Before leaving the clinic the following morning, Guzmán and I stopped to observe the routine. Two Spanish-speaking nurses were calling out the names of ambulatory patients so that each could be briefly examined and given their antibiotic treatments. I could see that the nurses were having difficulty summoning the patients by name. One nurse announced, for example, "Juana Aloy." When no one responded, he repeated, "Juana Aloy" several times more. After hearing the nurse shout, "Juana Aloy!" a few more times, I stepped in. My medical training suggested that the patient was "resistant" or "noncompliant"—that is, was refusing to take the required medication. I asked a couple who was standing in front of me what was going on. They merely shook their heads and said, "I don't know." I called Simón and asked him to investigate.

By that time the nurse had met with success. He discovered that the bearer of the name "Juana Aloy" was seated less than a meter away from him. As she came up to take her medicine, the nurse said, "You see how stupid these Warao are. They don't even know their own names!" Making pejorative comments about *indígenas,* a common practice in Delta Amacuro, is meant to amuse those who consider themselves *criollos.* Simón asked the woman in Warao, who was obviously deeply embarrassed, "What happened, sister? Had you fallen asleep?"

"No," she responded, "I was right over there."

"Then why didn't you come and take the medication when they called you?" The woman simply looked away, becoming even more ashamed.

At that moment, a community leader stepped forward and angrily addressed me. "Look, madam," he said, raising his hand in a gesture of authority and exasperation, "what happened is that these people arrived last night tired and suffering from diarrhea after paddling for hours. And then it turns out that you have to have a name here to get a pill."

Simón interrupted, "So who came up with the name—the woman herself or someone else?"

The leader continued, "That's what I'm telling you. Last night the nurse and the doctor gave them these names, and she has forgotten hers."

I asked, "You mean that Warao people don't have names?"

The leader answered, "Well, some do have names in Spanish, but others don't."

Simón added, "The ones who go to school and are raised in the mission do, but not everyone." At this point, the nurse resumed reading names off the list, shouting, "José Pérez! José Pérez!"

After some discussion, an adolescent emerged from a group sitting near us, and someone said, "This is him." The adolescent was also submitted to the gauntlet of laughter and taunts. Trying to justify a practice that he seemed to find demeaning for everyone, Guzmán muttered ambivalently, "We have to keep a register of patients," and we left the clinic.

Nearly a month went by before we left Pedernales. Our efforts bore epidemiological fruit within about three weeks of intensive work: the number of cholera cases in these communities fell by some 90 percent. The health education program was well received, which greatly pleased me. Nevertheless, the constant flow of insults directed at *indígena* patients by the residents of Pedernales and government officials, including those employed by public health institutions, wore me down to the point that I requested permission to return temporarily to Tucupita.

5 Turning Chaos into Control

Initial Responses by Regional Institutions

While medical personnel in Pedernales were struggling to keep cholera patients alive, officials in the Regional Health Service were faced with the need to transform an anti-cholera "campaign" that had died shortly after it was born in 1991 into a program capable of stopping the epidemic and convincing politicians and the public that the situation was under control—or at least would be very soon.

One of the first priorities was to control the explosion of information. Residents of Pedernales saw patients being carted to the hospital as they heard a new word, *cholera,* buzzing around the community. Soon delta residents were arriving in Tucupita and Barrancas, and their presence indicated that something big was afoot. It was impossible to keep these people hidden from the eyes of journalists and the lenses of their cameras. Reporters began showing up at MSAS offices in Tucupita and Caracas, asking officials to confirm rumors of a cholera epidemic in Delta Amacuro.

Ironically, one of the first tasks undertaken by health officials was to convince people that cholera was real and that it had arrived. Politicians, accustomed to turning a deaf ear to reports of *indígenas* dying, didn't believe Rodríguez or Romero. In characterizing these denials, Rodríguez said, "I don't know if it was because they didn't want to understand or because they really didn't understand—in other words, ignorance—but both things are bad."[1] Cristóbal Bayeh, the governor of Delta Amacuro, gave me (Charles Briggs) his side of the story: "The most difficult thing was that there were many different opinions when the problem started. . . . My job at that time was to make decisions, to make decisions at times even in the face of doubts. . . . At first we were persuaded that these were the famous diarrheas that come every year when the river goes down and when it rises, such that the water is more contaminated than in its normal state."[2]

Many Tucupita residents initially refused to believe that cholera was real or, at least, that it was really in the delta. Rodríguez noted that some people "said that they didn't believe in all that. And others said it was made up *[un invento]* to attack the government, and others stated it was a smokescreen, that is, [to cover up] living costs, so many problems with corruption that were going on." Many citizens and officials thought that national developments, good and bad, were never felt in Tucupita since it was far from metropolitan centers; accordingly, they believed that cholera would never reach the delta.

Some persons were never convinced that cholera existed. Stopping short of directly denying the existence of the disease, Capuchin priest Pablo Romero declared in 1994 that "among the Warao there have always existed diseases of the intestinal variety. When the river rises and they have their rituals—yes, they have their rituals to call the spirits, to invoke the spirits so that the disease that is produced by the spirits will go away."[3] Romero's view that a "normal diarrhea," not cholera, was responsible for the deaths was repeated by many. Andrés Fabian, an anthropologist who had worked in the delta for decades, commented to me, "It is hard to distinguish true cholera from what has been always around in the delta, called *'diarrea y vómito.'*"[4] Some anthropologists stated that there had always been periodic epidemics in the delta that killed a substantial proportion of *indígenas*. Devastating epidemics, it would seem, had come to be considered "traditional," a "natural" phenomenon that should not raise any particular sort of alarm. Eduardo Silva, the state director of tourism, blamed science. "The *indígenas* have always lived with that disease, which is diarrhea, which mystically gets called 'cholera,'" he said. "As I see it, cholera has always existed. What's happened is we give [it] this scientific name, saying that it erupted over there in Peru. But there has always been cholera here. . . . The *indígena* is proud when he is in the delta, and he or she is happy in the delta, fishing, dying of cholera or dengue, or maybe living happily throughout life."[5] These discourses racialized death, converting it into a local and natural phenomenon. They were so powerful that they led many people in the region to continue believing that the cholera narratives that had been circulating throughout Latin America since January 1991 had nothing to do with them, even when a massive exodus from the delta was packing the streets of Tucupita and Barrancas.

Public health authorities may have wanted to dramatize the situation, just as politicians initially wanted to minimize it. The word *emergency* became the dominant metaphor for talking about cholera in Delta Amacuro, just as in Venezuela as a whole. When an *emergencia sanitaria* (health emergency) was declared, MSAS officials were invested with special powers that could be enforced by the police and the military. Public health authorities constructed their relationships with regional politicians in terms of a narrative of modernity, casting themselves as representatives of science and hygiene who had been called upon to eradicate the premodern mentality of backward populations. Cholera was a potential catalyst for changing the attitudes of government officials as well as citizens and bolstering the status of reform-minded health officials. For Rodríguez, making cholera real and frightening seemed to provide the only viable means of inducing politicians—and his MSAS colleagues—to finally take the disease seriously. At the same time, however, officials knew from meetings in Caracas and from newspapers that MSAS was under fire as a result of the epidemic, and they were clearly aware that they had done very little to prepare for an outbreak in Delta Amacuro. They had a great deal to lose.

CONTROLLING THE FLOW OF INFORMATION

Producing information for media consumption was crucial to creating the image of a scientifically trained, effective, and bold institution capable of controlling a very real health emergency. Rodríguez and Magdalena Benavides, the two officials who had the right to release official information, held press conferences nearly every day. In Caracas, Rafael Orihuela, the minister of MSAS, and Luís Echezuría, the national epidemiologist, also made frequent statements to the press about cholera in Delta Amacuro. The statistics and explanations that these four officials provided largely shaped the way the press represented the epidemic. Their authority emerged primarily from their professional training and their legal status as the only individuals authorized to provide official information on the epidemic.

These officials augmented the credibility of their narratives by imbuing them with the sense that they had direct contact with reality: they were there.[6] Visiting the communities in which cases were said to be most concentrated enabled officials to provide eyewitness accounts that underlined the gravity of the situation. These accounts created the sense that they were directly aware and in control of what was happening. Eyewitness accounts also spatially localized the threat. When they witnessed the presence of the disease in the fluvial area, this suggested that cholera was *not* in Tucupita or on the mainland. Blanca Cárdenas, director of ORAI, told the local newspaper that she was leaving on 8 August "for the rivers of the Lower Delta in order to get a feel for [palpar] the situation."[7] This visit authorized Cárdenas's voice even before she left. Echezuría came to Delta Amacuro to "be at the head of the teams of public health physicians who are treating patients who are suspected or declared to have this terrible and fatal disease."[8] Echezuría suggested that Orihuela also might make a personal visit. Echezuría, Benavides, and other officials toured the delta in a Guardia Nacional helicopter, adding a sense of technological modernity and military might to the metaphysics of presence. The implication was that cholera could not hide from such a concentration of institutional and technological power. Three members of Congress visited Delta Amacuro "with the objective of verifying, on the very ground in which the events occurred, the cholera epidemic and the actions that the government is taking." Accompanied by Cristóbal Bayeh, the group took a helicopter tour of Pedernales and "ten communities that have been heavily attacked by cholera."[9] For modern politicians and officials everywhere, visiting the scene of a disaster is a political necessity.

Regional public health officials attempted to infuse their statements with authority by depicting their institutions as the sole locus for scientifically based information on the epidemic. Benavides, Rodríguez, and a colleague completed one study and reported it to the press by 11 August; it blamed the epidemic on the *indígenas* from Mariusa and other infected areas "who flee in terror from their habitat toward populated centers . . . trying to escape the JEBU (spirit) that is causing the disease among the Warao."[10] In the interview that I conducted with him in January 1994, Rodríguez noted that he had conducted surveys in the street during the epidemic to assess public knowledge of cholera and reactions to the epidemic. Nonetheless, ultimate knowledge of the epidemic rested on microbiological, not clinical or observational, evidence. Rodríguez asserted on 7 August that the cause of the epidemic was being studied "by way of all of the angles of the scientific vision," but that he would only be certain as to what was taking place once the initial laboratory results were in hand.[11]

Neither Delta Amacuro nor Monagas state boasted a cholera laboratory. Samples were sent to Cumaná in Sucre state. Searching for some means to transport samples quickly, Rodríguez turned to drivers of *por puestos* (intercity taxis). They proved to be unreliable, however, and many of the initial samples were lost. Rodríguez's authority was greatly enhanced when Luís Razetti Hospital in Tucupita installed a microbiological laboratory capable of analyzing the samples, particularly because the results were reported to him.[12] Although this monopoly did increase Rodríguez's control over the flow of information, it also increased skepticism. Stool samples were obtained for only a small percentage of cholera cases diagnosed by clinicians in Delta

Amacuro state, leading to massive underreporting in the official tallies. The massive gulf between the morbidity and mortality statistics produced by the laboratory and what people learned from friends and family members eventually led many to distrust MSAS statements.

The information that officials provided to the press needed to simultaneously accomplish several objectives: it had to generate sufficient concern to induce the public to take the matter seriously, prompt politicians to declare a health emergency, and motivate a wide range of institutions to provide material and other support. Yet these goals had to be met without undermining citizens' sense that the public health system was controlling cholera and that the disease did not present a real threat to any but the most marginal populations. Public health authorities achieved both ends by drawing on the parallel practices of racializing space and spatializing race—that is, making geographic designations in the region correspond to racial categories and infusing the terms *indígena* and *criollo* with spatial meanings. In particular, reporters, politicians, and public health officials spoke from a "here" that was *criollo* and relatively sheltered from cholera at the same time that *indígenas*, the space of the delta, and cholera were fused and placed at a distance. This spatializing scheme helped to cover up an ongoing reconfiguration of space in the region that was depopulating many delta communities and lining the streets of Tucupita and Barrancas with refugees (photograph 15).

This process of racializing and spatializing cholera was so powerful that it was evoked to explain its own failure—that is, when cases appeared in what were considered *criollo* spaces. When cholera was reported in Tucupita, reporters and officials placed it in Yakariyene, the *indígena* settlement outside town. Cholera cases among *criollos* and the death of a young *criollo* girl, which appeared in official statistics, were rendered invisible.[13] Similarly, a sizable number of *indígenas* were treated at a clinic in La Horqueta, a town near Tucupita, conveniently forestalling the possibility that they would seek treatment in Tucupita itself. When protests suggested that "there is some fear among the *criollo* population," officials told them that their fears of becoming infected were unfounded since "the possibility is very remote in view of the great effectiveness of the measures being taken."[14] Even when opposition politicians challenged official assessments of what caused the epidemic and MSAS's response, they did not question the way that authorities racialized and spatialized the disease.

Neither did the press. Reporters played a key role in naturalizing the dominant narratives by juxtaposing texts and evocative images that seemed to bring official words to life. The photographs published in *Notidiario*—

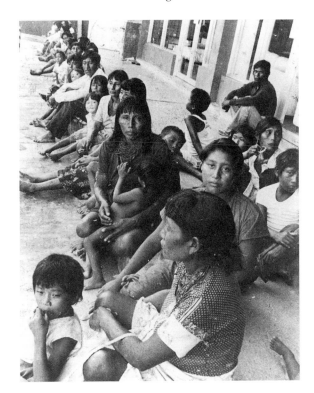

Photograph 15. *Indígenas* crowd the sidewalks of Tucupita during the epidemic. Courtesy of *Notidiario*.

usually several per day in August and September 1992—were of three general kinds: photographs of public health officials and facilities; pictures of delta communities and *indígenas* in Barrancas and Tucupita; and pictures of cholera patients. The photographs that appeared with the first articles paired pictures of Pedernales from the newspaper's archives with such headlines as "The Shadow of Cholera" and "Panic in the Delta."[15]

By 7 August pictures of dehydrated, seemingly lifeless *indígena* bodies began to appear. Photograph 16 is a fascinating example. The desiccated limbs, sunken eyes, and hollow expression of the man lying on the bed seem to identify him as a cholera patient, and the woman's dedication to weaving a basket out of moriche palm fiber mark her as *indígena*. The lengthy caption suggests that misfortune, including cholera, often befalls *indígenas* after they eat crabs. It describes "an *indígena* mother with her knowing hands weaving arts and crafts, who waits with her unaffected simplicity [*ingenuidad*] while her son, suffering from cholera, recovers."[16] Remarkably, the same photograph (with the mother cropped out) was reused the following day as the illustration for an article on *indígena* tuberculosis patients in the Luís Razetti Hospital. The disease apparently had mutated overnight.[17]

A photograph of a beautiful young woman dressed in a hospital gown and sitting on a cot, her hair bedraggled and her face bearing an expression frozen somewhere between terror and despondency, was used a number of times in subsequent editions and became something of a leitmotif for the epidemic. A photograph of a mother sitting in a hammock and cradling her dead child evoked a strong sense of tragedy (photograph 17). The long line of cholera patients, beds, and IVs in the makeshift hospital at Yakariyene was another image that was recycled frequently (photograph 18). Photographs of patients sprawled on clinic floors symbolized the chaos of the epidemic and portrayed *indígena* bodies as undisciplined (photograph 19). An image of a woman in Tucupita bearing sacks of belongings and leading several dogs came to embody the theme of migration to urban centers, and it appeared on a number of occasions (see photograph 20). Finally, another photograph that appeared frequently showed a woman cooking on the ground, with dogs in the foreground (photograph 21). In one instance a text regarding *indígena* belief in *hebu* appeared with this photograph, linking *indígena* disease etiologies with a scene reminiscent of statements by public health authorities regarding the lack of hygienic habits on the part of "the Warao."[18] What was left out, however, was that the woman had no home in which to cook. She might not have had to prepare food in such a space if housing or meals had been provided to refugees.

The bedraggled and often diseased bodies and the forlorn countenances shown in these photographs contrasted sharply with those of cleanly dressed, mentally focused public health authorities giving interviews, holding meetings, or organizing supplies. When the two types of images appeared on the same page of the newspaper, the racialization of roles in the epidemic was a natural by-product. These images reduced the terror of hundreds of *indígenas* to individual, irrational, automatic, or ahistorical reactions that were starkly opposed to the institutional, scientific, and modern responses of government officials, who were often accorded quasi-heroic roles.

Journalists and public health officials could have portrayed *indígena* nurses working against all odds to save hundreds of lives or reported the endless hours that many delta residents paddled to reach distant clinics, even as their bodies became progressively dehydrated. The images that were disseminated, however, cast the entire "Warao race," not just *indígena* patients

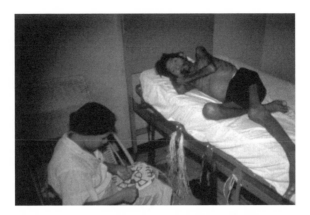

Photograph 16. Hospitalized patient and woman weaving a basket. The original newspaper caption identifies the woman as an "*indígena* mother" and her son as a cholera patient. Photograph by Freddy León, courtesy of *Notidiario*.

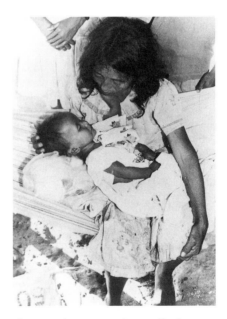

Photograph 17. A mother cradles her dead child. Courtesy of *Notidiario*.

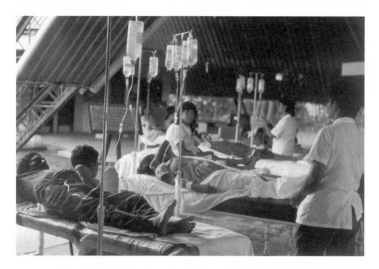

Photograph 18. Makeshift cholera clinic in Yakariyene. Courtesy of *Notidiario*.

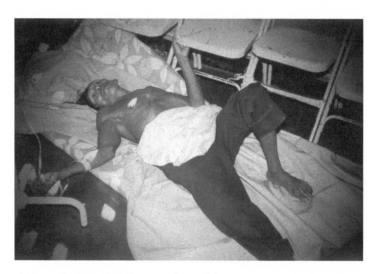

Photograph 19. Patient lying on floor of clinic. Courtesy of *Notidiario*.

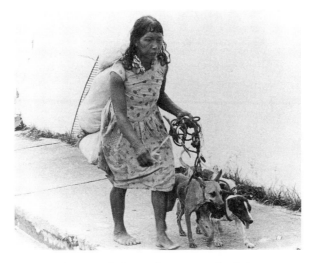

Photograph 20. A cholera refugee carries her belongings and leads her dogs on the streets of Tucupita. Courtesy of *Notidiario.*

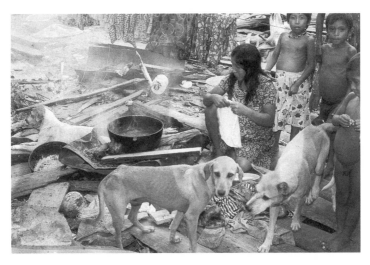

Photograph 21. Cholera refugee cooking. Courtesy of *Notidiario.*

and their relatives, as victims. Fear of contagion and death and rhetorics that drew on denigrating stereotypes to produce a class of innocent victims provided a volatile and potent combination. As Cindy Patton has noted, "Cultural narratives of perversion and contagion seem endlessly capable of turning apparently interpretation-proof facts into ammunition for media hysteria and individual discrimination."[19] The term *victim* constructs persons as lacking agency and voice, erases dimensions of their lives that do not accord with an image of powerlessness, and suggests that they are in need of pity, supervision, assistance, and representation.[20] Victim rhetoric served as a screen memory, blocking the production of other sorts of cultural memories. Press reports denied "*indígena* cholera victims" a complex personhood in favor of a one-dimensional, abject existence.[21] Particularly when joined to the discourses of superstition and filth and rendered not only objective but also powerfully affective through the use of photographs, these images placed a great deal of social and even historical distance between readers and the persons pictured. This distance precluded the possibility that some members of television, radio, and newspaper audiences might identify with cholera patients as sharing a common experience of poverty, exploitation, and disenfranchisement.

The media presented public health authorities as the only authoritative source of information on the epidemic. Nearly all other voices were relegated to echoing, extending, or criticizing official formulations. Nevertheless, journalists sometimes reflected critically on these official voices, creating intertextual gaps—that is, spaces where contradictions between different sources could be exposed.[22] One technique involved emphasizing the mode of transmission of official information. For example, the article titled "The Government Says That It Has Cholera under Control" called attention to the fact that the reporter's only source was the reported speech of one official. A second tool involved juxtaposing text and photograph in such a way that the latter called into question the veracity of the former: if, for example, Orihuela has a happy smile while Venezuelans are dying from dengue, malaria, and cholera, who can believe him?

Intertextual gaps were sometimes created between two or more statements made by the same official. Orihuela's contention that cholera was "under control" was juxtaposed to his admission that the rainy season could lead to floods, contamination of drinking water with sewage, and new outbreaks.[23] *Notidiario* sometimes juxtaposed contradictory statements that Benavides made at different points in the epidemic. These instances were rare, however. Officials attempted to avoid disagreeing in public about the epidemic, and restrictions on who could report official information minimized contradictions. MSAS was able to maintain a virtual monopoly over the production of information. When eyewitness accounts or rumors challenged official accounts, authorities could deprive the reports of credibility. Rodríguez told a *Notidiario* reporter that "at the level of the public, many rumors are circulating about cholera cases; as soon as this gossip becomes known [to us], we follow up on it properly, and it turns out in many cases to be without substance *[bolas sin fundamento]*."[24]

The press provided the greatest tool for discrediting reports of the epidemic that threatened MSAS jobs, policies, and resources, but it also constituted the greatest threat. Perhaps most worrisome was the possibility that the enormous media attention would reveal the ubiquity of death in everyday life in the delta. On 6 August 1992, the day that the first cholera article appeared in *Notidiario,* the newspaper also published an article titled "Hunger, Vomit, and Diarrhea Extinguish the Warao Race." The text was placed underneath a photograph of a woman seated on the ground and accompanied by two nearly naked children. The photo was an archival shot that had nothing to do with the specific content of the article, but it helped to elicit an emotionally charged response. The article reported a *denuncia* (accusation) by "the *indígena* Capitán Moreno Zapata" of Arawabisi, and it attributed the prevalence of illness to lack of medical care, poor health conditions, hunger, lack of economic and technical assistance, and corporate land theft. The press also used a rhetoric of extinction to criticize the government: "The *indígena* communities are slowly dying out since they are condemned to being abandoned, especially by the state government."[25] An article that appeared two days later advanced the same sort of critique by reporting that seventeen *indígena* patients with advanced tuberculosis were hospitalized in Tucupita. In short, even though reporters sometimes joined opposition parties in criticizing the government and questioning official assessments, they never challenged the racialization of the epidemic or the portrayal of *indígenas* as premodern, passive victims, nor did they disrupt the impressive degree of control over the flow of official information about cholera that Benavides and Rodríguez enjoyed. By helping to racialize cholera and by depicting cholera patients as helpless victims in need of state paternalism, reporters and opposition politicians collaborated in making medical profiling seem like a natural and necessary response to the epidemic.

FIRING UP INSTITUTIONS, FINDING RESOURCES

Institutions in Tucupita that served communities in the delta and received substantive funds from Caracas seemed to be perpetually bankrupt. Physicians and nurses who worked in the fluvial zone frequently had to turn away patients because they had no medicines. Often the frustrated practitioner who had to deliver this message got blamed for "not wanting to help." When community leaders showed up at ORAI to ask for assistance, staff members, virtually all of whom were *criollos*, usually shrugged their shoulders and said that the director was out. Through persistence it was possible to obtain an interview with the director, but nearly always the response was, "There are no funds available." Government employees who aspired to inaugurate projects in the delta were often told by their superiors that a lack of funding or transport made it impossible to launch any new programs.

Municipal, state, and national governments were the biggest employers in Tucupita in the early 1990s. Thousands of employees were paid from funds earmarked for helping *indígena* communities. Payrolls included many workers who never showed up for work but who delivered political support when it was requested. Some politicians and senior officials made personal fortunes by ensuring that little of this money actually reached the delta. The system worked as long as everyone played the game and nobody else was watching. But national officials and a national public started to watch as soon as the first cases of cholera were reported. Cholera threatened the game, shaking the centers of power in Tucupita.

In August 1992 a miracle started to unfold. Budgets that had been exhausted long ago suddenly had plenty of money. Boats that hadn't existed appeared in no time, and they had gasoline to spare. All at once piles of food were available for distribution in communities that had long suffered from some of the highest levels of malnutrition in the country. The notion that the country was near economic collapse had furnished an inexhaustible source of excuses for institutional poverty, but everyone knew that institutional and individual survival now depended on getting personnel and resources into the delta—fast. Reversing the situation that had formerly plagued the anti-cholera committee, once the epidemic began officials competed to see who, in the press's estimation, would be the first to act, provide the most resources, and be the most dedicated to helping the poor *indígenas*. The Tucupita airport, which had been defunct for years, was quickly readied to receive shipments of medicine, food, and equipment. National officials, who normally avoided visits to "the end of Venezuela," now vied for the right to show up in Tucupita, consult with state officials, tour the fluvial area, and promise support. All these players did their utmost to make sure that their efforts were adequately covered by regional and national newspapers and by Caracas-based television stations.

Suddenly the anti-cholera committee was the place to be, politically speaking. Formerly invisible members now wanted to take a leadership role. Exercising his authority as committee president, Bayeh declared "a state of health emergency."[26] Benavides assumed her position as general coordinator and took effective control of the committee, working closely with Rodríguez. Six subcommittees were formed, devoted to medical services, environmental sanitation, logistics, transport and communications, health education, and follow-up and evaluation, providing enhanced press visibility for their chairs.[27]

The governor focused on interinstitutional coordination and allocated resources that were not available from other institutions. Defensa Civil provided transportation, conducted censuses of refugees, assessed needs for food and other supplies, and donated some of its stockpiled comestibles. Although the epidemic occurred during the school holidays, which limited the participation of the Ministry of Education, bilingual teachers gave talks on cholera prevention in many communities. ORAI officials visited the delta and attempted to quell the panic inspired by cholera. The armed forces were extensively involved in the cholera control "campaign." In addition to providing helicopters and bringing materiel to the region in military planes, members of the Guardia Nacional worked alongside medical personnel in some regions. In the Pedernales area soldiers bearing machine guns often accompanied physicians on visits to communities.

A number of organizations provided personnel and resources. The Red Cross sent a contingent of fourteen persons, described in *Notidiario* as highly specialized professionals, to assist with health education in the delta.[28] Members of a national labor organization visited Curiapo and handed out medicine, food, and clothes. A private foundation, FUNDAFASI, was actively involved. While some owners and managers of fishing enterprises and sawmills placed profit ahead of the lives of their workers, as in the case of the Mariusan fishermen, others generously expended their own resources to save the lives of community members, whether employees or not. In addition to transporting cholera patients to clinics, some loaned their facilities to physicians for use as temporary clinics. Private citizens also cooperated, even across racial lines, to a remarkable extent. People donated food and other resources in a spirit of common cause. The responses in primarily *criollo* communities in the delta were not uniformly generous, but they contrasted sharply to the generally hostile reactions that emerged in Tucupita and Barrancas. Assistance was also provided by the European Economic Community, and the Dutch government donated $60,000 to help with cholera education.[29]

HEALTH EDUCATION
AND THE INDIVIDUALIZATION OF RESPONSIBILITY

Before the epidemic, two factors had kept investments in health education to a minimum in the delta. As microbiological approaches to medicine and technologically based interventions gained ground in Venezuela and elsewhere during the second half of the twentieth century, physicians' faith in the importance of their patients' social environment and even of clinically based knowledge and primary care accordingly diminished.[30] Although a countermovement that emphasized health education and health promotion arose, it was hard for techniques that rely on patients' ability to improve their own health status to compete with biomedical interventions that rely on the power of medical expertise, medications, and technology. Moreover, health education specialists have suggested that the effectiveness of health education is contingent on the target population's capacity to change their beliefs and behaviors.[31] Public health officials and other persons who designed and disseminated health education programs in Venezuela had to believe in people's ability to change. The region's racial economy augmented the power differential between doctor and patient in such a way that most of the physicians we interviewed strongly believed that *indígenas* were incapable of grasping biomedical concepts or incorporating hygienic and other bodily practices that reflect them.

Health education provided a shared focus for a number of agencies. Beyond the efforts of the Regional Health Service, hygiene talks were given by Red Cross volunteers, Defensa Civil personnel, ORAI representatives, bilingual teachers, fishermen, census takers, employees of nongovernmental organizations, and private citizens. Newspapers published information on cholera, and Radio Tucupita regularly carried programs and public service announcements. Caracas television stations also transmitted information about cholera prevention. Regional and national newspapers devoted articles to steps recommended by WHO and PAHO, including boiling water and storing it in sealed vessels to prevent contamination. Articles also included guidelines for preparing, consuming, and storing food, suggestions for general hygiene, reminders to avoid foods sold by street vendors, and statements regarding the need for oral rehydration and medical attention in case of infection.

MSAS and other agencies presented recommendations in illustrated brochures that were handed out on the street, in clinics, during health education presentations, and the like. Sometimes the information contained in these pamphlets was highly racialized. One leaflet intended for general—that

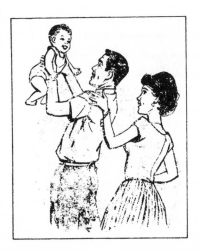

EVITAR EL COLERA
ES TAREA DE TODOS

Figure 2. Cover of an MSAS health education pamphlet on cholera. Courtesy of the Ministry of Health and Social Development.

is, *criollo*—distribution contained drawings representing a well-dressed, smiling, light-skinned family, parents and child (the cover is shown in figure 2). Each recommendation was accompanied by images: well-groomed, smiling children posing in front of a stove in a middle-class kitchen, a woman cooking and cleaning, a man spraying for insects and carrying out trash.[32]

Pamphlets designated for *indígena* populations, on the other hand, were different in a number of ways. *Indígena* languages were used in health education campaigns aimed at *étnias*, thus immediately signaling the racial classification of the target audience. By 8 August 1992, the ORAI staff had already translated recommendations into Warao and printed copies of a pamphlet for distribution in *indígena* communities. Officials in Caracas and Tucupita apparently assumed that all *indígenas* were fluent in Warao and literate as well. It never seems to have dawned on them that, given the dominance of Spanish, many bilinguals might have been more able to read texts in Spanish than in *indígena* languages.

Individuals who could read this pamphlet were unlikely to fit its illustrations. The cover features a young, somber *indígena* girl with an *indígena*

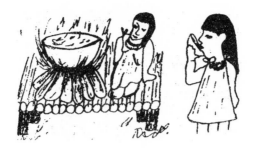

JO ISIA

— Oko jo jobikitane jo yakeraja ekorokitane jisabakitane ja.
— Jo ekorenaka jobinaka takine ja.

[Translation:
WHAT TO DO WITH THE WATER

— So that we can drink water, we must boil it well.
— If it isn't boiled, we can't drink it.]

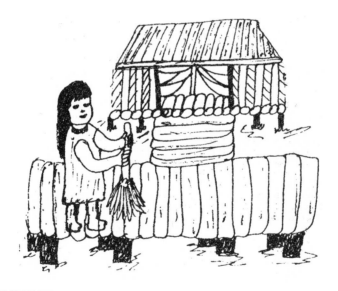

KA TEJO YAOROKI
KA BAJUKA YAOROKI

[Translation:
LET'S TAKE CARE OF OUR BODIES
LET'S TAKE CARE OF OUR HEALTH]

Figure 3. Drawings that appeared in an ORAI health education pamphlet.
Courtesy of the Regional Office of Indigenous Affairs, Tucupita.

house and hammocks in the background. The drawings that accompany the recommendations show houses on stilts with thatched roofs (figure 3). The women in the picture are wearing beaded necklaces and long, flowing dresses. They are preparing foods, using baskets, and cooking over an open fire. The text focuses on personal hygiene, food preparation and storage, boiling and storing water, and the need to seek medical treatment immediately if severe diarrhea occurs. The apparent audience for the pamphlet was homogenized. Some people classified as *indígenas* are doctors, nurses, and teachers, and many live in wooden, enclosed houses with metal roofs. Nevertheless, at the same time that the racialization of *criollos* seemed to suppress the fact that most are members of the working class, *indígenas* were lumped together in a way that depicted them as uniformly rural and poor and maximally different from *criollos*.

A pamphlet prepared by the Guardia Nacional racialized its target audience even further. An image of a well-groomed physician with a thick mustache (a feature not associated with *indígenas*), who bears both a stethoscope and the guard's insignia, is juxtaposed to drawings of nearly naked, beaded *indígenas*, who are shown defecating in the open, vomiting, and living in filthy circumstances (figures 4 and 5). In other drawings semi-naked *indígenas* are cleaning their homes, preparing food, picking up garbage, and going to the clinic. In short, they are aspiring to sanitary citizenship. The guard's insignia is prominently displayed on each page. Even though this text is in Warao and the document was produced for use in the delta, the figures do not resemble anyone who lives in the region. They are stereotypes, even caricatures, of *indígenas* that were modeled on residents of Amazonas state. The haircuts and loincloths are distinctly out of place in the delta. These depictions supported existing Venezuelan images of *indígenas* and created a stark contrast between the polished, professional, and confident *criollo* physician, who produces the messages of modernity, and the poor, dirty, helpless *indígenas*, whose lives depend on their ability to listen and to follow his directions.

Here we have a striking example of the way that images of cultural difference create powerful racial hierarchies. The side-by-side drawings grant "the two cultures" their own textual space, but the two illustrations are far from parallel. The physician is presented without a social or environmental context, but the *indígena* is framed by a rural landscape. The physician dominates the frame and looks the viewer in the eye, but the *indígena* is positioned back within the frame and looks at the ground. The physician speaks, naming the disease and the symptoms that the man is experiencing, but even though the squatting *indígena* appears to speak, he is not a speaking subject

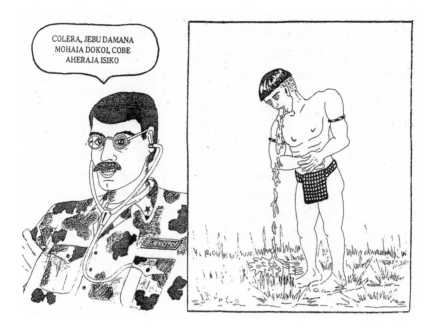

Figure 4. Drawings that appeared side by side in a health education pamphlet prepared by the Venezuelan National Guard. The doctor states, "If you get this disease, cholera, you will vomit, and your stomach will also hurt." The label on his shirt reads "Ejercito" (Army). Courtesy of the National Guard.

like the physician, whose open mouth and eye contact suggest that he is addressing the viewer. The physician speaks to potential *indígena* cholera patients, but the *indígenas* serve only as ventriloquists, projecting the same lines.

Insofar as *indígenas* rejected these stereotypical images, they were not likely to place a great deal of faith in the content of the accompanying text. On the other hand, if they accepted the denigrating images of themselves, were they likely to feel empowered to take the steps needed to avoid a local cholera outbreak or to save the lives of patients in the absence of ready access to medical care? Racializing images helped to defeat the best of public health intentions and to deprive poor communities of their potential benefits. The pamphlets directed at *indígenas* display a "politics of misrecognition."[33] In the midst of the 500 Years of Resistance movement of 1992, *indígenas* were actively seeking political and social recognition. Their leaders demanded an end to denigrating stereotypes and that subordinating practices be replaced and respect for the *indígenas'* collective self-images be represented. They sought to gain recognition for their attempts to shape the

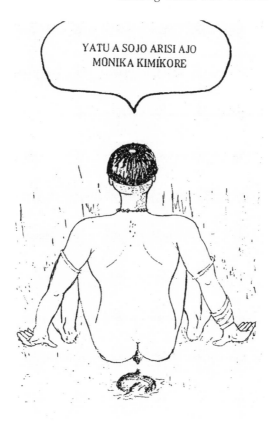

Figure 5. Drawing from Venezuelan National Guard pamphlet. The text reads, "You will also have rice water diarrhea." Courtesy of the National Guard.

course of social and political change in their communities rather than being characterized as uniformly "traditional"—as locked in unchanging cultural patterns. In the guise of being culturally sensitive, these pamphlets "misrecognized" or rejected *indígena* self-representations and, instead, presented *criollo* conceptions of *indígenas* as uniformly defined by "traditional" houses, baskets, and canoes. In the Guardia Nacional brochure, bodies are literally stripped of signs of insertion into "the national society." By invoking the cultural features of dress, bodily decoration, housing, cuisine, canoes, and language for *indígenas* alone, the brochure suggested that its viewers—the racialized population—were not sanitary citizens and could not be educated through modern, rational methods. By masquerading racial constructions as cultural difference, these practices of exclusion could be presented as a generous humanitarian gesture, a liberal response to problems that had been created by the culture of the unsanitary subjects.

The representations of middle-class *criollo* and poor *indígena* subjects in anti-cholera efforts also converged in important ways. First, patriarchal gender roles were imposed in the *indígena* scripts just as they were in the *criollo* versions: the women cook and clean while adult men are commonly pictured outside the house. Second, health education programs inaugurated in Caracas as well as the delta were concerned only with washing hands, boiling and storing water, preparing food, and obtaining treatment. These efforts are crucial in preventing cholera, but so are providing potable water and waste disposal, increasing access to medical care and education, and reducing social inequality. Exhortations that focused on hygiene and treatment individualized cholera, placing the burden of controlling the disease on individuals and families and pushing the role of nation-states and their institutions, corporations, international lending organizations, and the media into the background. A drive inaugurated personally by Benavides on the streets of Tucupita focused on soliciting funds for the "cholera campaign" from drivers and pedestrians, who were asked to place donations in tins, and distributing pamphlets.[34] A billboard that was placed prominently on the *malecón* (waterfront walkway) between Paseo Manamo and the river in Tucupita stated, "Prevention is everyone's task" (photograph 22). The billboard's silhouetted figures of men and women in various shades seem to be transfixed, held by the powerful gaze of the state, which is identified as the advertisement's sponsor by the phrase "Delta Amacuro State Government."[35]

Despite its worthy goals and its undoubted value in reducing cholera morbidity and mortality, this barrage of messages transferred responsibility for cholera prevention to individuals and families. A pamphlet produced by MSAS and Alcaldía de Delta Amacuro (the municipal government) exhorted, "'Don't die through ignorance.' Delta citizens, we are protecting you, contribute to activities for preventing cholera." This and other statements implied, "We've done everything we can and should do. If you get cholera and perhaps die, it's your fault!" The health education messages were metacommunicative, reaching far beyond the individuals whose hygienic practices needed improvement and conveying information about institutions, physicians, patients, and social relations in general rather than simply informing readers about cholera. The cultural representations in these brochures visually and textually racialized cholera; it just seems natural that the *criollos* pictured do not display cholera symptoms while the *indígenas* in the Guardia Nacional pamphlet defecate and vomit in images that rob

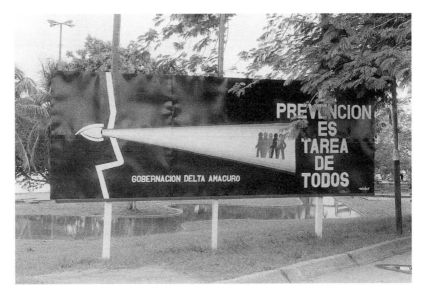

Photograph 22. Health education billboard next to the river in Tucupita. Photograph by Charles L. Briggs.

them of any sense of privacy. The materials targeted at *indígenas* seem to invite medical profiling. If *indígenas* get cholera, they can be blamed for failing to adopt the suggested prevention procedures, and stringent measures for containing these undisciplined bodies seem to be required.

The health education discourse that was produced collaboratively by journalists, officials, and politicians was condensed into a number of unforgettable images that shaped the cultural memory of the epidemic.[36] For those individuals who granted legitimacy to these representations, the frightening symptoms of cholera became enduringly linked to dirty, racialized persons. The health education programs provided public health and other institutions with a powerful screen memory that hid not only their own role in creating the conditions that fostered such high rates of morbidity and mortality—and deplorable everyday conditions—but also the role of national and international political-economic forces. The recursive quality of these images—they appeared across multiple media in a range of contexts on a daily basis—created a ubiquitous and unavoidable frame of reference for the production of cultural memory even for individuals who sought to resist them. The discourse could be ignored only by those who had no contact with radio, television, newspapers, health care facilities, or government offices—in short, by no one.

SUPPRESSING THE FLIGHT OF *INDÍGENAS*

At the time of the epidemic, the highest government official in Tucupita specifically charged to advocate for *indígenas* was Cárdenas, the director of ORAI. She is a strong woman with small, penetrating eyes. Her serious demeanor and careful, controlled speech lend her something of an aristocratic air. Like Benavides, she is a woman who has been accustomed to exercising power, both in ORAI, which is part of the Ministry of Education, and in party politics. When I interviewed her on the porch of her Tucupita home in 1995, she described herself in these terms: "I am an educator. I am from Curiapo and was raised in the village that they called Hohebura.[37] . . . I am good friends with the Warao. I like the Warao a lot, and I love to be in the delta, to share with them." Indeed, unlike most Tucupita officials, she made extensive trips into the fluvial area and stationed several of her employees there. She did not, however, focus on recruiting *indígenas* for positions within ORAI. Like most persons from the Curiapo area who are classified as *criollo*, she speaks Warao fluently, a skill that greatly aided her career at ORAI.

Cárdenas said that a crucial goal for the health education program was "to help the *indígenas* know how to grasp the recommendations and transmit them to their countrymen [*paisanos*] in their own natural environment." ORAI's job, she noted, was to work with other institutions "to make it possible to take care of the Warao in their own villages [*rancherías*]."[38] A compelling narrator, Cárdenas described the manner in which she and her staff attempted to keep *indígenas* from fleeing their communities.

Blanca Cárdenas, Tucupita, 10 March 1995

They were so terrorized that they just didn't know what to do. Their fear made them run around looking for help wherever they went. But after the cholera passed, everything came back to normal, and they carried on with their normal lives. They didn't continue to be terrorized by cholera, no. Because this is very important, you see. The *indígenas*, if you had left them alone and we had left, let's say us *criollos*, well, they would have fled from fear of cholera, and maybe the thing would have been even harder. . . .

They would say to us, "Aren't you afraid?" and [we'd say,] "Why would we be afraid?" And then they would ask me in Warao if I was afraid. "I'm not afraid!" So then that is something that helped them a lot to remain in the area, because if they saw us constantly visiting them in their communities and everything, that's a really big thing for them. Well—but if we had left, then perhaps they would have been even more terrorized and perhaps things would have been even worse. . . . And when we traveled here [to Tucupita] to run some sort of errand, someone stayed there. We never left them alone, because we were afraid that they would feel alone. So we played a really important role in this. . . .

It was in Winikina that [cholera] attacked so horribly. What happened is that it attacked rapidly and the crisis passed. But they took their Bactron [antibiotic] whether they had cholera or they didn't have cholera. And they asked us if we took it, and so that they would keep taking it we told them "yes," that we did take it. And right in front of them we took one or two tablets, understand, right, in order to help them understand that if they took it—they asked us, "Do you take it, too, in order to prevent cholera?" "Sure, we take it!" And we carried some here, we carried it in our wallets. And we took it and they would say, "We're going to take it too!" It was something that we—at least I—know well and speak Warao, and I knew that it would be necessary to teach them, because it wasn't going to be easy. And so I left it in their baskets. And when we came [and said], "Look, did you take it?" "Yes, the packets are all gone. Give us some more!"

Cárdenas racializes *indígena* responses when she implies that "the Warao" would give in to a seemingly irrational fear unless *criollos* were there to demonstrate a nonchalant demeanor. This patronizing attitude places Cárdenas in particular and *criollos* in general in the role of comforting parents while "the Warao" are cast as children given to uncontrollable emotions. Convincing people to take Bactron was the principal strategy used to calm these fears. Physicians often did provide the contacts of cholera patients with antibiotics prophylactically, but indiscriminate distribution of antibiotics is medically unsound. Note the power of pronouns in this narrative. Cárdenas's use of "we" unites a host of institutional actors whom she identifies as *criollos* at the same time that her use of the third person plural lumps together all *indígenas* as the recipients of official exhortations.

The key phrase in the narrative is "to remain in the area." A primary reason for dispatching teams of medical and other personnel to the regions where cases emerged was "to treat patients affected by the *Vibrio cholerae* 'in situ.'"[39] As Bayeh put it, "We needed to have them shut in [*encerrados*] in their communities, controlled [*controlados*], explaining things to them." He added that the large shipments of food to delta communities and the provision of hammocks, clothes, mosquito netting, and even outboard motors were intended precisely to induce *indígenas* to stay put.[40] When such carrot tactics failed, sticks were sometimes wielded, and government agencies forcibly returned *indígenas* to "their natural and traditional location."[41] These efforts reflected stereotypes of *indígenas* as nomads, wandering aimlessly in response to any sort of provocation.

Widespread efforts to keep people from leaving the fluvial area were spurred by the scandal that erupted when thousands of *indígenas* began to appear on the streets of Tucupita and Barrancas. The image of *indígenas* "fleeing cholera"—and bringing the bacteria with them—became a leitmotif for the epidemic, one visually encoded in media photographs (see photograph 15, earlier). Since reporters seldom ventured into the fluvial area, *indígenas* were largely invisible when they remained "in their natural habitat"; when refugees came to town, on the other hand, opportunities to obtain photos and brief statements abounded.

Treating *indígenas* in urban hospitals created political problems. Rodríguez told me that "because the people here worry more, public opinion is affected more when the hospital gets full of cases. It's not as if there weren't any in the delta, but just that they didn't see [patients who were hospitalized in rural clinics]. And since the population, the greatest population concentration is here in Tucupita, what affects [politicians] more is when the hospital is full of persons with that pathology or any pathology."[42] Pictures of *indígena* cholera patients in Luís Razetti Hospital elicited not only fear of contagion but also assertions of territorial rights in the face of "an invasion by *indígenas*." A hierarchy of citizenship that polarized *indígenas* and *criollos* was part of the system of political rights, responsibilities, and vulnerabilities that deeply influenced how public health institutions, no matter how much they were guided by scientific and humanitarian concerns, responded to the epidemic.

Efforts to keep *indígenas* out of town and invisible to reporters were also likely prompted by the hotly contested political campaign taking place at that time in Delta Amacuro. Opposition politicians looked for ways to attack the government, and the presence of *indígenas* on the streets of Tucupita provided an easy target. Their presence greatly complicated the political damage control undertaken by Benavides, Rodríguez, Cárdenas, and their subordinates.

FUELING CRITICISM

Cholera was used as a pretext for criticizing the state and its institutions from the start. Having long attempted to arouse public concern over health and other conditions in their communities, local leaders from the delta soon found that statements that contained the magic word *cholera* generated audiences and often government action in a totally unprecedented manner. Community leaders visited the press in attempts to demand their rights to health care, legal protection, and freedom from economic exploitation. The role of the press in deciding which *denuncias* to publish and how to present them greatly shaped their political force. Articles generally subsumed such statements within a familiar narrative of the plight of the defenseless *indígenas* and the government's failure to help them. The effect of leaders' efforts was thus contradictory and ironic: *indígenas* demanding citizenship rights were painted as helpless victims.

Even though public health officials tried to control the circulation of information, the racializing narratives that reporters told placed the epidemic precisely within the larger narrative frame that the officials were attempting to erase. Some stories focused on the lack of sanitary infrastructures and the shortage of primary care, which had been a problem long before August 1992. For example, when *Notidiario* reporters asked José Rivera why Mariusans had left the delta when people became infected with cholera, he was quoted as responding, "There is no infirmary nor any other species of institution that deals with health. . . . Living conditions in the area are unbearable *[insoportables]*, since we lack everything and there hasn't been a single state agency that has bothered to establish itself there."[43] His father's perennial protest over the government's failure to provide health and educational services in Mariusa thus finally made its way into the press. Nevertheless, the *Notidiario* reporter transformed the statement in such a way that stereotypes of the area as inhospitable were confirmed, and Rivera's words took the form of a stock phrase of opposition politicians (depicting government institutions as failing to make their presence felt in the face of calamities).

Other attacks on the government emerged in the voice of the newspaper itself. Here the line between reporting and editorializing was frequently blurred. One article intimated the role of corruption in creating conditions favorable to an epidemic by asking whether the budgets of the agriculture and education ministries, the Instituto Agrario Nacional (National Agrarian Institute), and the Governor's Office would be used in combating cholera. "Or could it be that the authorities will let the terrible forecast that cholera will lead to the disappearance of three-quarters of the Warao indigenous group come true?" The article stated, "The Warao have the right to live and to deny them assistance is a crime, for which one will have to appeal to Divine Justice."[44]

One of the ways government officials responded to these attacks was to assert that their efforts to bring cholera "under control" had been successful—that mortality was low and new cases were dwindling. As early as 17 August, Orihuela and Echezuría declared that the epidemic in the delta was "under control" even as Rodríguez was reporting new cases.[45] When authorities admitted in early October that there had been new outbreaks, criticism mounted anew. As the credibility of the cholera control efforts was tested again, a number of heads rolled, including those of Benavides and Cárdenas, who had served as the director of ORAI for a decade. Many observers suggested that once the initial scandal began to die down and the 5 December election approached, resources that had been set aside for the epidemic were reallocated to campaigning on behalf of ex-governor José María García Gómez[46] and that trips into the delta by government employees were geared more toward the body politic than corporeal bodies. Public health institutions were again placed under heightened scrutiny. The national Federación Indígena (Indigenous Federation) and Comando de Profesionales (Brigade of Professionals) demanded that the Comisión Indigenista (Indigenist Commission) of the Congress and the Comisionado de la Presidencia de la República para Asuntos Indígenas (Commission for Indigenous Affairs of the Office of the President of the Republic) visit the delta to assess the situation.[47] A national health commission came to the delta in November to gauge the effectiveness of control efforts and to push state officials to get the anti-cholera committee going again.

Some opposition candidates made cholera a focus of their attacks. Gubernatorial candidate Luís Cabareda asserted that "the cholera epidemic is directly related to the current low quality of life; extreme poverty joins bad hygiene and impoverishment [depauperización] and the poor quality of public services, especially sewers and potable water." Painting a sympathetic yet demeaning picture of indígenas, Cabareda argued that the epidemic could easily embrace Tucupita because of the lack of an adequate sanitary infrastructure.[48] As the epidemic wore on and the election neared, gubernatorial candidates embarked on quick, vote-and-photo-op-oriented tours of the delta. Even though the press and opposition politicians largely echoed official racialization of the epidemic, government officials accused them of foul play, self-interest, and lack of patriotism.

Cristóbal Bayeh, Tucupita, 17 May 1995

There were even a lot of political games being played. There's an epidemic on, and so the political parties try to take advantage [sacarles provecho] in an electoral year. . . . Regarding all the attention [the press] gave to this subject, I'd say it was to exploit the news. They brought out the news more to draw attention, not to inform people—they did it simply to promote their newspaper. For the politicians, it was only to promote themselves, not to look for and find solutions to a problem. I visited the media in Caracas, I, as governor, went to *El Nacional*, I went to *El Universal*, I even went with the only *indígena* physician, I went with [Vicente Medina], and we declared Delta Amacuro to be in a state of emergency, we made an appeal for help, we explained the situation—it was as if nothing had happened. . . . And the press, instead of advancing a request for aid, to make these issues evident, they rather presented it in the news as an epidemic, something dreadful that is finishing [people] off.

In his righteous indignation Bayeh apparently forgot that at the time he too was part of a party organization similarly locked in a rather brutal and acrimonious electoral campaign. He suggests that health issues should have been kept apart from the political power struggle that entered into most arenas of public life in Delta Amacuro. Patriotism, a powerful discourse in Venezuela, was mustered to squash attempts to debate the politics of health rights when they were most obvious and inescapable.

Some individuals accepted the moral weight of Bayeh's position. One of these was an individual generally referred to as "the Warao physician," Dr. Vicente Medina. Medina was born in Nabasanuka and educated at the Capuchin mission. After receiving his medical degree he returned to the delta, where he was employed by the Regional Health Office during the epidemic. Medina was, however, politically aligned with the Partido Movimiento al Socialismo (MAS). He was a leading critic of public health officials at the same time that he was helping to create some of the dominant epidemiological conceptions of the epidemic. In December 1994, after MAS leader Bernardo Alonzo became governor, Medina was serving as a substitute delegate to the lower house of Congress and pursuing advanced medical training in Caracas.

Of medium height and sturdy build, Medina is given to infectious smiles. His voice transmits his passionate commitment to his work, an awareness of the political complexities of public health institutions, and the pain and uncertainty born of the constant need to defend himself in the face of slights and outright attacks by officials and others who would, it seemed, rather not see an *indígena* in a position of power and prestige. When I interviewed him in Caracas, Medina criticized his own use of the epidemic as a political tool. "I include myself among those who attacked such targets as the Regional Health Service, its director, as having failed to govern," he said. "And I even presented an accusation or took as a point of departure that there was a disaster and previously there had been an appropriation [that is, a misappropriation] of the budget earmarked for indigenous issues. These things happened, and I took advantage of these disastrous events." Medina then contrasted his own actions to those of persons who used scientific principles to control cholera. The criticisms that Medina directed at public health authorities in 1992 were more muted than his public declarations the previous year about the racialized and substandard character of health care for *indígenas*. Benavides reportedly charged him with professional misconduct in the Colegio de Médicos (College of Physicians and Surgeons) of Delta Amacuro, and, as a result, he came close to losing his license to practice medicine.

The view that public health should be above politics—as plausible and high-minded as that seems—protected the status quo of oppressive health conditions in two ways. First, it made it more difficult to perceive and challenge the politics of health care except when they intersected explicitly with electoral politics. Second, it suggested that only partisan political interest can motivate criticism of government health policies. The attacks mounted through the media by community leaders, reporters, and opposition politicians actually helped to reveal deplorable everyday health conditions, challenged the dominant interpretations of the epidemic, and opened up spaces for new representations and interventions.

I do not want to romanticize these critiques as thoroughgoing challenges to the status quo, however. None presented substantive plans for transforming health infrastructures or improving primary health care in the fluvial area. Nor did any challenge the narratives that placed *indígenas* in the role of powerless and generally voiceless victims while assigning physicians and institutional officials the role of scientifically informed and sympathetic saviors (although some critics did suggest that these actors did not play their parts very well). Indeed, debates regarding institutional responsibility for deplorable health conditions provided contexts for sharing racialized accounts of the epidemic. Politicians and health care workers often traded accusations that the other party was responsible for "corrupting the *indígenas*." Oscar Rendón, a young nurse from Tucupita, described a confrontation he'd had with a politician from the Santa Catalina area.

Oscar Rendón, Tucupita, 5 August 1999

He told me that in the indigenous communities the *indígenas* were dying of hunger and they got sick a lot and all that. And I asked him, "Well, who was the one who brought that way of living to the *indígenas*? Politicians!" Because when [politicians] needed something, they needed [support] for their campaigns so that they could win a particular office, they took, they offered them two packages of food, two or three cases of rum, they held a party for them. And because of their ignorance, *indígenas* believed that this was going to last all of their lives. And when this round of electoral campaigns was over, they forgot about them. They left them even worse off than they had found them before. I think that they are the ones who brought them to prostitution, to all this robbery, and shamelessness and laziness, and everything. Because the *indígena* in his environment used to be able to subsist. He planted, hunted, fished, and in that way lived off his environment.

Politicians and MSAS health workers shared a romantic vision of the life of the *indígena* prior to the coming of the *criollo*. They thought that the power of *criollos* to shape the lives of *indígenas* and the passivity of *indígenas* were indisputable. They believed that the result of *criollo-indígena* interaction was a complete and irreversible fall into a pathetic moral, economic, and political state for the *indígenas* alone. The violence of racial constructions—their pervasive, denigrating, and sometimes fatal effects—was seldom questioned. Public debates thus operated within limits that prevented the government's foes from effectively challenging the status quo.

HEALTH AND THE INDIGENOUS SOCIAL MOVEMENT

In 1992, the year that cholera "erupted" in Delta Amacuro, the politics of inequality were exploding all over Venezuela. Neoliberal policies and the growing desperation of the poor, which had entered public awareness during the 1989 uprising in Caracas and other cities, came into sharp relief in 1992, when Chávez framed his attempted coup as a blow at neoliberalism and the political system on behalf of *el pueblo* (the people). In some communities, however, race was the most important issue. A hemispheric social movement based on pan-indigenous identities turned the projected celebration of the Columbian Quincentennial on its head and provided a highly visible stage on which to raise questions of human rights, constraints on access to government services, environmental degradation, and land expropriation. Leaders of indigenous communities traveled widely through the Americas, and Venezuelan activists visited regions where there were populations classified as *indígenas*. Although cholera was not a major focus of the indigenous social movement in Venezuela, the two phenomena intersected in powerful and unpredictable ways in Delta Amacuro.

For many delta residents the most pressing issue of the day was land expropriation. The displacement of *indígenas* was certainly nothing new. The establishment of plantations for the production of coconuts, cacao, and other products and the creation of cattle ranches had claimed substantial areas of the upper delta. Rubber tappers engaged in brutal labor practices and placed pressure on lands south of the Orinoco. In the late 1980s and early 1990s, residents of the southeastern part of the delta were concerned about losing their rights to lumber concessions. By 1992 the growing aggressiveness of the palm hearts factories, particularly the ones located at Merehina and Hobure, had become the greatest concern. One thirty-foot manaca palm usually yields enough palm hearts to fill only a single sixteen-ounce can; the product is destined for expensive restaurants in Europe and the United States as well as the domestic market. About one hundred trees must be felled in a single day to provide a living wage. This dangerous work conferred no benefits such as disability pay or medical insurance. The boats that picked up the palm hearts sold food, axes, tobacco, and other goods to workers at high prices, and workers were often told that their wages were less than the value of the goods they purchased. Residents were thus trapped in a system that resembled debt peonage.

Land expropriation, labor exploitation, environmental degradation, and exclusion from political office were the main foci of *indígena* protests, which were increasing in size and organization, and they figured among the chief concerns of the Unión de Comunidades Indígenas Warao (Union of Indigenous Warao Communities), formed in 1990. Activists sought to obtain motorboats and other resources needed to organize throughout the delta. In the face of the protests the government ordered the Instituto Agrario Nacional (IAN, National Agrarian Institute) and others to hold meetings in the delta, hoping that they could assuage concerns and halt the growing discontent. Vague offers of title to the land on which communities were located were offered, but activists soon realized that this system would set residents against their neighbors and that all but a tiny fraction of land in the delta would thus be ceded de facto to the government and corporations. Activists demanded title to the entire delta on behalf of "the Warao people."

It was almost inevitable that this struggle would intensify in 1992, as *indígena* and *criollo* activists joined in the "500 Years of Resistance." One of the largest demonstrations took place in November, less than a month before the election (photographs 23 and 24). As a "*criollo* ally," I was asked to participate. Because it was known that I had a video camera, I was asked to tape the event. Some two hundred participants, including national leaders, representatives from the Kariña *étnia* of Monagas, and several political candidates, marched from the outskirts of Tucupita to Plaza Bolívar. They carried large banners and shouted, "Land or Death!" to advance accusations of genocide against the Corporación Venezolano de Guayana (CVG), a government agency charged with development and public works projects in the region. At the concluding rally, activist and educator Feliciano Gómez called for a moment of silence in honor of Guaicaipuro, the colonial "*cacique*" who

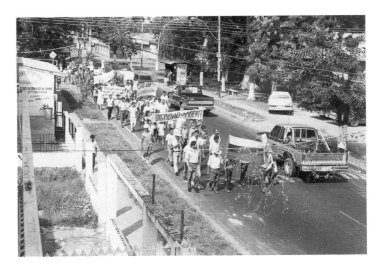

Photograph 23. Protest march held in Tucupita in November 1992. Courtesy of *Notidiario*.

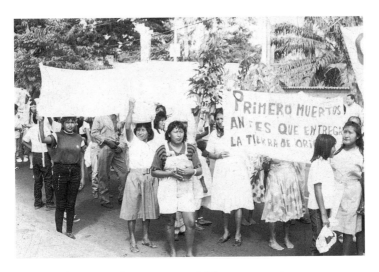

Photograph 24. March participants with banners accusing government institutions of genocide. Courtesy of *Notidiario*.

symbolized *indígena* resistance to the Spanish conquest. He then addressed the crowd.

Feliciano Gómez, Tucupita, 18 November 1992

The desire of all indigenous people has always been to continue living as an aboriginal community *[pueblo aborigen]*, as authentic sons and daughters of this land called Delta Amacuro, preserving our identity. We are here to protest the plundering of our lands that began five hundred years ago with the Spaniards. Now it continues in Delta Amacuro state, and is present in the Venezuelan state in the form of the Ministry of Defense and the Instituto Agrario Nacional, the state government, the CVG, and their staff, who act as pimps by taking away the lands of the Warao here in the Delta Amacuro. Today we are particularly in solidarity with the nearby communities that are having their lands taken away by a corporation named Agrodelca, with the complicity of the CVG, the Instituto Agrario Nacional, and the state government of Delta Amacuro. For this reason the affected communities and the Warao communities present here declare that the above-mentioned institutions are the mortal enemies of the Warao. In solidarity with the affected communities, we are going to defend their rights with all our resources. To take the land away from the Warao people is to kill the Warao people. We ask all of our Tucupita friends who are present here that they join in solidarity with their Warao friends, because the death of the Warao would destroy the cultural inheritance of Delta Amacuro state. We are not asking for anything that is not ours, we are demanding something that is ours— our property—and they have taken it from us. But we are here on the land and these are the renewable natural resources that should be given to the Warao.

We Warao say that we have experience with death, with pain, and with the development that has come to Delta Amacuro, as in the concrete case of the damming of the Manamo River, which caused death and continues to cause hunger and poverty to the Warao, the true sons and daughters of this land. That's why we say that no development can be real development that comes at the cost of hunger, poverty, and death. This is what Agrodelca is going to bring to, to ensure for [the people of] Playa Sucia and its environs. We also denounce the pitiless exploitation of the Warao by the palm heart and lumber industries. For the Warao, the worst of all is that the Warao are exploited, are poorly paid even under the calm and indifferent gaze of the institutions whose job it is to prevent this. We, the Warao people, say that we are not just going to think about this—we are going to take advantage of this opportunity to solve what is the greatest problem for all indigenous peoples, the problem of land tenure.

The Warao people, united with all of the other *étnias* in the country, declare our great desire to take our Indian liberator, the Indian heroes, the great Guaicaipuro, to the Panteón Nacional [National Pantheon]. They are just as deserving as the Venezuelan liberators, and for this reason they have the right to a place of honor in the Panteón Nacional. In memory of the great Guaicaipuro and our other Indian heroes, in defense of our lands, the Warao understand, and we demand the defense of our lands. We demand collective title to the lands of the lower delta and that the Warao become the masters of our community and the riches of the forest and the other renewable natural resources for the benefit of the Warao. Long live Guaicaipuro! Long live the Warao! CVG out of El Garcero! Death to the invaders! Thank you, ladies and gentlemen.

A central focus of magical healing in Venezuela, Guaicaipuro had become a symbol of the *indígena* social movement in Venezuela. Gómez evokes Guaicaipuro as he links the national indigenous social movement to struggles taking place in Tucupita. He places development schemes that favor commercial profit, especially lumber mills and palm heart factories, at the expense of small-scale producers alongside "the plundering of our lands that began five hundred years ago with the Spaniards."

Gómez then introduced María Luz Figueroa, an activist who came from the community that lay at the heart of the CVG controversy.

María Luz Figueroa, Tucupita, 18 November 1992

Okay, brothers and sisters, we are here for the reasons that our brother Feliciano just expressed. I'm not going to say too much, I'm going to be brief, but what I want to say is this: In '89 they sat down in Caracas, together with the governor of Delta Amacuro, the regional IAN office, and the CVG, to sign a document regarding the future of us Warao. They have always thought that we are zoo animals, they have never thought that we are human beings, just like them, with five senses, brothers and sisters. Without taking us into account, they sat down behind a desk to sign the sentence of the Warao, of us Warao of El Garcero, signing a twenty-five-year lease that gives away our lives to the CVG, so that the gringos can come, just [like] the Spaniards once again, so that they can finish the task of killing [us], just as they did in 1960 by damming the Manamo River. But now we are a people that has woken up. We are a united Warao people, we think just like they do. We can't just sit down to debate them behind a desk, jointly with them, to decide what will be the rights that belong to us as Warao. We, too, are human beings. We think now, we aren't zoo animals as the Venezuelan *criollos* have thought. Up with the Warao!

Today we think for ourselves, we made this banner by ourselves, we have been able to organize by ourselves, we have now woken up, brothers and sisters. Now we are going to fight against those invaders, those criminals who have just signed this sentence. We are going to show them that we have courage and dignity. Better death than to lose the land of one's origin! . . . When they establish the Agrodelca corporation, everything will be over for us, because soon planes will come to fumigate us, believing that we are pests [plaga]. They will come to pollute the river, they will come to destroy us, the forest, and our animals. Our children will die, little by little. Now they speak of cholera and will continue to do so, as if the indígenas were not poisoned but died from cholera or some other thing, but they will never say that they were poisoned. They are still dying and they will continue to die, thanks above all to Agrodelca. And I hope that you, as delta residents, as local representatives, won't allow the rice-producing Agrodelca corporation to come to our community. You young brothers and sisters and students, you professionals, in the solidarity that you show in coming with us, let's stop this. I end by asking the Liberator, our Father, to help us as he always has helped us and will help us with our lands.

Although Gómez had enjoyed higher visibility in indígena activist circles for a number of years, Figueroa was not widely known at this time. Nearly ten years later, a prominent indígena leader who helped organize the protest told me that it was this speech that had first demonstrated Figueroa's rhetorical and leadership capabilities. She became a key aide to the three indígena representatives to the National Assembly who were elected following passage of the 1999 Bolivarian Constitution.

Both speeches are heteroglossic, meaning that they drew on multiple vocabularies and social contexts.[49] The speakers incorporated discourses of cultural heritage (Gómez: "cultural inheritance of Delta Amacuro state"), the language of community organizing (Figueroa: "we are a united Warao people"), and ecological discourses (Gómez: "renewable natural resources"). Both speakers used pronouns to distinguish two audiences: "us Warao" and "you criollos." This suggests that Gómez and Figueroa were speaking as racialized subjects, sometimes as indígenas in general and sometimes as Warao in particular, to other racialized subjects, criollos. All criollos are referred to in the third-person plural. Activists supporting their causes are distinguished from the "pimps" who occupy offices of the nation-state. Figueroa accused institutional officials—along with "Venezuelan criollos" in general—of racism, claiming that they think of "Warao people" as being "zoo animals."

Standing at the feet of the statue of Simón Bolívar (photograph 25), Gómez drew on the anti-colonial rhetoric of the national hero by describing institutions of the nation-state as being on the side of the despised losers of the War of Independence. He asserted that these "new Spaniards" were less interested in addressing citizens' needs than in the "the plundering of our lands." The new colonialism that these institutions served, both actively

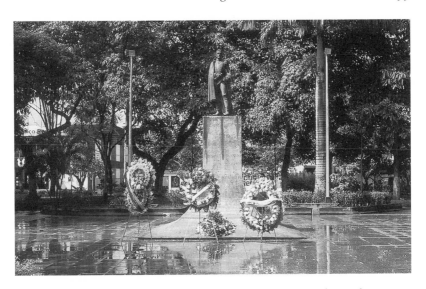

Photograph 25. The statue of the Liberator, Simón Bolívar, on Plaza Bolívar, Tucupita. Photograph by Charles L. Briggs.

and in the guise of their "calm and indifferent gaze," embraced land expropriation, ecological destruction, and economic exploitation at the hands of corporations, both Venezuelan and transnational. The state, in short, had become the enemy of Venezuelan nationalism. A "solemn" offering of baskets and products of the forest, representing "Warao culture" and the natural environment of the delta, were placed at the feet of "the Father of our Country." Figueroa and Gómez inverted the ideological underpinnings of racism when they constructed *indígenas* as true Venezuelan nationalists who were defending the national space against foreign penetration and domestic treason. These two Delta Amacuro activists were not alone in invoking the anti-colonial rhetoric of Bolívar. In 1992 Chávez also used Bolívarian rhetoric, construed in terms of class rather than race, as a basis for a coup attempt. The way that Chávez was racialized as black suggests that issues of race were also present in the larger political scene.[50]

Where does cholera fit into this picture? The remarkable thing is that it doesn't, at least not directly. The protest took place in the fourth month of the cholera epidemic. Although the number of cases and deaths had diminished, people were still dying from the disease, and delta residents and hundreds of cholera refugees were still living on the streets of Tucupita and Barrancas. The epidemic was only mentioned briefly toward the end of Figueroa's remarks. Building on her assertion that Agrodelca would threaten the health of her community by spraying crops with pesticides and polluting the river, she incorporated the hypothesis that the epidemic was caused by some sort of poison that was released into the river and that reports of a cholera outbreak constituted a government cover-up. This brief and cryptic remark was the only allusion to the worst public health crisis that had emerged in delta communities in recorded history. No criticism was directed against the regional health system.

Why didn't activists place cholera on their agenda? In an interview that I conducted with Gómez in July 1995, he recalled that when the cholera outbreak began they were "really scared, right, scared." He continued: "And we stuck very close to the clinic [in Nabasanuka]. We couldn't go very far away, we stuck very close to the clinic."[51] At the same time that he criticized himself for not doing more to save lives during the outbreak, he admitted that he had been constrained by the terrible fear of contracting cholera. I suspect that the monopoly that public health professionals had on the dissemination of information about the epidemic played a telling role here. Questions of health were medicalized to such an extent that neither cholera deaths nor highly visible medical-profiling strategies became part of activist agendas.

Medina, as a physician, could have spoken authoritatively about cholera in such a context, but his position was less radical than that of Gómez and Figueroa, and he seldom participated in these public protests. Although he made public statements that criticized government institutions, including MSAS, he was employed by the Regional Health Office and he had already come close to losing his license as a result of making critical public statements. Efforts by politicians to discredit *indígena* activists were intense, and people learned to pick their issues.

This is not to say that activists never challenged MSAS during the epidemic. When cholera cases still filled the clinic at Nabasanuka, a physician arrived from Caracas and immediately ordered all patients who no longer exhibited acute symptoms out of the facility. Gómez and other community leaders challenged the decision, accusing the physician of acting like Christopher Columbus because he thought he had the right to throw people out of a facility located in an *indígena* community. The physician apparently saw cholera as a purely biomedical phenomenon; when symptoms disappeared, the case was closed. Furthermore, the clinic was an MSAS facility, and the physician undoubtedly believed that hierarchies of institutional authority should rightfully control who was there and what they did.[52]

Gómez and other Nabasanukans placed cholera within a larger narrative that included questions of land loss, limited access to government services, community empowerment, racism, and the fear and dislocation produced by the epidemic. They also perceived that the physician's order reflected assertions by MSAS employees that *indígenas* were remaining in clinics after recovering completely so that they could get free food—a recontextualization of racist stereotypes of *indígenas* as perpetually lazy. On a practical level, the effect of the order was to require Nabasanukans to feed and house scores of individuals who were still too weak to return to their homes in other communities. No one had asked whether residents were willing to take care of the ex-patients or had the resources to do so. Fear of cholera and MSAS's monopoly on the circulation of official information may have kept the disease off activist agendas, but incidents suggest that delta residents did sometimes challenge the way that MSAS authorities represented and regulated cholera patients in relation to specific circumstances that arose in predominantly *indígena* communities.

PROTECTING THE RACIAL ECONOMY

Institutions of the Venezuelan nation-state, such as public assistance agencies, courts, schools, and clinics, largely create the categories through which race-based social inequality is defined. They formulate the rules that determine where individuals are placed, and they make this process seem rational, fair, and even natural. Indeed, the mission of ORAI is based on a dichotomy between *indígena* and non-*indígena* subjects. Some institutions receive funding earmarked for *indígena* communities, some treat *indígena* clients differently. When newspapers and television news programs across the country reported that a massive cholera epidemic in the delta was decimating its *indígena* residents, the depth of social inequality became deathly apparent. The revelation threatened the racial equilibrium that helped regulate access to power and resources in the region.

Rather than recognize the way that race-based inequality permeated everyday life in the region and constituted the major "risk factor" responsible for high morbidity and mortality in the fluvial area, officials and journalists operated from the start on the premise that cholera was racialized. Gómez succinctly summarized this situation when he explained why institutions suddenly committed an unprecedented amount of resources to fight cholera: "The government . . . acted like that only out of fear—they said, 'No, we've got to help, because if the Warao die, we're going to have a problem.'"[53]

Institutional responses to the epidemic constituted a racial project in that they deepened the racial inequalities of the region and redistributed re-sources accordingly.[54] At the same time, these agencies depicted their ef-forts as valiant, race-blind attempts to save *indígena* subjects from them-selves. This racialization of cholera enabled national and regional institutions to maintain their legitimacy and their resources in the face of the threat to their legitimacy posed by the heightened visibility in 1992 of the emergent social movement that championed the rights of *indígenas*. The government was criticized, but not for sustaining a system of racial inequality. It was faulted only for failing to play the game adequately—that is, for failing to save the lives of poor, helpless *indígenas*. Treating cholera control as a racial project served a purpose that extended beyond regulating an *indígena* pop-ulation. By racializing cholera as an *indígena* disease, the nation-state's fail-ure to achieve modernity could be made to seem natural and inevitable. Racial difference posed an epistemological and social barrier that even the most dedicated institutions could not be expected to surmount.

The outcome could have been different. The opening weeks of the cholera epidemic witnessed a huge infusion of supplies, transport, and personnel into the delta. It was undoubtedly the most widespread and successful interinsti-tutional project that had ever been undertaken in Delta Amacuro. It had the potential to provide Venezuelans with a model of how national and regional government institutions, civil and religious groups, businesses, and private citizens could cooperate effectively in meeting a collective goal. Government agencies competed with one another in attempts to build new, positive im-ages as "can-do" institutions with heroic leaders. Some of these efforts even crossed the lines that separated races, classes, and occasionally—and perhaps most remarkably—political parties. The epidemic could have become a model for challenging the racial economy and building a new society.

Unfortunately, this possibility was precluded from the start by the short-term nature of the goals that directed responses to the epidemic. No one proposed creating and maintaining chlorinated water systems in the delta, even for large communities. No one considered the possibility of doubling the number of type-II clinics and thus significantly decreasing the distance that patients would have to travel to secure a physician's care. Efforts did not focus on providing economic resources to end the malnutrition that kept infant mortality so alarmingly high. Although Venezuela's financial deci-sions were constrained by its debt to international lending institutions, the willingness of the European Economic Community to provide economic as-sistance and PAHO's desire to use the epidemic as a means of transforming sanitary infrastructures in Latin America suggest that the moment was ripe for beginning a truly remarkable transformation. Unfortunately, as Gómez suggested, the need to protect the racial economy—and the political economy it sustained—seems to have prevented even imagining another course of action. The contradiction that lies at the heart of state institutions— between the democratic rhetoric that promises equal access and treatment to all citizens and practices that enforce inequalities of race, gender, class, and sexuality—had to be protected from the challenges represented by *indígena* protests and popular insurrections.

6 Containing an Indigenous Invasion
Quarantine in Barrancas

What became of the Mariusans after their exodus from a place that they had come to identify with death, terror, and uncertainty? They were fated to remain at the center of the storm; indeed, catastrophe seemed to follow them wherever they went. Some, about one hundred, traveled to the clinic in Nabasanuka, but most headed directly for Barrancas, their most frequent stop on routine trips to the mainland. With a hospital only a relatively short walk from the Orinoco River, Barrancas spelled safety. The Mariusans hoped that *criollo* physicians would know how to cure their strange new sickness.

The Mariusans anticipated finding support from friends in the *indígena* village and from Antonio Bustamante, the fisherman with whom they had worked for so long. Exhausted, frightened, and desperately hungry, they were dumbfounded by the welcome they received when they climbed the steps that led from the water's edge. The *criollo* residents of Barrancas were horrified. Government officials asserted that hundreds of the "least civilized" *indígenas* had suddenly "invaded" Barrancas. Many Barranqueños contended that thousands had arrived. Until this moment many residents had dismissed news reports about cholera, thinking it was just another smokescreen concocted by the government to deflect attention from the economic crisis. The arrival of the Mariusans convinced them that cholera was altogether too real.

Barrancas del Orinoco is in Monagas state, which boasts some of the most intense agricultural and petroleum development in Venezuela. Barrancas and its some 10,000 residents are viewed as a vestige of the premodern world by other Venezuelans, as is also true of Tucupita.[1] Government officials sent from Caracas or Maturín, the state capital, see themselves as emissaries of modernity, enlightened embodiments of the nation-state charged with bringing civilization to a barbarous region. Barrancas was apparently the point where the cholera epidemic of 1854–1857 began in Venezuela, but since the disease had not been reported in the country again until 1991, the previous outbreak had disappeared from collective memory.[2]

Ramón Rivera, a younger brother of María Rivera, was one of the Mariusans who traveled to Barrancas. In 1992 he was about thirty-five years old. An extremely kind and good-hearted fellow, he decided while quite young that he did not want to marry, and he chose to work "as a woman," cooking, raising children, and weaving hammocks. He is one of our closest friends in Mariusa. In October 1994, Rivera, with the help of Diego González, the eight-year-old boy he was raising, recalled the flight to Barrancas:

Ramón Rivera, Mariusa Akoho, 12 October 1994

When the *wisidatu* died, we headed off, each in his or her own direction. There were no canoes and there were no motors. As we left one was seated here, one there, one there, one there—we couldn't even move our legs. . . . We were headed for Barrancas in a small canoe, without the others, without our nets, without any of our belongings—with nothing, with absolutely nothing. We had to leave so much stuff behind, and it got stolen. I myself still had not gotten sick. We couldn't eat; we ate only the tiniest amount. [We thought,] "If we eat, won't we die? Won't we get diarrhea?"

By dawn, I was nearly dead. I was very close to death when dawn came. I was so tired. I was so tired I could have died. I just couldn't go on. We were all near death as we tried to sleep on the way to Barrancas. Just when we arrived, the National Guardsmen, the National Guardsmen came out of their car. They grabbed us and took us and threw us inside cars and took us away. There were lots of us inside.

Here Diego González interrupted to tell us that they had been inside the school; then Rivera continued.

They threw everybody inside there, all the people. The building was packed. There were lots of people; everybody was there. They threw all the people who had come from here in the forest inside there. But instead of being able to eat, we had to live almost without food. They gave us only a little food. They gave us only starch, no meat or fish. And we didn't beg for anything more, either. They kept us inside there for two weeks.

Diego speaks some Spanish and had spent much more time in town than his adoptive father had. The boy seemed to have a keen appreciation of the irony of being held captive in the Eloy Palacios High School; the building in which *criollo* children attended school had become a prison for *indígenas* who had been denied access to education for decades. About 260 Mariusans were housed in the cafeteria of the school (photograph 26).[3] The Mariusans were held in quarantine by local police and the Guardia Nacional in this cordon sanitaire, where they were attended by physicians and nurses from the

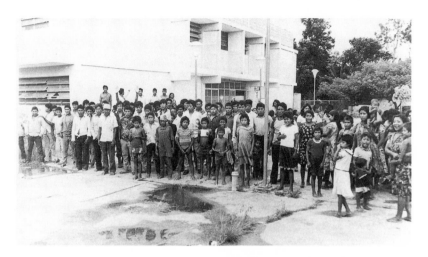

Photograph 26. Mariusans lined up in front of the high school in Barrancas. The original newspaper caption reads, "The new contingent of *indígenas* who have arrived in Barrancas, fleeing cholera, placed in the high school." Courtesy of *Notidiario*.

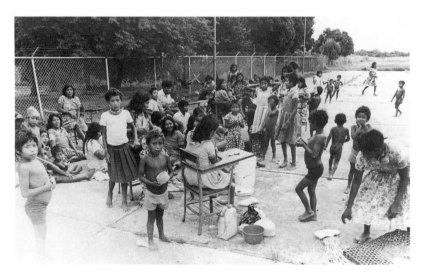

Photograph 27. Mariusans on the grounds of the Eloy Palacios High School in Barrancas. Courtesy of *Notidiario*.

local hospital. The barbed wire around the school that usually kept vandals and thieves from getting in now kept the Mariusans from getting out. A *Notidiario* photograph showing women and children in the school courtyard carried this caption: "The majority of the migrants are women and children, and they walk around the streets looking for anything" (photograph 27).[4] The caption and the illustration contradicted each other—these women and children could not wander the streets because they were locked in the schoolyard. The Mariusans had found the medical assistance they so badly needed, but at the cost of their freedom and human dignity.

I spoke with a number of people about this experience in February 1995. José Rivera offered this recollection.

José Rivera, Nabaribuhu, 16 February 1995

After leaving from here [Mariusa], we arrived in Barrancas. As soon as we arrived in Barrancas, we were in a school, a high school. We were there thirteen days. It was horrible—we suffered a lot. We had to sleep without hammocks, on the floor. It was horrible. All of us got really angry. We got angry. We said to the government officials, to the mayor of Barrancas, "How did you come to be the boss of the Warao people? Give me permission to go to Tucupita so I can speak to officials there and tell them what has happened."

"No," [they said,] "not even a single one of you can go. Every single one of you will stay here, locked securely inside."

"Okay, if that's the way it is, I'm going to call the director of ORAI."

Back then, the director of ORAI was Blanca Cárdenas. And the director of civil defense arrived with her. His name was Ricardo Salas. I spoke to them. . . . We said, "We're suffering horribly. We're sleeping on the floor. There are lots of children, lots of pregnant women; they have to sleep right on the floor. This is horrible. Okay, you're in charge. With whom can we speak? We want to get out of here. Even though we're in Barrancas, even though we arrived here, we want to get out of here. We want to leave this building."

"No," [they replied,] "you have brought too much [cholera] with you! If you come out with all of your people, all [the *criollos*] will die. You must stay here two weeks, taking medicine so that the doctor can watch all of you, can vaccinate everyone. If you don't do this, all of you will die."

Well, they kept us in the same place constantly for thirteen days.

Rivera uses a powerful device to tell his story, one that scholars often refer to as reported speech. Reporting not only actions but also conversations provides a powerful means of inserting snapshots of a character's beliefs, emotions, and motives into a narrative.[5] Rivera uses this device when he portrays the Mariusans' sense of outrage and the depth of their determination to obtain their liberty. In reporting Cárdenas's and Salas's words, he conveys the shock and sense of outrage that the Mariusans felt when they suddenly realized that others were blaming them for the spread of the disease. This new relationship to the nation-state was experienced in bodily terms, as hunger in the gut and the press of cold concrete against the skin.

To deal with the power of the nation-state, the Mariusans tried to exploit the fissures that existed between competing governmental institutions. They were able to prompt a visit from ORAI director Cárdenas, whom they regarded as a potential ally, but they were surprised to find that this strategy failed. Despite the tension that generally exists between officials in Tucupita and Barrancas, Cárdenas and Salas presented a united front, aligning themselves with Barrancas officials against the incarcerated Mariusans. This interinstitutional cooperation was an important development in the relationship between the government and *indígenas*. During the epidemic and its aftermath, it dealt a significant blow to the emergent political presence of delta communities.

The Mariusans were beginning to develop a consensus that the pathogen was not the product of sorcery but was a *criollo* disease, that it had come "from outside," possibly carried by a fisherman. They soon learned that the physicians, politicians, bureaucrats, and other *criollos* who had taken control of their lives saw things differently. The people in Barrancas racialized cholera as an *indígena* problem. "The Warao"—specifically, the Mariusans—were threatening "the people," the *criollo* residents of Barrancas. Officials believed that continued incarceration was needed to save the lives of the "Indians," who were considered to be incapable of helping themselves, and to keep them from "spreading the disease." The epidemic was spawning a new geography of blame, and the Mariusans learned to their horror that they had been placed at the center of it.

The Mariusans also were surprised by the effectiveness of the effort to isolate them. They frequently came to do business in Barrancas, staying several days at a time. The Winikina population that lived next to the river included a number of their friends. Everyone in town knew that the Mariusans were being held in the school, but no one came to see them. Bustamante's two Mariusan wives waited for him at the high school, but he did not come. Bustamante's "real wife" lived in Barrancas, and she would not be seen with her *indígena* counterparts. Another Mariusan woman had anticipated a visit from Bustamante's son, Jacobo, because they had been living together in Mariusa. These women and their relatives gained insight into the very different way that race, class, sex, and gender operated in town. The lesson was as cold and hard as the high-school floor.

One of the most fascinating aspects of José Rivera's account is the shift in his narrative from first person plural, which positions him as a member of the collectivity, to first person singular—a sole voice that represents the others: "*We* got angry. *We* said. . . . Give *me* permission to go to Tucupita so *I* can speak to officials there" (emphasis added). Rivera does not tell us how he came to speak for other Mariusans, but Cristóbal Marcano, Busta-mante's foreman in Mariusa, commented explicitly on this issue. A fellow with a stocky figure and a somewhat nervous disposition, Marcano's close association with the fishermen and his origin in Macareo, a neighboring area, made him feel like something of an outsider in Mariusa.

Cristóbal Marcano, Mariusa Akoho, 12 October 1994

Our suffering was the fault of the officials, we suffered because of what they said. Then they asked, "Who's your *cacique* [leader]?"

"We have no *cacique*, our *cacique* died. We have no *cacique*, we have no *cacique*."

In order to name a *cacique*, they asked, "Who is in charge back along the [Mariusa] river? Who is in charge back along the river?"

"The fellow who was in charge back along the river died."

"Okay, where are the sons of this fellow who was in charge, who died?"

"Well, his sons are here. There's one, and over there is another."

"Okay, is there one among them who speaks Spanish, who speaks Spanish well?"

"Yes, there is one."

"Where is he?"

"That's him."

"He's the *cacique* now." They called him. "Are you the one?"

"I am."

So he became the *cacique*. They said, "Damn, you're the *cacique* now, we're making you the *cacique* right now, because you can speak [Spanish]. Okay, you're it."

This act of investiture was quite a departure from the way that leaders had been chosen in Mariusa. Every year during the *nahanamu* celebration, all aspirants to leadership roles gathered around the dance floor. After the *wisidatu* danced, senior men determined the order of male dancers for the year. The first to dance would be the *kobenahoro* for the coming year, the next man would assume the role of *kapitán* (captain), and so forth, in diminishing order of rank. Women were neatly excluded from any direct role in the selection process and, of course, from these leadership positions. Santiago Rivera's authority as a healer, storyteller, orator, and political strategist had kept him in power for some thirty years. All of a sudden one of his youngest sons, a man of about twenty-five years of age who lacked experience as a healer or as a leader of any sort, was thrust into the most important political position in his community on the basis, primarily, of his ability to communicate with monolingual Spanish-speaking officials of the nation-state. Bureaucrats, politicians, and missionaries had often complained about the elder Rivera: he had frequently outmaneuvered them, and he had been a hard guy to push around. By killing Rivera and displacing the community, cholera enabled government officials to achieve what they had long sought—the installation of a man who would be easier to talk to and, they hoped, control.

Government officials appointed the new leader of a local community in much the same way that nurses assigned names to patients in delta clinics. They even gave him a title, *cacique,* that was used only for *indígena* leaders, thereby erasing the position of *kobenahoro,* the name that they had conferred on *indígena* leaders in previous generations. Democratic ideologies are powerful in Venezuela, and they crucially shape conceptions of the nation, the state, and its citizens. Here we see how democratic practices could become deeply racialized. Official representatives of an elected government never even considered consulting Mariusans about their preferences, let alone "allowing" them to democratically elect their own leader. And, one might add, José Rivera, as surprised as he was at the time, did not challenge their decision. He walked right into this role, immediately speaking on behalf of "his" community.

Stories told in the media about the Mariusans' internment contained three recurrent themes that sustained common racial stereotypes. One was the uncontrolled and uncontrollable fertility (and hence promiscuity) of "*indígena* mothers" and their inability to keep their children alive. Another was "breastfeeding babies" *(lactantes),* which was often represented by photos of women breastfeeding in public. This image powerfully suggested that *indígenas* were both erotic and repulsive. The third theme was trash—sacks of beer and soft-drink cans collected for sale to recyclers—which marked the *indígenas* as homeless and poor.

On 17 August, toward the end of the internment, *Notidiario* ran an article on the "truly worrisome and frantic" situation "that has been created by the arrival of Indians from the delta in Barrancas." The article described the Mariusans as "seeking medical attention, medicines, and food," and as people who "fled the terror that the presence of cholera has caused among the Warao ethnic group." The article both reported and reproduced connections between public health policies and racial stereotypes: "In the face of the sudden influx *[afluencia]* of *indígenas* from the delta, Barrancas officials placed some of them in the high school, causing a tremendous problem with the *criollo* population, but the majority is wandering around the streets and next to the port with all of their belongings, some toddlers and cans, and an astounding quantity of children of various ages and breastfeeding babies."[6]

This passage spatializes the racial opposition between *indígenas* and "the *criollo* population" by contrasting the people who came from the delta with the residents of the city. Residents more commonly referred to the arrival of Mariusans and other cholera refugees as an "invasion." This equation of race and space is, of course, belied by history: people have always traveled frequently from the delta to the mainland and, in the case of commercial fishermen, vice versa. Taking a step back in time, one might say that it was the *criollos* who "invaded" the delta. Nonetheless, the metaphor transforms an *indígena* in Barrancas into matter out of place, a condition that is deeply connected with defilement, desecration, and taboo.[7] The article also describes immigration as a river or flood that can damage the sovereign terrain inhabited by citizens, a common metaphorical system.[8]

MODERNITY ARRIVES IN BARRANCAS

Unlike Tucupita, Barrancas is not a state capital. Senior public health authorities for Monagas state work in Maturín. Accordingly, the key player in shaping how Barrancas officials reacted to the epidemic was Dr. María Vargas, director of the hospital. Vargas had recently been transferred from Barinas, a small city located in the plains of central Venezuela.

Unable to contact Vargas by telephone, I (Charles Briggs) took the bus to Maturín one morning in March 1995 and walked across the street to an MSAS office. Although she worked at another location, Vargas graciously made the drive across town to meet me. We conversed for two hours. A poised and articulate woman of about fifty-five, with graying hair and a slender figure, Vargas has an outgoing and generous manner coupled with a powerful sense of duty. She mentioned that her decision to become a physician had been motivated by her uncle, a high MSAS official and a well-known public health physician.

Vargas focused intently on the story that she told, transporting us back in time and place to Barrancas in August and September 1992. Vargas remarked that she had long looked forward to the chance to recount these events—and, seemingly, to put her version on record.[9]

Dr. María Vargas, Maturín, Monagas, 31 March 1995

The experience helped me to gain a foothold in Barrancas. The experience was very good.

The first boats came with a massive quantity of sick patients, a population of approximately 279.[10] And what we did with them was that within moments we hospitalized 10 patients, of which 4 were in really bad shape at first. Patients in shock, [or rather] nearly dehydrated and nearly in shock—we had 4 patients almost in shock.

We formed a cordon sanitaire, taking over the Barrancas high school. We isolated the patients who appeared to be healthy there. . . . We then immediately made the announcement—we notified [officials in Maturín]—and we began to take the preventative measures that were needed in connection with the hospitalized patients. The hospital was declared to be in a state of emergency. And then I called the maximum authorities, the mayor of the community, so that they would begin to work as a team with the cordon that we had formed. And the whole thing was successful—the medical team, the whole thing. . . .

We gave the patients whom we isolated in the high school their respective outpatient treatments, twenty-four-hour-a-day medical attention. I recall a colleague from Caracas, Dr. María, a marvelous person. She was the physician who was in charge at night, she had that shift. She was very attentive to those patients. Since they were like that, they were her children. She would get up at dawn and go and give them their medication, along with the nursing personnel and the army. She was the physician. I had another colleague who cooked for them in her house—she cooked for the Indians. A marvelous woman. They formed a team, you see, and I will never forget it. The army also helped us a lot. They were there with us [in the high school], and then they helped us maintain order inside, to guide those people, because it's not easy to manage [manejar] that kind of population. Oh, they also helped in terms of cleanliness. Or let's say that the mayor's office took responsibility for bringing them clean water. Then the army helped maintain order; and when we were going to give the medical treatments, they helped us too. And we gave them their three meals, and we managed everything. Everything went well. . . .

Well, I personally am truly grateful for the medical team that we formed. When I first arrived, I had problems with them because of the way I presented things in the beginning. I consider myself to be a most exacting [estricta] person because I like to have things done well and all that. I always encountered stumbling blocks because there were certain vices here. [Administrators] had not straightened out [the medical practitioners in Barrancas] the way they should have. And so they saw me as the really bad boss, [but] afterward they understood. When [the epidemic] came, they saw that what I wanted was best for them—to take preventative measures, to straighten out [orientar] the physicians, and all that. [The epidemic] succeeded in doing that, and it also succeeded in uniting us more and in letting them truly understand that the things I wanted to do were really for them. And they even offered a tribute to me.

We worked—at least I myself worked—twenty-four hours a day in the hospital in order to avoid leaving [the medical staff] alone, so that they wouldn't feel alone, to give them all the support they deserved by being there. I remember that one day a patient was in shock, and a colleague was really frightened—and this is normal. I myself had that experience. This is normal, and a person gets frightened. Well, the patient was an Indian woman who was completely in shock. The doctor took me aside, and he was really frightened, and I shouted at him. Well, afterward he kidded me, "I go and hope to find solace with you [*buscar aliento en usted*], and what you do is to reprimand me."

I told him, "I wasn't trying to reprimand you, my son [*mi hijo*], but I have more experience than you do, and I am not going to sit down and cry with you. Didn't you see that the Indian survived? She survived because all of us acted." . . .

Well, I'm going to tell you frankly that I even abandoned my son, the only one I have, the thing I most adore. Well, when there was cholera, my son fell. He hurt himself, and I went to get him the next day so that the nurses could take care of him. They wanted to suture him for me, and they really spoiled him. And I really felt terrible, because I knew what I was going to be up against, and I made my decision and I brought him here [to Maturín]. When I called him on the telephone, he would cry. But he had to stand up to it, he had to understand. I considered this to be my responsibility, and I couldn't abandon these people—not here or anywhere else that it could have happened, whether it was here or not. I gained a profession that I love, and I love it because it took me a great deal of sacrifice and study to gain it. And I took my oath, specifically to help the poor and the people who have nothing. Sure, I have needs like anybody else, but that doesn't mean that I can think that "I'm not going to do this." . . .

It's hard to believe how difficult it is to work in rural communities. No matter how many good things we physicians do, sometimes they never recognize them. For example, [the beginning of the epidemic] created a huge emergency that fell directly on the shoulders of all the physicians, not just on mine. Well, they used to say that I was crazy, because I would explain to them that the community was not accustomed [to modern sanitary practices], right? In Barrancas the population has always considered itself to be marginalized. And I have talked with this population, and they suggested to me that no one is concerned about them. And [officials] really *are* concerned about them, even if that seems untrue. But here at the state level and at the national level there is a lot of concern with this population. As you know, the country is in crisis, right? And sometimes we would like to give everything to one group, but that's impossible. And we parcel things out in accordance with the necessities and the characteristics of each area. . . .

We implemented a checkpoint over there, what's it called? where the boats come in. With the inspectors we had to examine the condition of the fish to see if they would allow them to proceed or not. This was along with the mayor's office, and the army helped us and the police helped us.

The army offered us a great deal of support. . . . And I took advantage
of this opportunity to inspect all of the businesses in Barrancas and to
close them down. And that's why I consider myself to be very exacting
[*estricta*]. . . .

I became the head of this entire region, of Temblador and Barrancas.
Well, they gave me this reward [*premio*] for helping them out with
the cholera. Yes, I see that, okay, I won it for all the work that I did, the
things I did.

Vargas's narrative is anything but equivocal. She characterizes her decision to place the Mariusans in the school as the imposition of a "cordon sanitaire." Individuals who had cholera symptoms were hospitalized. Then the
"healthy" Mariusans were "isolated" to prevent the spread of the disease.
Having declared a health emergency, Vargas used the special powers thus
involved to institute a wide range of measures in Barrancas.

In suggesting that Barranqueños mistakenly believed that they did not
figure in national or regional agendas, Vargas distances herself from the
townspeople and positions herself within the collective voice of state and
national officials who had the power to determine priorities and distribute
resources. Vargas reports that such efforts, before the epidemic, had met
"stumbling blocks," resentment, and resistance. By taking command, quite
literally, Vargas added the power of the municipal government and of the
military to that of public health institutions. Unrelenting in her efforts—
"I consider myself to be a most exacting person"—her position became
nearly untenable: "They used to say that I was crazy."

Officials often helped businesses get around cumbersome rules, including sanitary regulations, particularly when the parties requesting assistance
had economic or political clout. Remuneration in cash or kind was often
given to these officials as a token of gratitude. Later in the interview, Vargas suggested that local physicians had helped to sustain such arrangements
by signing sanitation permits for fishermen without conducting inspections.
Many of the fishermen who worked in the delta operated out of Barrancas,
maintaining homes there and either selling their fish near the river's edge
or in the market or using the town as a take-off point for wider markets.
Vargas attempted to put an end to this process of circumnavigating sanitary
regulations. At first, she performed the inspections herself, single-handedly,
and she refused to approve any more permits until substantive changes were
made. The situation provoked a politically charged confrontation with the
fishermen, their union, and local officials.

In Vargas's narrative the epidemic becomes part of a crusade to bring
the metropolitan world of public health from Caracas to a backward area.

Vargas casts herself as the successor to her uncle's path-breaking efforts, inserting her narrative into a history of public health in Venezuela. This broader narrative gives her cholera story its specificity and coherence—the epidemic makes sense once it has been constructed as a breakthrough in overcoming vicious resistance to an inevitable transformation. Her knowledge of events and conditions that were baffling and terrorizing leads Barranqueños to make a cognitive breakthrough—they finally understand and accept the logic of her actions. The professional disaster that threatened to emerge was transformed *tout coup* by the epidemic into a resounding success story.

Cholera provides a crucial moment of triumph, not just for Vargas but for modernity and modern health. The physicians who had so doggedly resisted Vargas came to see "that what I wanted was best for them." According to her narrative, physicians weren't the only ones to come around. Vargas was able to fully implement her plan for inspecting the fish brought to market, and the police and army installed a checkpoint. She used the power that cholera conferred on her to inspect all of the businesses in Barrancas and to close down establishments that did not meet her standards. During the interview, Vargas framed this transformation not simply as the victory of one ideology over another. It was, rather, evidence of the transcendent power of "experience," which leads less-seasoned practitioners to accept the perspective of their superiors. Literally embodying the biomedical order—disciplining one's own body and emotions as well as those of physicians, patients, and even communities—was what was needed to save lives. The modern hygienic order instituted by Vargas left no space for emotions, such as her colleague's reaction to a patient's symptoms, or for personal circumstances, such as her relationship to her young child.

Toward the beginning of the interview, Vargas asserted that it was the instruction she received from her professors in medical school, her previous experience as a physician, and the advice she received from her mentors that had enabled her to succeed in Barrancas. She, too, had laughed at the wisdom proffered by her professors, just as the Barrancas physicians initially laughed at her, but her perspective changed: at another point in the interview she noted that "when you become a professional and you live that reality, you understand." Modernity, according to this way of thinking, is both singular and concrete; it is not a social construct but just unfolds naturally from experience in the world—provided you have the proper sort of biomedical training. All other perspectives, the full range of views that she found in Barrancas, simply became obstacles on the road to modernity. In her narrative the power of the nation-state, as represented by the voices of high officials in Maturín and Caracas, is removed from the realm of partisan conflicts, individual agendas, and economic interests and is reborn as the modern voice of science.

In modern society rulers usually impose their will through a diffuse and often implicit process in which institutions shape identities and social relations.[11] Vargas tried to mobilize exactly this sort of power when she arrived in Barrancas. Her uncle embodied the authority of national officials to structure space in social and political terms—for example, by creating sanitary districts—and thereby enhance their ability to regulate how national policies were carried out in "local" areas. Assuming her uncle's mantle, Vargas envisioned herself as a prophet of modernity who had been entrusted with a mission to transform a backward rural region. "Vices" were evident not only in the "local population" of Barrancas but also in the hospital staff itself, and direct, even confrontational tactics were required.

In her narrative the epidemic constitutes a temporal rupture—the definitive point at which modern biomedical order became less a question of coercion than one of voluntary acceptance and the assimilation of ideas and practices. Hegemony was achieved when the perspectives of the officials of Maturín and Caracas—who represented metropolitan modernity—were internalized by socially and politically peripheral citizens. The image of machine-gun-bearing soldiers marching Mariusans off to receive antibiotic tablets and blocking the exits from the Eloy Palacios High School complicates this tale, suggesting that coercion was just as important as voluntary acceptance for the internalization of authority, given that the population to be disciplined was racialized.

Vargas's narrative is a classic heroic tale: in it she stands alone in her valiant struggle to bring modernity and professionalism to Barrancas in the face of hardships and incredible odds. Not only did local politicians, who possessed some power but had questionable commitments and motives, rebuff her first attempts to secure help from them, but she found that her very existence, professionally speaking, was threatened. When cholera magically revealed the scientific and social superiority of her message, her adversaries turned into allies. Her account glosses over the presence of scores of other officials who came from metropolitan centers to the periphery, the roles they played in the cholera epidemic, and the tremendous similarity of the heroic tales that they tell.[12] The dedication that Vargas demonstrated during the epidemic is clearly laudable, but it is important to point out that this experience became a means of claiming that only one vision of modernity—of the way that lives, communities, and institutions should be ordered—was valid.

In fact, Vargas's claim to the mantle of modernity rested on a somewhat shaky foundation. The involuntary confinement of Mariusans appeared to be in accord with MSAS's *Manual of Norms and Procedures for the Prevention and Management of Diarrheal Diseases and Cholera,* which combines recent medical findings on cholera with public health legislation on quarantines that had been adopted over half a century earlier.[13] The manual states that public health practitioners are charged with "the active surveillance and control of the sources of infection," as supported by "the natural leaders of that community and other organizations present in it." Steps to be taken in connection with the "surveillance of persons" include:

1. To prohibit persons suffering from Obligatorily Reportable Diseases to circulate by way of public roads or to change residence without the required written permission granted by Health Authorities, which will specify the terms and conditions of relocation.

2. Health authorities, through Epidemiological Offices, will be able to create cordons sanitaires [*podrán acordonar sanitariamente*] in regions or localities in order to prevent the propagation of transmissible diseases.

3. To restrict those who suffer from Obligatorily Reportable Diseases, or who are proceeding from places where there are persons with this type of disease, from visiting places where several people come together to remain overnight (high schools, institutes, universities, factories, theaters, movie theaters, churches, etc.) when the possibility of propagation of the disease is presumed.[14]

What MSAS promulgated as modern public health policy, however, was construed by international health authorities as the failed practices of the past. WHO, the paramount international public health institution, issued a manual entitled *WHO Guidance on Formulation of National Policy on the Control of Cholera,* which takes a different position:

> Cholera is spread from place to place largely by infected persons, most of whom have no signs of illness. These are called "healthy carriers." There is no practicable way of identifying all healthy carriers, and it is not feasible to prevent their movement by restrictive measures. . . . Additionally, measures to control the movement of individuals and populations are costly in manpower and other resources that could be used better for effective control activities. *For all of the above reasons, WHO recommends that countries should not use cordon sanitaire, quarantine, or frontier controls in their efforts to prevent the spread of cholera.*[15]

PAHO, the international public health organization for the Americas, similarly discourages the use of quarantines in cholera epidemics.[16]

Moreover, even the MSAS *Manual* does not grant authority to round up "apparently healthy" persons and to detain them against their will. And it is hard to justify keeping anyone in isolation for two weeks when the *Manual* clearly states that the period of incubation is from hours to five days, usually two to three days.[17] It seems ludicrous to suggest that they would be likely carriers of *Vibrio cholerae* after five days of confinement, particularly after the population was forced to take antibiotics. Incarcerating the Mariusans in the high school may have had less to do with modernity and public health norms than with the racial economy of Barrancas and the anticipated reaction of Barranqueños to the presence of potentially infected *indígenas*. This situation points to another good reason why quarantines are problematic: they can easily become radical extensions of everyday practices of medical profiling.

My goal here is not to condemn Vargas for violating WHO guidelines. Indeed, although the most recent WHO and PAHO cholera control bulletins arrived in MSAS offices in Caracas, only MSAS publications generally were sent to regional offices. A hospital director in a small city would be very unlikely to have access to WHO or PAHO publications. Nor do I claim for myself the right to sit in judgment on Vargas, MSAS, or WHO. My goal is to reveal the situated and contingent character—and the social and political force—of constructions of modernity and modern hygienic norms. What is deemed to be rational and modern is deeply shaped by the position of individuals and institutions within the very social hierarchies that these concepts supposedly legitimate. Vargas saw herself as a quintessential embodiment of modernity, yet she relied on a technique that international epidemiologists saw as the epitome of the failed practices of the past. The imposition of modernity and rationality is a powerful way to construct social and political hierarchies and to position oneself within them. Although modernity and rationality give us license to dominate the people we succeed in placing below us, they simultaneously subordinate us to individuals and institutions that lie above us in imagined hierarchies of modernity.

APARTHEID, BARRANCAS STYLE

Shortly after the Mariusans arrived in Barrancas, the mayor of the Sotillo municipality (within which Barrancas is located), Diego Escalante Castro, noted that a state of emergency was declared and that "the multitude of *indígenas* who have landed among the population of Barrancas" would receive all needed assistance, "thereby bringing under control the current situation that has alarmed this community."[18] Barrancas residents believed that the Mariusan "invasion" was part of a larger and more persistent problem. The sense of alarm and the image of an invasion by a "multitude" of *indí-*

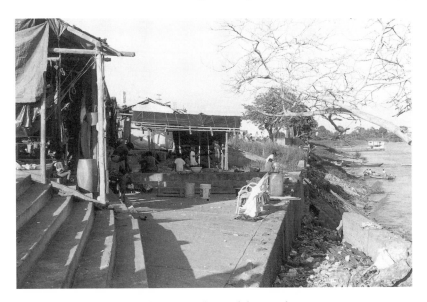

Photograph 28. Houses of former residents of the Winikina region next to the Orinoco River in Barrancas. Photograph by Charles L. Briggs.

genas triggered associations with other *indígena* residents of Barrancas: several hundred former residents of the Winikina and Arawabisi areas had lived in the city for nearly two decades. Their location on the *malecón* (photograph 28), the street that runs parallel to the Orinoco, provided them with access to their boats and the river, which was their source of water for drinking, bathing, and washing. But the *malecón* is Barrancas's prized scenic area, and it is frequented by tourists and residents during their leisure hours (photograph 29).

A prominent member of the Partido Acción Democrática, Escalante is a slender man with an angular face and a self-assured manner. When I (Charles Briggs) telephoned him from Tucupita, he generously agreed to meet me if I could come the next morning at seven o'clock sharp. I arrived bleary-eyed, having taken the first *por puesto* (taxi) from Tucupita. I found the mayor conversing with a number of men in the first rays of light, which were striking the front of the municipal building. Friendly and articulate, Escalante seemed open and defensive at the same time. He was anxious to tell a professional identified with Tucupita what he saw as Barrancas's side of the story. At the same time, he was concerned that I might be looking for more evidence to support the contention that Barrancas officials were violating the rights of *indígenas*.

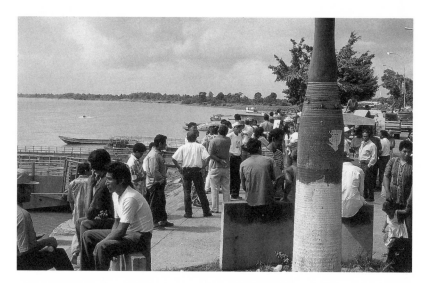

Photograph 29. *Barranqueños* relaxing on the *malecón*. Photograph by
Charles L. Briggs.

Diego Escalante Castro, Barrancas, 15 November 1994

When I arrived ten years ago in Barrancas, what really caught my attention was seeing people walking barefoot around town. I come from Caripe,
and Caripe is totally different from this town because Caripe has a lot of
European influence—Spaniards, Italians, Portuguese. And logically it has
a culture that is totally different from that of Sotillo. That's why it really
catches my attention when I see people walking barefoot and things like
that. A group of *indígenas* from Barranquillas were encamped *[acantona-
dos]* along the riverfront walkway *[malecón]*. The national government
had made them some huts *[chosas]*, but of concrete. They came and did
their business there, sold their arts and crafts, their *ocumo chino* [a root
crop], their fish. And then they went back toward the lower delta. But
then some of them began to stay, some were born here, more stayed,
more stayed.

Now there are *indígenas* encamped [in] Barrancas who have been here
eighteen, nineteen years. So you can understand that it has become very
unlikely that they would want to return to the lower delta, the ones who
were born here. But then a conflict emerges in that they aren't *criollos,* nor
are they really *indígenas,* do you understand? And they're people who
haven't received any sort of education *[formación],* so just imagine how
serious the problem is. What sort of identity can these *indígenas* have
when they aren't *criollos,* because the *criollos* don't accept them as such,
and they're not *indígenas,* because—logically, sure they're *indígenas,*

since they are living there within the group, but they can't leave because they're not from [the lower delta].

Well, as a result of this situation and in addition to this there is a series of bars near where the *indígenas* are encamped. The *indígenas* go to the bars and pick up the bottles. They drink what's left, get drunk, and make a scene there [*forman un espectáculo*], and this goes on all the time. The children who are being born are, of course, adapting to this and absorbing all this activity. . . .

In the face of the serious [health] problems that existed [because of] the influence of the bars, we invited the anthropologist Benjamín Suárez, a young man from here, born here in Barrancas, Benjamín Suarez. And we suggested that he do a study—do a project to see if we would be able to get them out of here, to see if we would be able, since this habitat is not theirs, to locate them in a place that would really be favorable for them. It was then that we came up with the Chivera project. We went to the lower delta, and we saw how they lived there and all that, and the anthropologist came up with the Chivera project. We moved them there with their consent, we took them to Chivera [Island] and they themselves made their dwellings and all that there in Chivera, fourteen dwellings. . . .

That was in 1986 or 1987, around there. Unfortunately, an election was near, and politics killed that project because a commission came from the national congress. I remember that Congressman Luzardo came, Adrian from Maturín came, Congressman Rodríguez Acosta came, and others who at that time were part of the Comisión Indigenista of the Congress came. Well, that really caused a riot [*alboroto*]. Since it was an election time, they brought out the little *indígena* children with oozing sores [*ronchitas*]—they brought them out and that meant cameras and photographs, press, and they started that riot, do you remember it? They started the riot that killed this project for all practical purposes. They brought the *indígenas* back again from over there and they brought them where they had been located. But we had destroyed those huts, right, and so they picked up the palms they had over there and all their manaca palms and brought them here and they made those things that they had all over again.

Escalante begins the interview by drawing a strong racial contrast between the European—meaning "white"—cultural character of Caripe and the barefoot *indígenas* roaming the streets of Barrancas. This juxtaposition of images is ironic in the extreme. The *indígenas* provided his first impression of Barrancas and were the quintessential symbol of its racial and cultural difference. At the same time, the overall thrust of his comments is to characterize *indígenas* living in Barrancas as people who do not belong in town and should be excluded from it, supposedly for their own good.

Escalante paints a familiar picture of "the *indígena* problem." Unlike *crio-*

llos, who live in towns and cities, *indígenas* are likened to animals who dwell in a "habitat"—the use of the term reveals a biological view of life in the fluvial area. Since this connection between race and space is seemingly so natural, *indígenas* who move to town necessarily undergo a pathological process that strips them of their "Warao" identity but does not enable them to "become *criollos.*" Rather than embracing modern identities or being bicultural, *indígenas* who live in Barrancas for an extended time, particularly children, are portrayed as acultural, developing without "any sort of education *[formación]*" whatsoever. *Formación* refers to much more than formal education or training; it suggests that *indígenas* born in Barrancas have not been socialized. They emerge as intrinsically pathological or perhaps not fully human.

Escalante did not attribute this situation to the municipality's failure to provide schooling for *indígenas,* although education is a constitutional right. When the municipal government did decide to provide schools in 1994, the *indígenas* were segregated from other schoolchildren and placed in the local ethnological and archaeological museum, where they were given an inequitable education: some seventy children were assigned to one teacher. Nor did Escalante seem interested in reflecting on the racism that largely deprived *indígenas* of all work except picking up beer cans or infrequent stints loading and unloading trucks. For Escalante, society was not the problem, and the actions of the municipal government, which he headed, were not the problem. The difficulty was the departure of *indígenas* from their "habitat." Following Malcolm X, one might counter that the problem is not really so much an *"indígena* problem" as a *"criollo* problem" or, more accurately, a problem with widespread racism and its institutionalization by national, state, and local governments.

Escalante's account of the confrontation at Chivera Island compares national with regional sites of power and liberal with pragmatic perspectives. The national government, in its desire to help the "poor *indígenas,*" provided permanent housing, which he discredits as *chozas* (huts). Barrancas did not want to provide any services to *indígenas.* Escalante explained during the interview, "What is our fear? . . . In the lower delta there are twenty-five thousand or twenty thousand more *indígenas,* and so after we relocate these ones, the others will come here, seeing the benefits that the ones who are here are receiving." The Chivera project constituted official, coerced segregation based on an anthropological construction of culture and space. Backed by "studies" of how "the *indígenas*" lived in the lower delta, anthropological authority was used to impose an idea of what sort of environment was favorable for them—how they *should* live—off the mainland. The island that was chosen is flooded each year during the rainy season, which is undoubtedly why it is unoccupied. A liberal discourse on human rights upset the deal offered by the municipality, a deal Escalante considered generous. He reduced concern over coercion and residential segregation, which violate the Venezuelan constitution, to a matter of political games played in an election year.

Diseased bodies that were out of place seemed even more in need of exclusion than healthy ones. Still angry over the government's failure to expel *indígenas,* many Barranqueños were enraged when they witnessed "a massive invasion" from other areas and learned that "Warao" were being treated for cholera in two of the central institutions of the town: the hospital and the high school. Suárez, the anthropologist, recalled that "because cholera came to Barrancas through the *indígenas,* this heightened the way they rejected them, such that [people said,] 'Why are they next to the port? Why are they bringing that disease? They're going to infect everyone!' Because of the geographic space that they are occupying next to the port, 'the wind will carry it into the middle of town!'"[19] Escalante, Vargas, and other officials were under the gun to get "the invaders" out of Barrancas quickly.

Although they criticized their counterparts in Barrancas for devising segregationist policies, Delta Amacuro officials also made great efforts to keep *indígenas* "in place" during the epidemic. Manuel Mato, who served as the resident physician in Curiapo during the epidemic, noted, "*Indígenas* really are very intelligent and hardworking in their environment. I think that the *indígenas* are compromised when they come to the city, where the politicians have taught them to beg, have taught them things that are not part of their culture."[20] Tourism director Eduardo Silva compared *indígenas* in the delta, where they were "owners and masters of this geographic space" and were united with its flora and fauna, with town-dwelling *indígenas.* The latter he portrayed as prostituted and disease ridden, "like little snakes dancing drunk." According to Silva, going to school, living in town, and participating in politics created "the lazy, shameless Warao, product of democracy."[21] Officials and residents who wanted to exclude *indígenas* from the mainland employed a skewed logic: If it was natural for *indígenas* to live in the lower delta, then it was just as natural to exclude people classified as *indígenas* from living in town; if moving to the mainland automatically led to alcoholism, prostitution, and pathology in general, then it was easy to justify violations of democratic ideologies and constitutional principles as humanitarian efforts to protect *indígenas.* The parallel to apartheid policies in South Africa is striking.

Narratives of modernity, democracy, and the nation-state suggested that *indígenas* living in the delta died from cholera and other diseases and could not enjoy the substantive rights of citizenship because they were not "civilized," not part of "the national society." Some people moved from the delta to Barrancas and Tucupita precisely because they believed that otherwise they would never gain access to modernity and the state. In doing so, however, *indígenas* discovered that as racialized subjects they were excluded from modernity by fiat. Rather than becoming part of "the national society," urban *indígenas* were designated as *less* fully human than their "uncivilized" kin back home.

To be sure, Escalante did not invent this argument; it emerged frequently in institutional discourses in the region. Indeed, the notion that modernization produces an interstitial, pathological state in racialized subjects was a recurrent feature of colonialism, one that often was used in the social construction of colonial medicine.[22] The results were residential segregation, second-class citizenship, and violations of basic human rights. National protests are easier to squash and international scrutiny easier to evade when the nation-state is racialized implicitly through the way it defines citizens and the seemingly unintended effects of institutional practices.

FINAL LESSONS FROM BARRANCAS

Public health officials shaped the cholera story as a tale of a valiant battle waged by medical science against superstition, ignorance, and disease, yet Vargas admitted that the epidemic forced her to accept some departures from modern practices. She used an outbreak of tetanus to evaluate the source of the blame for the eruption of cholera.

María Vargas, Maturín, Monagas, 31 March 1995

In the days before cholera we were worried because two cases of tetanus had appeared. And I in particular was worried because the epidemiologist who had trained me would never accept the appearance of cases of tetanus. He had taught me that there shouldn't be even a single case of tetanus if the human resources, the materials, and all that were available. I came [to Barrancas] with that norm, and for me this was like—it was like something sacred, something that was very demanding, understand? What worried me was that here [medical personnel] took it—I see that they thought it was funny when I was confronted with these cases of tetanus in Barrancas before cholera appeared.

And I was really worried, but afterward I myself did an analysis. Okay, but it's not our fault, it's not my fault, because of conditions there. Well, it was a population that—it wasn't that they didn't receive medical attention. We, at least, did everything that fell on our shoulders. We had just finished a sweeping vaccination campaign, a sweeping one. Because you know what their customs are like. For example, in the case of the *indígenas*, for example, when they give birth they cut the umbilical cord with any old object; sometimes they use razor blades, anything that will cut, and all that. And you know that this produces tetanus. But it wasn't because we wouldn't take the preventative measures. I asked myself all those questions, and my responses worried me. But later when [the cholera epidemic] came, I realized, I said, "Well, I went and visited them." But it's also the conditions in which they live, what they eat. I tell you honestly that I just don't see how this population can be getting tetanus since we are vaccinating them. But, well, we are going to study the other factors involved, diet and all that, and living conditions.

At this point I asked a question: "And especially in which areas [or] facets of the diet of the population?" Vargas replied:

What they eat the most is fish, which they acquire right there, next to the river. And they eat that kind of bread, they make *arepas* from, those dumplings that they make with wheat flour. That's what they eat, by and large. In any old part or, let's say, in the shacks in which they are located, they would make a fire there and they would put their fish right in it. And they only partially cooked it, they didn't cook it well, you see. And that's the way they ingested it. . . . I personally went at six in the morning, at twelve o'clock in the day, and at six in the evening to see what they were eating and how they were eating and how they prepared it. At that time, I took on the role, I acted as if they were my children. I would scold them and I would make a scene.

Vargas's story can teach us two additional lessons. First, what she recounts directly contradicts stereotypes of Third World officials that suggest they lack professional standards and are unconcerned with the welfare of the populations they administrate—we hope that public health officials in the United States and Europe pay careful attention to her story. Vargas is a credit to her profession, as self-sacrificing and dedicated a practitioner as one could find. She holds the medical personnel she administers to "very strict" standards, and she is even more demanding of herself. The image of public health, and of MSAS as an institution, that she brought to Barrancas allowed no room for incompetence, corruption, or inaction. The standards that she established for scrutinizing individuals and institutions were based on epidemiological data. The presence of tetanus prompted her to establish a policy of zero tolerance. No excuses were acceptable: if a single case appeared, it was the public health practitioners who had failed. Second, Vargas projected herself as heading in the opposite direction from that taken by Barrancas residents. The gap between the public health norms she brought with her and health outcomes in Barrancas initially left Vargas racked with anxiety because she was not measuring up to the rigid requirements of modern public health. Her experience taught her that outbreaks of tetanus and cholera did not necessarily signal any sort of institutional failure.

Why could public health standards be relaxed in this environment? Barefoot *indígenas* on the streets of Barrancas changed everything. How could officials accept lower standards for a racialized population? How could the presence of tetanus and cholera not provide an objective measure of the failure of public health institutions? Vargas accepted deplorable health conditions and excused herself and the public health system from culpability once she had acquired proficiency in using a language of culture to racialize disease and to assess blame. Barranqueños learned to accept modernity and public health norms as ultimate, exacting standards; Vargas learned to be comfortable with a very imperfect realization of the modernist project in areas such as Barrancas. When racial inequality lies at the heart of social relations, different rules apply.

In her narrative Vargas uses denigrating images to characterize *indígenas*. She infantilizes them ("I acted as if they were my children"), supervising and scolding her dirty and ignorant charges. She clearly notes that this is not the vision that she brought to Barrancas. She was initially shocked at the attitude that "they"—presumably medical personnel from Barrancas—adopted when the tetanus cases appeared. It is crucial to note that Vargas learned to reformulate public health norms in this fashion in Barrancas. This is not to say that she did not bring racial stereotypes with her. Moreover, this is not to say that a logic of blaming the poorest and most politically marginalized subjects is antithetical to conceptions of health and hygiene. Blaming the poor for their sanitary plight has been part of modernity since the nineteenth century, and physicians are hardly alone in this regard.[23] But everyday racist practices are shaped by regional economies, socially and politically specific categorizations of people, and ways of treating them.[24]

Venezuelans who come from areas in which there are few people classified as *indígenas* are often shocked at the racial logic and practices that prevail in Barrancas and Tucupita, just as Vargas was. Here experience—that is, social and cultural practices—is once again key.[25] At the same time that institutional practices internalized modernity in different ways, physicians, municipal officials, and other Barranqueños taught Vargas to reconceptualize public health through a racial lens. Experience—that is, the experience of dominant subjects in a region that is penetratingly racialized—taught even extremely well-trained and amazingly dedicated public health professionals to accept unconscionably high morbidity and mortality from preventable infectious diseases as a situation that could not be changed. Vargas learned not only a set of racial categories but how to put them together with public health practices. She learned, in short, how to incorporate medical profiling into policy decisions and everyday practices.

This resocialization process exposes a fundamental contradiction. One of the precepts of public health that Vargas brought to Barrancas was its universality—the idea that it applies to all people at all times. To accept lower—or less inclusive—standards would contradict the democratic ideologies that shaped the way these norms were institutionalized in MSAS. Culture came to the rescue. Mayor Escalante hired an anthropologist to project the cultural patterns of *indígena* life in the delta onto the model hamlet that would racially segregate Barrancas. Vargas learned to play anthropologist herself. When she visited *indígena* houses in the port area, she did not just scold the women; she investigated "what their customs are like" and "the conditions in which they live, what they eat." Both officials used the logic of culture to justify exceptions to the constitutional guarantees of a democratic state. Rather than challenging the segregationist policies of the municipal government that denied adequate housing, education, legal protection, employment, and sanitary services to residents of the portside communities, Vargas naturalized the cultural intractability of *indígenas*.

It is important to make sure that we do not racialize the outcome by suggesting that the impacts of public health policies were felt only by *indígenas*. Nothing could be farther from the truth. When poor urban dwellers or *campesinos* (peasants) posed a problem, the logic of culture or the discourse of poverty could be extended to them as well. In this way the experiences of a tiny population of *indígenas* in Barrancas ultimately could legitimate a wide range of institutional shortcomings. The epidemic prompted Vargas to scrutinize the customs of the *indígenas* and to accept the shortcomings of the public health system, not to push for long-term projects that would improve sanitary infrastructures and increase accessibility to health care, thereby benefiting all Barranqueños. Everyone pays for racism.

POSTSCRIPT

The state-sponsored Museum of Yupari,[26] which is a few blocks from the port, clearly lays out the *indígenas'* situation. It has exhibits reflecting the culture of the Caribs who, according to archaeologists, once inhabited what is now Barrancas, and it also presents the history of the Warao through artifacts and text. Present-day contributions of *indígenas* to the delta are nowhere to be found. In 1992, the year of the Columbian Quincentennial, the Fundación

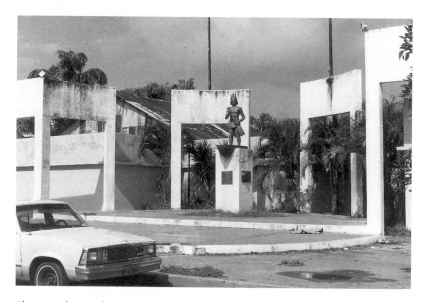

Photograph 30. The Plaza del Indio next to the *malecón* in Barrancas, with a statue of "the Cacique Oyapari" standing in a canoe. Photograph by Charles L. Briggs.

Pro-Barrancas decided to recognize the town's *indígena* heritage in its 462nd year of existence by creating the Plaza del Indio (Plaza of the Indian) in a prized and contested area—the *malecón* (see photograph 30). In the center of the plaza a statue was erected to "the Cacique Oyapari," who, according to Suárez, "at the time of contact in 1531 was the community representative." Barrancas thus simultaneously undertook two contradictory acts: it placed healthy *indígenas* in a sort of concentration camp and dreamed of further segregating the town by expelling the *indígena* residents who had "invaded" it, and, at the same time, it honored the *"cacique"* who was in charge when the conquest and enslavement of *indígenas* was inaugurated in the area. A dead colonial *"cacique"* apparently could be an object of civic pride and historical memory while real, live *indígenas* were the object of ridicule and official policies of segregation.

7 Exile and Internment
The Mariusans on La Tortuga

Barrancas officials did not succeed in sending back the *indígenas* who were living along the *malecón* "to their communities of origin." But the case of the Mariusan cholera refugees was different. They were identified as reservoirs of the disease, even after they had ingested antibiotics for two weeks, and Barranqueños didn't want them in their city. No one, other than the Mariusans themselves, seemed to be very worried about their constitutional rights. To stem the protests, Mayor Diego Escalante Castro found a way to get the Mariusans out of Barrancas and away from the probing gaze of reporters.

Escalante and hospital director María Vargas collaborated with Delta Amacuro officials to "return" the Mariusans to the delta. They and other state and local officials decided that the Mariusans' new home would be La Tortuga ("Turtle") Island, which is in the middle of the delta (see map 1, page 2). Escalante announced that a cordon sanitaire had been installed to halt "the movement of *indígenas* who are carriers of the cholera *vibrio* toward the southern part of Monagas."[1] The Mariusans' stay in the Eloy Palacios High School had been only the beginning of their confinement. The cold, hard cement floors there were the most hospitable conditions they would know for some months.

Neither the residents of La Tortuga nor the Mariusans were told of the plan, and nothing was done to prepare for their arrival. As José Rivera tells it, the Mariusans learned on the morning of 14 August 1992, their fourteenth day of confinement, that their fate had been decided. Although they would have liked to reject the plan, the presence of the Guardia Nacional made the deal very hard to refuse.

José Rivera, Nabaribuhu, 16 February 1995

Okay, they came to see us again. "You people are no longer in danger of dying, you no longer have any disease."

"We want to leave."

"Well, okay."

"We have truly suffered a lot. We want a motorboat."

"We'll give you everything you want."

"Where are you going to dump us?"

"In La Tortuga. There is a clinic, there are medicines, there is a nurse."

"Well, as you say."

"You aren't going to Mariusa. If you go to Mariusa, you will die."

"We don't want to go to Mariusa, either. It's really dangerous for us there. When we were there, it was really bad."

The official said, "Well, okay. Come on, hurry up!"

From there, they took us over to Volcán [a small port near Tucupita that provides access to the Orinoco]. There they put us aboard a freighter [*chalana*].

I asked if they had been taken against their will, and Rivera relied affirmatively.

Against our will. We didn't have even a single mosquito net. The plain truth is that here on the [Mariusa] coast there are no mosquitoes, so we don't have mosquito nets. We all said, "No, it would be terrible for us to have to go to La Tortuga. We have no mosquito nets, and there are lots of mosquitoes there."

"We'll give everything to you there. There are mosquito nets in the freighter."

"Well, if that's the case, okay. Hurry up, let's go." We left.

It was about this time, about eleven [in the morning], when we arrived at Volcán. There were no mosquito nets, but there were lots and lots of officials, lots and lots of soldiers. They talked about us. "The people from Mariusa have too much cholera. We don't want them to stay around other people. We have to take them to some place where they will be by themselves." We couldn't say anything—there were lots and lots of soldiers. So we left. We, who had believed them, saw that there were no mosquito nets, none. [As soon as] we arrived [at Volcán], we left for La Tortuga. It was about six in the evening when we arrived [on La Tortuga]. . . . It was already getting dark. We believed that we would have houses. But there were no houses for us. Well, we were in bad shape. Just like that, "You'll stay here!"

At that time there was a priest there. That priest, that priest—his name was Father José. I said, "Well, fine, we're going to suffer here! I'm going to talk to the governor!"

[Father José said,] "Well, stay here, sleep well. Even though it's true that there are no houses here to sleep in, it's very close [to Barrancas] here. It's too far to go there to Mariusa." We stayed. We were there a week and a half without being able to sleep at all—there were too many mosquitoes. It was really terrible.

The other priest, Father Simón, arrived. He said, "No, why hasn't the governor come here? And why hasn't the director of ORAI come here?" Two days later he left for Tucupita, and in two days the freighter came with some food, a lot of food. The freighter was full.

Again we said to [Father Simón], "We're dying, there are too many mosquitoes here. Why haven't they given us mosquito nets?"

"No, there are still no mosquito nets." A letter was sent. Then the people who fumigate also came, and they used the treatment for mosquitoes, they sprayed a little. The mosquitoes were no longer so impossible. There were many fewer. Although there were still some around, it was better. There weren't too many. When [Father Simón] came back, they gave us mosquito nets. They gave us mosquito nets and hammocks.

We asked for forty sheets of zinc [roofing] and a motorboat. [We wrote] a good letter, and the priest took the letter to Tucupita. In three days the governor came. At that time Cristóbal Bayeh was the governor. He came with Father Simón, and we all spoke with him. He gave us a used outboard motor. We asked him for forty sheets of zinc. "Fine." He gave us everything: hammers, shovels, and nails. We asked for everything we would need to make houses. . . . We all worked there.

But the people [nebu] said, "No, we can't live here. The people who live on the Araguaito River are bad, they wreck everything for Warao. We don't like this at all. We can't set our nets because they'll steal them. We can't leave our motorboats unguarded, we can't leave them alone. The people from Mariusa, from Araguaito, the Warao people of Tortuga keep fighting, they quarrel with one another." That's what they said to me. I didn't like that.

In this narrative Rivera describes how the Mariusans' release from incarceration in Barrancas led to more confinement, suffering, and humiliation. Interviews that I conducted with officials suggested that Ricardo Salas, the regional head of Defensa Civil, selected La Tortuga in keeping with an interinstitutional mandate to get the Mariusans out of Barrancas and back into "their natural habitat." During the interview, Rivera reported overhearing a conversation that branded the Mariusans as cholera carriers and as needing isolation—even after they had been quarantined and treated with antibiotics. The officials clearly had decided that the Mariusans were quintessential unsanitary subjects and thus lacked the right to decide where and how they would live. Rivera resentfully reports that they were tricked into leaving the high school. His apparent acquiescence to the plan

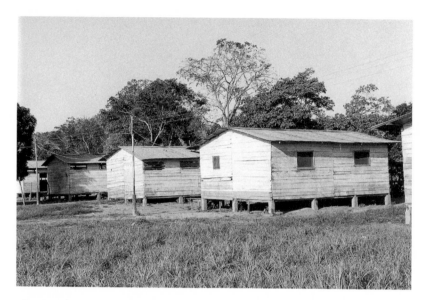

Photograph 31. Government-built houses on La Tortuga Island. Photograph by Charles L. Briggs.

constitutes recognition that no options were open to them at that moment. Once again, military might enforced decisions made by public institutions in a medical emergency. The vessel that took Mariusans to La Tortuga normally is used for transporting cargo and livestock. The Mariusans felt like cattle.

La Tortuga is a frequent stopover on the journey from Mariusa to Barrancas, so it was well known to the Mariusans. The island is near the headwaters of the Mariusa River. Much of the forest has been cut down to make way for agriculture and cattle. The farms and ranches are operated by *criollos* who have moved into the area from the mainland and from Margarita Island, which lies north of Sucre state. Just downriver from La Tortuga are a store, a school, and a rural clinic staffed by a nurse. The land on which the officials unceremoniously placed the Mariusans was adjacent to a series of wooden houses built by the government for a community of about one hundred *indígenas* (photograph 31)—they were a small island of *indígenas* in a predominantly *criollo* area. Tortugans, as they are called, say that they moved from the Mariusa region some forty years ago.

The Mariusans were not the only ones caught unprepared for their exodus to the island. The Tortugans had not known that 250 persons would arrive late one evening in mid-August. There seem to be more mosquitoes than air at that time of night, and people hate to open the doors of their tightly sealed houses for more than a split second. The Tortugans had not been consulted as to whether they would be willing to share land that they considered their own with a community nearly three times as large. There was no place for the Mariusans to hang their hammocks; they had no shelter from the rain and mosquitoes.

THE CLARETIAN MISSIONARIES

Salas had selected La Tortuga because it was sufficiently near to Tucupita to enable government institutions to keep an eye on the Mariusans and provide them with necessary resources, yet sufficiently far to avoid problems with *criollos* on the mainland. Tortuga seemed perfect—an expanse of "vacant land" on an island inhabited only by *indígenas*. There would be no *criollos* to protest. Then Salas discovered that a group of missionaries had, unbeknownst to the government, set up shop on the island. Who were the priests that Rivera mentioned, and what were they doing in the middle of this scene? Every summer Claretian seminarians who are studying in Caracas spend August getting experience and performing community service. Purely by chance, the site selected for community service in 1992 was La Tortuga. Six seminarians were supervised by three priests: Simón Mato, Gabi Gutiérrez, and José Nóbrega.

Gutiérrez, who was in his early thirties when we (Clara and I) interviewed him in November 1994, spoke extensively about the Claretians' experience on La Tortuga. Hailing from the Andean region of western Venezuela, he is a stocky man with a jovial face and bespectacled eyes that burn with intensity and dedication. Gutiérrez's stay on La Tortuga, which came at the beginning of his pastoral career, was clearly the formative experience of his life. Articulate and confident, the priest obviously had reflected deeply on what he would say, and he acknowledged that he had been looking forward to having the chance to tell his story. The three of us sat in a tidy, sedate pastoral office—a surreal backdrop for the tale that unfolded.

Father Gabi Gutiérrez, Caracas, 10 November 1994

When cholera came, when it exploded, there was a team of seminarians there, students of philosophy in their first and second years of Claretian training. They began their missionary experience on the first of August. They moved to La Tortuga, and they were going to work with a very small group of one hundred persons. They were going to give them—to live with them, to observe, see how they lived, and share with them intimately, when suddenly they [were] confronted by the invasion of Mariusans to La Tortuga, who were looking for somewhere to go, trying to establish themselves there in the face of the cholera outbreak. So suddenly we saw that on La Tortuga what had landed on top of us was more than three hundred people in a very small place.

The fellows said that, well, they operated on an emergency basis— it was even raining when they arrived. That was the first blow-up. The Mariusans got into conflicts. There were conflicts between the Mariusans and the inhabitants of La Tortuga, because it was like a kind of invasion. So there were very tense moments at first, and we didn't know what to do. Even the seminarians looked a little tense. A kid who has hardly begun [his training] suddenly finds himself in the midst of three hundred persons who are fighting for their lives—one very ill over here and another one sick over there and the children. . . .

As I see it, they should have spoken with them. The government should have sent someone first to view the situation there, should have constructed some temporary houses or what have you, of palms or moriche palms or what have you. But having them come at nine or ten at night, dumping a group of people like animals, like dogs, and [saying] to those already there, "Take care of them"—that was serious. And that brought, could have produced truly bad consequences. And who knows what might have happened if we hadn't been there. A small war could have erupted. . . .

During those first days, things were tense because we were waiting for help and it never came. We didn't have anything until more Claretians arrived. Then the first help from the government arrived, but I'll tell you, more than ten days went by, more than ten days.

The contradictory language Gutiérrez uses to describe the Mariusans' arrival is telling. On the one hand, he uses exactly the word that many people in Barrancas used when the Mariusans arrived there: *invasion*. In suggesting that the Mariusans were "looking for somewhere to go," he echoes the claim made by journalists and government officials: that the Mariusans had asked for permission to live on La Tortuga. On the other hand, Gutiérrez implies that he knew people had been transported against their will when he states that they had been dumped "like animals, like dogs." By all accounts the first ten days were impossible, but the Tortugans and the Mariusans spoke very favorably about the Claretians. The missionaries decided that the Mariusans had become their responsibility, and they helped the new arrivals explore possible courses of action. Claretians and Mariusans alike were angered by the government's failure to follow through on promises of material support. When reporters were not beaming images of bedraggled bodies onto television screens or plastering them on the front pages of newspapers, officials did not seem to think that any action was required.

EMBODYING RESISTANCE

Rivera said in his interview that the situation on La Tortuga was desperate. Conditions were so miserable that he could not keep Mariusans on the island, and the only course of action was to violate government orders and head back to Barrancas. Getting away from the mosquitoes was only part of their motivation. People understood quite clearly that catching the attention of journalists was the only way to force the government to keep its promise to provide adequate resources. The result was a remarkable political event, an incident that articulated the rights of delta residents and expanded the range of possibilities in the region for *la política indígena*— indigenous politics.

First to greet the Mariusans when they returned to Barrancas in late August was José Guevara, one of the most interesting and enigmatic figures in the cholera narratives. Guevara, who is tall and muscular, was raised in the delta and is fluent in Warao. His angular face has been weathered by years of exposure to the intense light reflected off the waters of the Orinoco's tributaries. He seems to defy the pervasive system of racial classification that assigns a single and immutable identity to each resident as "Warao," "*criollo*," "Trinidadian," "Guyanese," and so on. *Criollos* sometimes refer to him as an *indígena* and sometimes as *criollo*; most *indígenas* see him as a *criollo* who has some *indígena* ancestry. Guevara is the commander of the Escuela Forestal (Forestry School) of San Félix, a division of the Guardia Nacional that is charged with defending the region's forests. Although he wears a military stripe on his shirt, he is not one to travel in pressed fatigues, piloting a large motorboat with machine-gun-toting soldiers at his side, as do most officers in the Guardia Nacional. He is much more likely to be found in the delta, cruising in an old canoe powered by an outboard motor. He goes from community to community, selling oranges or mangos brought in from San Félix and swapping stories with everyone. He is an activist for environmental, political, and human rights in the delta. He has taken on the owners of sawmills and palm hearts factories, undaunted by their political and economic clout.

We ran into Guevara in October 1994 when we were visiting Tekoboroho, a small community close to Guayo (see map 1, page 2). He was selling oranges, which were manna after weeks of delta travel. Standing in a palm-thatched house, looking out over the river, Guevara related his account of what happened when Rivera and other Mariusans arrived in Barrancas.

José Guevara, Tekoboroho, 22 October 1994

When the people arrived in Barrancas del Orinoco, there were already more than three thousand persons gathered there and a shortage of food, a shortage of housing, a shortage of assistance. So I felt an obligation to leave on foot with three thousand persons from Barrancas del Orinoco as far as Tucupita. We went on foot, we went on foot to Tucupita! Well, nobody was organizing things at that time, but, rather, the Warao went to Tucupita because here [in the delta] people were dying of hunger, and in Barrancas there wasn't any kind of support coming from the government. So they [said], "No, let's go to Tucupita!" [he repeats in Warao]. What [the government] wanted was for the people to stay there. They had taken them to La Tortuga. Nobody can live in that place, because that's where the mosquitoes live. I spoke with [José], whom they had made the leader of Mariusa on La Tortuga Island. He's the one.

So, just think of the confrontation that we had with them, with that woman from ORAI, and with the people from Civil Defense. Because they sent [the Mariusans] forcibly—no ifs, ands, or buts. They wanted to require those people to keep living there on La Tortuga, isolated, far away, hidden, without work, a frightened people, a people that was still disoriented, that was still going around aimlessly from place to place as a result of having seen so much death. Suddenly they [took] them to that place, as if taking them to a concentration camp. So then they didn't want to stay there, and that was when we went to Tucupita.

I asked him who had agreed on the march.

Everybody, absolutely everybody was in agreement; no one disagreed. They were united, the people from Winikina, and the people from Mariusa, and all the *indígenas* who were there at the time were all in the same boat. We went on foot to Tucupita. That was about a month or a month and a half after cholera first hit. From where all those people had amassed in Barrancas, we went from Barrancas to Tucupita. And the governor, the governor they had at the time, well, he gave us food. He sent us a truck full of food and hammocks, and he gave them to the people from Mariusa and the people from Winikina. He gave them two outboard motors, a twenty-five [horsepower] and a forty [horsepower] outboard motor.

Okay, the people, all the Warao, we went back again to Barrancas. And some of them wanted to go fishing, but not to stay there. Rather, they took the outboard motors in order to fish and then come back quickly, not to stay. They didn't stay more than five days or six days in Winikina and in Mariusa. They left with the outboard motors, fished, and came back quickly to Barrancas because they didn't want to live there because they were afraid.

So then the situation just went on, because not everybody benefited from the outboard motors. There were very few—two outboard motors for three thousand people. And that's when they said to me, "[José,] what can we do? Let's go to Tucupita—no, let's go to San Félix!" We left at five o'clock in the morning on foot for San Félix, and we arrived at ten o'clock at night there in San Félix, in Los Barrancas. There a friend of mine gave me—he took me and bought me seven thousand *Bolívares* worth of bread and juice and gave them to the people.

And the next day we went to look for the news media to ask them for help. So that they would report that we were in San Félix protesting because we didn't have any kind of help whatsoever. . . . And the news media helped us, or rather they reported the motive that brought us there. And so that was the second day. And the next day the governor went by and waved, and then a little while later some five patrol cars [came] to pick up everyone, and they threw us out of San Félix. [The governor of Bolívar state] said, "I don't want to see any Warao here, because they're not from here. They belong to the Delta Amacuro." And they threw everyone out of there, they threw all of us out of there. They sent buses, several packed buses, to Tucupita and placed us in the hands of Governor [Bayeh]. The governor didn't pay attention because he was used to seeing Indians. He said, "No, I'm used to seeing Indians—leave them any old place." And they dumped us off, and everyone went off on their own.

These marches were born from widespread desperation and frustration. There are no reliable counts of the number of people who left communities in the delta to take up temporary shelter in Barrancas, Tucupita, and smaller communities on the mainland near the delta. Guevara's estimate of three thousand participants seems high, but regardless of the number, the march along the sixty kilometers of highway between the two cities was an event that caught officials in Tucupita by surprise, particularly after it was reported in *Notidiario* (photograph 32). The article related that persons connected with the Defensa Civil beat some of the marchers with fists and clubs in an effort to stop the protest in Barrancas and noted that Mayor Escalante followed the march in a pickup truck "to prevent any new aggression on the part of the authorities." The reporter, who merged his own words with extensive quotes from Guevara, added that Escalante also sought "to be sure that we left his jurisdiction. That would rid him of a headache."[2]

The article described what happened when the marchers arrived in Tucupita. They stopped in front of the office of the state government of Delta Amacuro, an unpretentious building on the corner of Bolívar Plaza. "Some

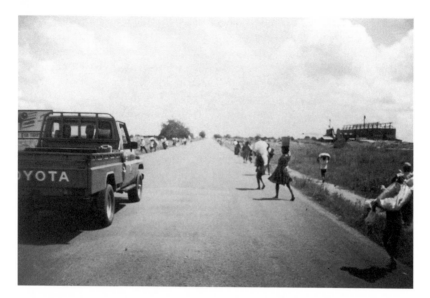

Photograph 32. Marchers, carrying their belongings, on the road from Barrancas to Tucupita in September 1992. Courtesy of *Notidiario.*

indígenas" then entered the building, and Bayeh attempted to persuade Guevara to leave. In a remarkable rhetorical about-face, the journalist, who seemed to be aligned with Guevara and the marchers, suggested that the story had a happy ending: the governor "ordered his staff to give them two outboard motors, blankets, hammocks, food. With all of this in their possession, they went away convinced that nothing is better for them than Mariusa and Winikina, their ancestral lands."[3] The delivery of material goods, the article implied, had wiped away the fear of cholera that drove people to the mainland, paving the way for contented *indígenas* to return to "their ancestral lands." The actual situation was different. The epidemic was still very much in progress on 4 September 1992, and the marchers were, by their accounts, using their actions to make it clear that they would *not* return to the delta until their safety could be assured. Moreover, some former residents of Winikina had been living in Barrancas for more than a decade, and they had no intention of returning "home" at that point. The reporter provided the happy ending envisioned by Barrancas and Tucupita officials.

RACIALIZED CITIZENSHIP

The recurrent cycle of making promises, presenting goods, and exchanging accusations regarding the failure to keep bargains was a crucial facet of the process by which *indígenas* were denied political agency. When *indígenas* criticized government policies and demanded change, officials reconfigured these actions as demands for material items: food, money, motors, and the like. The success of this strategy depended on widespread stereotypes. Characterized as backward, ignorant, and lacking the will and ability to fend for themselves, *indígenas* were purportedly always begging and therefore always dependent on the government and *criollos. Indígenas* were generally excluded from all but the most menial and unreliable forms of employment. Nevertheless, when a "Warao" asked for a handout, the action confirmed a racial stereotype rather than calling attention to the racialization of economic opportunity. When unions, neighborhood organizations, students, opposition political parties, or other groups staged protests, these actions conferred political strength and legitimacy. When invoked by *indígenas*, however, protests became acts of collective mendicancy. The march to Tucupita was deprived of its political content and dismissed as more evidence of the well-known *indígena* penchant for begging, decadence, and dependence on *criollos.*

Citizenship in Venezuela had long been defined as the right to a decent standard of living, made possible by sale of the nation's oil.[4] In Delta Amacuro, however, access to a share of the state's largess was racialized. Devising extra-official means of securing a chunk of the nation's oil reserves conferred an aura of astuteness and active citizenship on persons classified as *criollos*, but it confirmed only subaltern status, political impotence, and stigmatized identity for *indígenas.*[5]

Residents of Delta Amacuro were expected to know how race, politics, and economics came together. Father Gutiérrez explained how he acquired this knowledge.

Father Gabi Gutiérrez, Caracas, 10 November 1994

You had to be very careful when living with the *indígenas* because there were people who organized them in order to be able to get more things from the government for their own gain. You know who I'm talking about, that there was an *indígena* among them, let's say an *indígena* who was better educated. And he liked to create disturbances, stir things up against the government, basically to foster discontent. So they told you that you had to keep your eyes peeled to see who's in command of them. But I never saw that person over there [on La Tortuga]—you know who I'm referring to. So when I was a newcomer in the delta, [they told me,] "Be careful! There are some troublemakers over there and they want to take advantage of that cholera business. Keep your eyes peeled." There was a gentleman over there in San Félix, [José Guevara]. I don't know, that guy is sure smart, he's no fool. He knows what he wants.

Gutiérrez frames this political assessment of *indígena* politics as reported speech, suggesting that he is relaying the words that were passed along to him when he arrived in the delta. When I met Escalante in Barrancas in 1994 he similarly warned me about Guevara's ability to "stir them up."[6]

We remember the many times that people made these kinds of comments when we were new to the delta. We received advice from politicians, bureaucrats, missionaries, merchants, taxi drivers, neighbors, and friends. In short, just about anyone who considered himself or herself *criollo* was anxious to teach a newcomer what things were really like. As activists, we subsequently became the *objects* of such comments. We were sometimes targeted as troublemakers ourselves, accused of "stirring up" our collaborators in projects on health, land, and human rights—and, believe it or not, of being witches who used our supernatural powers to harm our adversaries. Such comments created a reception field that led observers to construe even concerted political action as an effort to manipulate the gullible masses for their personal gain. Even Gutiérrez, who was quite critical of the "schema of domination" and "exploitation" that placed *indígenas* in a "subaltern" position, internalized this racialized view of political and economic relations.[7] He accepted the narratives that cast Guevara as the leading protagonist in the drama of "Warao" political manipulation, and he simply presumed that we believed them as well.

Beyond talk of mendicancy, another rhetoric also denied *indígenas* the ability to take serious political action and served to counter the political content of their march. *Notidiario* commented that the marchers regarded the event as an "adventure," implying that they were interested only in frivolous entertainment.[8] This rhetoric often emerged during the epidemic through the juxtaposition of photographs showing laughing and smiling individuals (many of which were archival shots taken before the epidemic) with articles that described the catastrophic effects of cholera.

Another rhetoric was used to explain the participation of Mayor Escalante. One of the principal rationales for expelling the Mariusans from Barrancas was that they "belonged to Tucupita," meaning that their "places of origin" were within Delta Amacuro.[9] *Notidiario* suggested that Escalante supported the march in the interests of returning the people en masse to their proper jurisdiction.[10] Guevara similarly suggested that the governor of Bolívar state rounded up the people who walked to San Félix "because they're not from here" and that he symbolically placed the people "in the hands" of the governor of Delta Amacuro. Human beings were cast as the property of state governments, chattel tied irrevocably to the lands on which they or their parents were born. These simultaneous mappings of race and space bespoke a legacy of conquest and colonialism that is still very much alive in the region.

Indígenas are generally regarded as remnants of Venezuela's racial and social roots, persons who still dwell in a prior historical realm. For them, citizenship is not a present and given reality but a status that is deferred; it lies in a future that can be accessed only once *indígenas* become modern. Of course, to become modern, they have to stop being *indígenas*. Protesting, blocking roads, and making demands on the state are key means of demonstrating citizenship in Venezuela. However, as their sanitary shortcomings confirmed the failure of *indígenas* to measure up to the image of the modern citizen, even the same actions were read in a diametrically opposed fashion.

MEMORIES OF LA TORTUGA

The Mariusans' stay on La Tortuga was inscribed in cultural memory through very different narratives. For Bayeh, it represented the anti-*indígena* policies of heartless Barrancas politicians, a bold attempt to provide a beleaguered population with a new beginning, and a failure on the part of Mariusans to adapt to a new climate when they were overwhelmed by mosquitoes. Many Mariusans remembered their stay on the island as a time of intense physical suffering, when they lost their right to freedom of movement and were denied their human dignity. José Rivera stressed that La Tortuga became a symbol of false government promises and outright misrepresentation as he recounted the promise that food, hammocks, and mosquito netting would be waiting on the freighter. José Guevara referred succinctly to the Mariusans' placement on La Tortuga as equivalent to imprisonment in a concentration camp, and this phrase was often repeated by activists in Tucupita.

For activist and educator Feliciano Gómez, these events encapsulated the discrimination experienced by "Warao" at the hands of *criollo* populations on the mainland. Others told stories of the huge loads of food and other supplies that left Tucupita for the island but were sold, at least in part, along the way. For them, La Tortuga provided a language for talking about government corruption. In the story of Monsignor Ramón Rodríguez, head of the Capuchin missionaries and bishop of Tucupita, discriminatory practices were wielded by government officials while salvation was offered by mis-

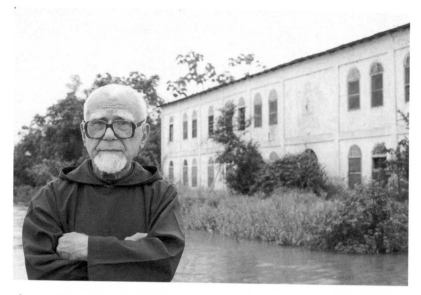

Photograph 33. The Arawaimuhu Mission with Father Basilio Barral. Barral, who worked in the delta for some fifty years, died before the beginning of the epidemic. Photograph by Charles L. Briggs.

sionaries: "When the Mariusans came here, those people threw them like some garbage, like cattle, there on La Tortuga. That is precisely where the priests from Sierra Imataca had set up camp that year with some kids from Caracas. And they did an extraordinary job there, the Claretian priests."[11] Rodríguez placed La Tortuga within a debate between the Venezuelan state and the Spanish missionaries over who were the abusers and who the saviors of the *indígenas,* an argument that stretches back to the War of Independence. The image of a brown-robed Capuchin priest and the mission station were icons of modernity in the delta for over half a century; Father Basilio Barral, who is pictured in photograph 33, worked there for some fifty years. Monsignor Rodríguez uses the story of the Claretians to reclaim the idea that missionaries continue to be a principal life-support system for *indígenas* in Delta Amacuro.

Stories of the Mariusans' stay on La Tortuga particularly provide a site for debating images of the state and its institutions. Can government officials be rightfully represented as agents of paternal benevolence who labored on behalf of a helpless, resistant, and ungrateful population? Or can they be best described as a motley collection of corrupt, politically opportunistic charlatans who used hunger and the threat of physical force to squash the will—

and the bodies—of the people? Did missionaries play a key role in the state's game, get in the way of progress, foster dependency, or (as they generally suggested) buffer the violent impact of the state and capitalism on *indígenas*? Were Delta Amacuro officials, regional representatives of national institutions, and missionaries seeking to bring the delta into the modern world? Or were they the greatest obstacles to its arrival?

Gutiérrez positioned himself as a mediator between the forces of a heartless civilization, represented by the state, and people who had been left behind by modernity. Although he portrayed himself as bringing civilization to the wilderness, in material and cultural as well as spiritual terms, and as preventing a human disaster, he did not seem to feel that he was able to change the racism and economic exploitation that characterized the way *criollos* treated *indígenas* or to achieve long-term changes in the precarious way that Tortugans and Mariusans had been inserted into modernity. Gutiérrez argued that although European colonialism was finished, a colonial attitude lingered, such that "we *criollos* in Venezuela and especially in this region dominate the *indígena* without meaning to do so," and he accused the government of being thoroughly "paternalistic." His strong social-justice agenda did not prevent Gutiérrez from learning one racial stereotype: when he recounted the many trips that he took to Tucupita to request assistance for Mariusans from state agencies and businesses, Gutiérrez stated that "they told me I was a real beggar *[era muy pedigueño]*."[12]

Insofar as he identified (or was identified) with the Mariusans, Gutiérrez became "a real beggar" rather than an equal partner in a collective struggle against racism. When he learned to racialize the anti-racist struggle itself, Gutiérrez became blind to the importance of the massive protest marches on the mainland and the Mariusans' key role in them. By learning a discourse that denied political consciousness and agency to *indígenas*, Gutiérrez distanced himself from actions that challenged the very postcolonial schemes that he excoriated and resigned himself to the sense that racism, in the end, is implacable.

The protest actions and Rivera's account of them suggest that the Mariusans actually held very different theories about the workings of political and institutional power. Appeals to officials in a number of institutions and in three Venezuelan states showed a keen awareness of political and institutional rivalries and an interest in exploiting them. Through his conversations with activists who lived in Tucupita and elsewhere, his discussions with Guevara, and his participation in other actions, Rivera was quite aware in 1992 that a national movement that promoted the rights of *indígenas*, one that enjoyed international support, had challenged political subordination and economic oppression. Mariusans viewed their resistance to confinement on La Tortuga as part of this larger struggle. They saw their actions as progressive, as attempts to promote adequate living conditions and to expose efforts to keep delta residents backward and poor.

What could be more modern than using democratic practices to call the attention of the mass media and a range of public and private institutions to a massive violation of human rights? Gutiérrez imagined Mariusans and Tortugans as the objects of a modernizing agenda who had to be taught the importance of hygiene, but Rivera and other Mariusans claimed a place beside him as agents of modernity who were challenging an anti-modern government.

Public health authorities, who enjoyed much greater access to the press than did either Gutiérrez or Rivera, were largely successful in elevating their narratives of La Tortuga to the status of an official story. Many voices angrily proclaimed an alternative version of brutality, corruption, false promises, and the actions of benevolent and even saintly missionaries. These two narratives formed a shell game in which two small objects, one representing modernity and the other barbarism, were switched rapidly under a set of institutional shells. Both narratives denied political agency to Mariusans and portrayed them as mendicants. Images of the march were projected by *Notidiario*, but the stories confirmed that Mariusans and other *indígenas* had learned the art of political protest only in order to obtain bigger handouts, such as outboard motors.

The confinement of Mariusans on La Tortuga revealed the racialization of citizenship in Venezuela and the legal rights that citizenship supposedly confers. The marches demonstrated that the *indígenas* were willing to go to great lengths, literally, to protest this racialization. In the end, all of these events were construed in such a way as to simply acknowledge the racial divide and confirm the *indígenas'* subordinate status.

8 Medicine, Magic, and Military Might
Cholera Control on La Tortuga

The narratives told about the Mariusans' stay on La Tortuga often focused on hardship, the denial of constitutional rights, corruption, and protest, but it is crucial to keep in mind that their confinement was officially framed as a cordon sanitaire, a public health measure needed to eliminate a medical threat to the *criollo* body politic. The medical effects of the quarantine were, at least for the target population, exactly the opposite. La Tortuga was in the middle of an area where cholera cases were spreading. The Mariusans initially were not provided with medical care, and their only source of drinking water was the river. Moreover, the cordon sanitaire required other *indígenas* heading for the mainland—including symptomatic individuals seeking medical attention—to stop at Tortuga, which quite possibly created a cholera "hot spot" in the vast circulatory system of the Orinoco delta. Predicting the outcome of this equation is hardly rocket science: government officials had condemned the Mariusans to another round of cholera infection.

When the Claretians first called for medical assistance in coping with cholera cases, María Vargas "loaned" them a young physician for a few days. Two Claretian physicians also visited for a short time. Benavides and luck collaborated to provide a solution that was more durable. Just as the first cholera cases were being reported on the island, Dr. Ricardo Campins was calling the regional health office in Tucupita in search of work. Campins, a tall, confident, handsome man, is from central Venezuela. He is an excellent storyteller. Campins's wife, Yuleima López de Campins, is young, dark-haired, and attractive; her girlish face is graced by large eyes that light up when she speaks even as her voice maintains its refined and modulated tone. Both are physicians who performed their year of service in the delta, although López de Campins, who graduated six months after her husband, did not work at La Tortuga.

We visited Campins and López de Campins, and together we spent a delightful morning in a small restaurant in the mountains overlooking a fertile agricultural region. Campins's account was dramatic and detailed, and it portrayed him as a complex character in the story.

Ricardo Campins, 13 November 1994

The truth is that when I graduated I saw how terrible it is to graduate and then find oneself unable to work because there's a political racket, right? So then I called the director's office [of the regional health office in Tucupita], and they immediately directed me to "come, doctor." And I go there, and what I find is that cholera had been breaking out right at that very moment. . . . But the truth is that I was scared, without even knowing why. First of all because I had never treated a cholera patient, right? The diarrheas that are known here [in central Venezuela] are diarrheas caused by gastroenteritis, that's all, which are easier to treat, right? And the etiology is less aggressive. We arrive there, and the first thing they tell me is that I'm not going to one of the traditional clinics, but I'm going to be in the middle of the Delta Amacuro, right in the middle, on an island called La Tortuga, blocking the entrance of cholera from the ocean toward Venezuela, right?

I first got to know La Tortuga because a physician who had been loaned from another state had been there—they had taken him on loan. And, well, it was frightening. Nothing but jungle, with no type of services— there were no lights, there was no potable water. And we were in *indígena* communities, with just the minimum, right, in terms of material things needed to live—the minimum that a person needs to live. The thing that was closest to civilization was a plastic or galvanized tub. That's it, right? So I established myself there for a month and a half. What really surprised me was how the *indígenas* from Mariusa Island, from the mouth of the Mariusa, returned, how they arrived—really worried, scared, incredibly panicked, because their families were dying. Dying from a *hebu*—what they call a *hebu*, a malignant *hebu*. What they call a Warao curse [*un mal warao*], right? A *hebu*. And, well, what— I begin to see what a terrible disease cholera is. I wasn't familiar with it. I had known it only through books, and I never imagined the quantity of liquid that a person can lose in diarrhea, you see? Never, never. I still remember the fear, panic, and terror I felt with that first patient. . . .

When I arrived in the delta, I had gotten the impression from my colleagues that it was a terrible disease. And there was an incredible panic among the paramedical personnel, as much among the physicians as among the nurses, who were from the same population that was suffering from cholera. At first we operated under the hypothesis that it was highly contagious—and in fact it is, in fact it is, but not that much. At first we took precautions not just with the food but in the way you handled the patient. There were three buckets, one with almost full-strength chlorine, the next with a lesser amount of chlorine, and the last one had hardly any chlorine, so that you could wash your hands in three stages in order to go from patient to patient, right? At first they used facemasks, but then they realized that this was not necessary. And they even stopped using gloves, because people realized that as long as you kept your hands clean before eating, there was no problem. And you could even touch the secretions, just so long as you didn't pass them along to your mouth, right?

And I got cholera in La Tortuga! It was terrible! . . . My symptoms were identical to everyone else's. Really strong abdominal cramps. And the diarrhea. At first I had lots of watery bowel movements, but they had some color. After cleaning out, let's call it washing my intestines with the quantity of liquid that is produced, you begin to have watery bowel movements that are much clearer. I didn't take any stool samples, right? I didn't take any stool samples because we didn't have the specimen tubes, the special specimen tubes that [the Ministry of] Health was giving out. They never came during the month that I was on La Tortuga. During the first month and a half of cholera I never saw a specimen tube. I only saw them at the very end, right? So it was just logical—the Ministry of Health says that there is no cholera as long as there are no specimen tubes that come out positive, understand? The [regional] epidemiologist can be watching an *indígena* die from profuse diarrhea and he will say it's not cholera until he sees a positive result from a specimen tube. But whenever you come across an intestinal diarrhea that is that frenetic, with that volume—you don't find them in other cases—it must be cholera, with violent dehydration. You can have an intestinal diarrhea that produces an important reaction, but it doesn't become severe in less than two hours, isn't that true?

Okay, so it began. That [my cholera infection] was right at the end [of my stay on La Tortuga], because of course one takes all the precautions at first. But one gets, how can I put it, underdeveloped in the end. And it's also that one trusts. As physicians, we come to trust in what we observe in the course of treatment. That it is indeed possible to cure, that as long as you take certain steps absolutely nothing will happen to you. Well, you start putting behind you that terrible fear that you had, right?

And at some point, I don't know when, I became infected. During the day I started having bowel movements. At first they were profuse but with color, with the normal color. But then in the afternoon, the diarrheas were clear, right? And like I told you, I couldn't take any samples in order to confirm [that it was cholera], but what I did was to begin to take a combination of Bactron with tetracycline, right? I combined them just in case. And at the same time rehydration, plenty of oral rehydration, right? I drank plenty, plenty of liquid. And the next day my bowel movements were lesser in quantity each time, but they kept on being watery. And an incredible depression, that is really terrible. On the second or the third bowel movement, I felt as if the world was slipping away from me. I didn't even have the strength to get up. On La Tortuga there are some latrines that—yeah, that's another thing. The *indígenas* go poo-poo in the river, right? But the state made them latrines behind each of the houses, and they are still like new—the latrines are new. Nobody used those latrines, just the physician while he was there [referring to himself]. Well, that was where I was, dying in one of those latrines because I didn't have the strength to get up. I had to call for someone. I couldn't get up. They had to take me out, get me up, help me get up.

In an echo of Father Gabi Gutiérrez, Campins tells the story of La Tortuga in terms of his coming of age as a professional. Like Mr. Kurtz and Marlow in Joseph Conrad's *Heart of Darkness,* Campins had traveled from a familiar environment to one that was foreign, overwhelming, primitive, and racially Other. The only evidence of civilization was a tub used for washing clothes. (Somehow, the medical gear and two-way radio he took along did not evoke the modern world.) The journey produced an epistemological transformation from knowledge gained from books to a concrete, immediate, and, one might add, visceral understanding of disease and treatment. Cholera became simultaneously powerful and terrifying, controllable and safe.

Campins was one of only a few physicians or nurses who spontaneously reported that he or she felt strong emotions—fear, panic, and terror—on seeing the severity and rapidity of the dehydration that cholera can produce. Many practitioners insisted that their professionalism made them so focused on taking medically appropriate measures that fear and repulsion never entered the picture. In their accounts fear pervaded *indígena* responses, but it was carefully expunged from those of *criollo* professionals. (Recall how Vargas scolded one of her staff physicians for displaying emotion, even in private.) In his narrative Campins allows himself to become a more complex subject, combining fear and professionalism. Over time, for Campins and most of the other health care personnel, cholera became commonplace. It came to be understood as another problem easily solved through established medical procedures.

Interestingly, in his narrative Campins links himself to the Mariusans affectively, sharing the same sense of fear and panic. But he immediately distances himself from the *indígenas* by characterizing "their" fears as magical—"a Warao curse." Here Campins racializes the way that people on La Tortuga were talking about cholera. He off-handedly reduces a complex array of explanations and uncertainties to a simple, homogenous, unquestioned belief in spirits. By this time, Mariusan cholera narratives already incorporated information provided by physicians and nurses, but he seems to have been oblivious to the complex and unstable ways that people perceived the disease. When race explains all, exegeses are simple, clear, and powerful.

Campins's candor is striking. No other institutional practitioner with whom we spoke ever admitted having had cholera symptoms. Campins breaks down the physician's distance from and authority over patients: his symptoms "were identical to everyone else's." He speaks of being overtaken by the sense that "the world was slipping away from me" *(que el mundo se me iba apagando)*, his voice dropping considerably in pitch and volume, taking on the sort of ethereal tone that is often used to speak of otherworldly experiences. Medical authority disappears for a moment as he evokes the words that so many cholera patients used to describe the overwhelming feelings of weakness and the loss of bodily and mental control associated with rapid dehydration.

At the same time, Campins inserts a medical perspective into this experiential language. Keenly aware of the sensation that his guts were being flushed out and that he was growing weak, he reports that he was monitoring changes in the quantity and color of his own diarrhea just as he would with his patients. He similarly reports the course of treatment he prescribed for himself, specifying both the combination of antibiotics and the type and quantity of oral rehydration solution. What is perhaps most interesting is that he never surrenders the power to cure. Even though a nurse was working with him, he limited her role to taking the tops off the bottles of rehydration solution, which he was too weak to do. "I cured myself," he asserted during the interview. The role of women on La Tortuga once again disappeared.

Campins interrupts himself when he alludes to the latrines, initiating a commentary regarding the hygienic practices of *indígenas*. The residents reportedly so steadfastly resisted the efforts of the state to promote modern hygienic practices that they refused to use the latrines. Even in the face of an illness so powerful that it produced "an incredible depression," the physician retains his status as a modern subject by making the trek to the outhouse. There he becomes a prisoner of modernity.

Campins's story contains three substantial asides. Although the lack of sample tubes may seem a rather trivial detail, it raises the issue of a major limitation on his right to diagnose cholera, which compromised his authority as a physician. Although Campins was certain that he and his patients had contracted cholera, only the regional epidemiologist had the authority to decide what constituted a cholera case. Campins paints a biting image of the epidemiologist watching an *indígena* die from cholera-like symptoms during the outbreak (rather than intervening clinically), all the while denying that it was cholera. Here we see a powerful confrontation between the role of the clinical practitioner, whose knowledge of the disease is mediated by his or her visual and tactile contact with the bodies of the sick, and the much more distanced role of the epidemiologist, who views cholera primarily through the lens of statistics and laboratory tests. Campins's assertion is provocative: if only "laboratory-confirmed cases" count as cholera and sample tubes are not available, both clinical and microbiological perspectives become meaningless—if powerful—illusions.

Campins also interrupted the narrative to explain why he became a patient. He describes a gradual process in which practitioners moved from the use of strict and elaborate procedures in response to the construction of cholera as a "terrible" and "highly contagious" disease to the relaxed sense that "you could even touch the secretions, just so long as you didn't pass them along to your mouth." Campins suggests that the focus shifted from prevention to treatment, from standing in awe of the power of the disease to a faith in the power of biomedicine to cure it. The physician, in this story at least, came to believe so strongly in his power over the disease—his own agency—that he got infected.

There is more going on here than the performance of a cautionary tale for medical students. The parallel with *Heart of Darkness* goes farther than the riverine passage into an uncivilized world inhabited by racial Others; just as Mr. Kurtz loses contact with his modern self, falling into backwardness, Campins, sliding into backwardness, depicts a gradual loss of conscientiousness regarding the bodily practices of the modern world. As he spoke, our own experience with cholera patients enabled us to follow his movement from dipping his hands in chlorine solution to touching the diarrhea and vomit teeming with *Vibrio cholerae*. Immersion in this "frightening" place, where there was "nothing but jungle," in the middle of "*indígena* communities," seemed to strip away the veneer of modernity and expose the "underdeveloped" quality beneath.

Campins's rich story resonates with Venezuelan narratives of modernity. His account parallels President Rómulo Gallegos's famous novel, *Doña Barbara*, which pits an urban lawyer, representing the force of modernization, against a barbaric tyrant of the wild plains, Doña Barbara.[1] Although Campins's tale seems to be influenced by Gallegos's text, his reflections on Tortuga go beyond a simple confrontation of premodern and modern forces to play with the border that separates uncivilized and civilized worlds. His story suggests that even the physician, who is the embodiment of Venezuelan modernity, can fall subject to the vices of an uncivilized environment and reveal the "underdeveloped" self that lies within, although the modern subject and the techniques of modern medicine overcome the "terrible" disease of backwardness that wells up from within: the physician cures himself. Campins seems unconvinced that civilization is capable of defeating barbarism in an environment that is "nothing but jungle."

MAGIC MEETS MEDICINE

Campins went on to describe how he embraced this ambiguous region between opposing worlds by attempting to appropriate the power of both magic and medicine.

Ricardo Campins, 13 November 1994

I recall one of [the shamans], I don't remember his name, he sure was ugly. The man is from Mariusa, he speaks oddly—Alvarez, that's the one! Yes, the man is a good guy. . . . I really saw him engaged in his practice as an *indígena* healer, with a huge rattle full of parrot feathers on top. Really. But I couldn't take pictures, he wouldn't let me.

I treated a child, a little girl, who had been polytraumatized [creating an inflammation or possible rupture of the intestines] by him. He polytraumatized, traumatized her with his hands and with a rock, I think it was, because he wanted to rid her of the cholera *hebu*, right? This cholera *hebu*. And she had faringoamigdalitis pultacea [an acute inflammation of the throat], right? And she had cholera, too. And he wanted—he said that he had to cure this. The girl cried. She was polytraumatized, and I had to send her to [the hospital in] Tucupita. I think that they had to operate on the patient afterward. But she had reflexive abdominal pain, which means that she had an acutely inflamed abdomen, right? And this was due to the trauma that the shaman himself inflicted on the girl, you see. To be sure, he felt impotent in comparison to me, you see. What I did is to not fight with him. I invited him into the examining room, into the improvised clinic that we had, so that he would see how I worked. And he spent the entire day seated, just watching me work. It was a true exchange, because later on I was able to see him. But he told me not to use my camera. . . .

Okay, the truth is that I had to use the technique, I had to observe their shamans, their healers, and see how the healer himself knew that he was fooling the Mariusans, the Warao. Their belief is so deeply rooted that when someone gets sick, he knows he's fooling them, but he cures them just by the act of seeming to take out some object. I grabbed a screw—the *bahanarotu*, that's what they call the guy who takes out objects!—and I would suck on the abdomen and make believe that I was looking for something in the abdomen. And it's traumatic, too, it produces trauma.

That belief is so deeply rooted in them that I had to use it too. I would all of a sudden take a screw out of the abdomen, and I would say that this *wisidatu* business is really great, really great. I used the pills and I used their kind [of medicine] as well with cholera patients. And you'd see, it's hard to believe, but [I used it] with parasites, colds, faringoamigdalitis too. And the people didn't say anything; they watched me keenly and they sought me out—this belief is really deeply rooted.

Campins provides us with a compelling account of relations between institutional and lay medical practitioners. Most physicians in the delta kept their distance from their *indígena* colleagues, and some denied treatment to patients who were also seeing "witches" *(brujos)* or "quacks" *(curiosos)*. Campins characterizes the world of medical practice on La Tortuga at this time as consisting of three practitioners: himself, José Félix Alvarez (of Mariusa), and Diego Castañeda (of La Tortuga). This construal of the dramatis personae denies significant roles to the nurses who worked there and the women who cared for cholera patients.

In his narrative Campins recapitulates an important chapter in the history of modernity: the victorious struggle waged by science over magic. He begins with an unflattering portrait of Alvarez. The visual motif, the "huge rattle full of parrot feathers on top," evokes the stereotype of the "shaman" as exotic Other. Campins dramatizes his claim that the "shamans" recognized their impotence by describing Alvarez's failed attempt to treat a patient and subsequent decision to place the sick in Campins's care. Campins's authority is underlined by the medical terms he uses to identify the child's illness. Campins stresses Alvarez's defeat by relating that the healer "felt impotent" and was fascinated by the unfolding world of medical science.

A magnanimous victor, Campins not only encourages the gaze of his colleague but returns it, observing the tricks of Alvarez's trade. Crossing the great divide, Campins adds magical practices to biomedical techniques. The result is not a hybrid form of knowledge or a relationship of equality between medical and vernacular epistemologies. Campins constructs medicine as precise, objective, and authoritative knowledge and Alvarez's practices as a set of "deeply rooted" supernatural beliefs *(creencias)* that do not even deserve the term *religion*. Alvarez's role is presented as disingenuous: Campins asserts that even the shaman did not believe in what he practiced. The hocus pocus of "shamanic" practice is so simple and transparent that Campins is quickly able to learn all he needs to know.

Alvarez, an old friend of mine (Charles Briggs), is one of the most knowledgeable and versatile practitioners of vernacular curing in the delta. He was around sixty years of age at the time of the interview. Alvarez is heavyset.

His features are broad and his hair is cropped. He has two wives, and he has not met with success in repeated attempts during the past decade to find a third. Jovial and sincere, he is one of the most emotionally expressive men I have met in the delta—he always hugs me powerfully and kisses my cheek numerous times when we meet after a prolonged absence. When Manuel Torres decided to teach me techniques of *hoarotu* curing, Alvarez aided in the instruction. There are three primary categories of healers in the delta: *wisidatu, hoarotu,* and *bahanarotu.*[2] Each works on a distinct class of pathogens, and each involves a specific epistemology, mode of training, and curative practice. This classification oversimplifies the diversity among practitioners and specialties, but it forms a widely used shorthand. Alvarez is highly unusual in being a skilled practitioner of all three varieties.

Alvarez is also a remarkable storyteller, so I was somewhat shocked to discover that, when I discussed the events that had occurred on La Tortuga with him and six other men, he had little to say about his time there. People generally relished these opportunities to exhibit their skills as narrators, but Alvarez offered next to nothing in the course of the exchange. He did enjoy recounting one incident: "Cholera hit again—it hit me! I just shitted and shitted, it was nothing but water. Damn, there was nothing left of me. I didn't know what was happening. When I shitted nothing but water, it really hit me. I almost died." He also drew attention to his friendship with Campins, whom he described as "a good fellow" who "did good work there."[3]

Alvarez also emphatically denied that Campins had learned how to incorporate *bahanarotu* practice into his interventions: "Oh, no, no. He doesn't know any of that—he's just telling lies, telling lies. He did learn a little bit about how to treat cuts." Here Alvarez invoked the hierarchy that orders the epistemologies of vernacular curing. *Bahanarotu* practice entails a lengthy apprenticeship and the mastery of a large body of specialized knowledge, but learning to cure cuts is a much less powerful and much more easily acquired skill. Alvarez was implying that he had taught Campins the rudiments of this introductory practice—he was pulling rank. The possibility that Campins could, through observation, learn enough about the *bahanarotu's* practice even to fake the extraction of foreign objects from patients was no more credible to Alvarez than the possibility that Alvarez had learned the rudiments of biomedical practice would be to Campins. When I asked him about his attempts to cure cholera patients, Alvarez simply noted that he was unable to divine the "name" of the disease. His silence spoke eloquently about the experience of watching helplessly as an epidemic decimated his community.

SEPARATING THE "UNCIVILIZED"
FROM THE "SEMI-CIVILIZED"

My first impressions of the Tortugans were influenced by what Mariusans had told me about them. The many trips people make from Mariusa to the mainland nearly always include a stop at La Tortuga. I got to know a number of Tortugans, including Diego Castañeda and his wife, Sol María Aranguren, a silver-haired, full-figured, outgoing, and witty woman of about sixty-five. I also became acquainted with Julio Romero, a strong fellow then about fifty who has a distinguished manner and a kind face. Campins and Gutiérrez referred to him as "the *cacique*" of Tortuga. His wife, María Teresa Salazar, was about fifty. She has a kind face, sturdy features, and gracious demeanor. Romero was promoting Vicente García, a slender, handsome, and serious man of about forty, to the state government as a prospective *comisario* (local official). These individuals, along with half a dozen of their neighbors, spoke in February 1995 about the differences that distinguish them from "the Mariusans." The Tortugans stated that their "roots" were on the coast near Mariusa, but they constructed time in such a way as to create a deeper cultural divide.

The concept of spatial fixity, of living in and being from a particular place, was a curious and powerful construct. Romero suggested that although his parents may have been from *akoho*—the "mouths of the rivers" along the coast—*he* was born in La Tortuga. He said that he frequently returned with his parents to the coast to collect moriche palm starch and other forest products, to hunt, to harvest crabs, and to participate in festivals, but that these visits did not have any bearing on his identity.

García used the question of food production and consumption to create a temporal divide, arguing that the Tortugans used to eat the forest food. Although that way of life was only a cultural memory for Tortugans, it was everyday life for the Mariusans. It was his past but their present. And even this connection was disappearing from cultural memory, he claimed, as *idamotuma* (the old ones), the members of his parents' generation, died. García used cultural memory not to create social connection but to deny it.

Although the Tortugans implied that they no longer ate *yuca, ocumo,* plantains, or corn, they did grow these foods. In Tortuga, agricultural products and fish are generally sold to *criollos* who live nearby or, when transport is available, sold in town to pay for wheat flour and sugar. Unfortunately, the floods that come during the rainy season often destroy the Tortugans' crops. García mentioned an additional component of their diet, one that led to another contrast with the Mariusans: "We eat everything.

But those people, even if they're dying of hunger, they won't eat beef. . . . Their food is grubs, moriche palm hearts, and moriche starch."[4] *Criollos* frequently make fun of *indígenas* for refusing to eat beef or pork, suggesting that "they" would rather starve to death than eat what any rational person would recognize as highly desirable food. There was a bittersweet element to this claim, however. García also noted that the forest foods make one strong, while a diet of flour and sugar leads to weakness, disease, and death: "That's why there are so few of us here." Indeed, selling fish and crops to secure the capital needed to embrace modernity—commercially produced flours—had created significant health risks in many of the more "civilized" delta communities by lowering protein intake and decreasing nutritional balance.

When I asked where cholera had first appeared, Aranguren placed it squarely at the mouth of the Mariusa, claiming that the Mariusan "sorcerers" brought the disease from the Mariusa coast. The story gives the Mariusans agency: they are seen as actors with malevolent intent, who took cholera to the island "so that it would infect us." The Tortugans, on the other hand, never become identified with cholera, never become agents of transmission. The narrative casts them as innocent bystanders who had the misfortune to be on the path taken by the Mariusans.

Note that cholera, people, and culture follow the same path in this account, one that leads from Mariusa to Tortuga. The two places differ in terms of time, in that Mariusa continues to be the locus of a previous way of life, at the same time that the premodern world coexists with its modern counterpart.[5] They also differ in terms of space, such that one becomes the quintessence of the premodern world of forest gatherers while the other is cast as a more modern realm of agricultural production and sale. Mariusa and Tortuga are chronotopes—fusions of space and time—and the origin narratives that the Tortugans told about themselves and cholera are linear movements along this time-space continuum.[6] The Tortugans claimed that they lived in, if you will, a different time-space zone, thereby creating a powerful sense of social distance from the Mariusans.[7] Scholars suggest that space is not just a physical or cognitive fact—"Both the material space of physical nature and the ideation space of human nature have to be seen as socially produced and reproduced"[8]—and the same argument has been made for time. In the Tortugans' account, however, Mariusa becomes naturalized as a space that existed apart from how Tortugans, *criollos,* or government officials conceptualized it and related to its residents.

How does this production take place? Clearly, telling stories such as the Tortugans' account helps people to imagine these time-space worlds, but something else is also going on. A clue lies in the Tortugans' statement that they sold *yuca, ocumo,* plantains, corn, and fish to *criollos* in Tucupita and the surrounding area. The sense that Mariusa is remote and not part of the modern world was produced both by racialization, which painted it as the quintessence of the *indígena* world, and capitalization, which located Tortuga as part of the market economy and Mariusa as lying off that map.[9] The Tortugans were able to make themselves modern by consuming flour and sugar, which integrated them into the market economy. Because they had little capital and little ability to defend their economic rights against *criollo* exchange partners, achieving this position had come at a formidable cost—their diet had become impoverished, which, they admitted, weakened them physically.

As producers and consumers—of both food and culture—the Tortugans participated actively in the production of these distinct senses of place. The creation of temporal-spatial distance through schemes of racialization and capitalization is the core of colonialism, which reaches its endpoint in the displacement of racialized Others from space, through land expropriation and forced removal, and from the contemporary world, through genocide. As they imagined themselves in terms of this linear process that led from a premodern, *indígena* time-space to a modern, *criollo* one, the Tortugans internalized the very practices that racialize and subordinate them. And they helped racialize cholera as a disease that springs from the *indígena* heartland.

To be sure, this schema is not solely of the Tortugans' making. Campins similarly distances the Mariusans vis-à-vis a time-space continuum when he distinguishes the two communities.

Ricardo Campins, 13 November 1994

I found an island with vegetation that was approximately two meters high, where there were some barracks made of wood by the state for the *indígenas* who were there. They are, quote, "civilized," unquote, right? We're going to use that term because the Mariusans are not civilized. The Mariusans are quite pure—even if they have been influenced by civilization because they use motors, they use nets. . . . But on La Tortuga, the influence of civilization, of our civilization, is truly much greater. . . .

The *indígena,* I suppose, who behaves like an *indígena* is the one who I call a "purer" *indígena* because he has the face of an *indígena,* the eyes of an *indígena,* and all of the characteristics of an *indígena,* and he lives like an *indígena.* But [the Tortugan] lives like a, quote, "*indígena,*" unquote, because he has plastic plates, plastic or metal silverware, pots and pans. He knows how to use flashlights, he knows what a battery and a radio are. Obviously, he is not a pure *indígena,* not as pure as in the case of the Mariusan, who uses boats that are very similar to the ones that his ancestors always used, the type propelled by paddles. . . . And [the men] wear only trousers, with no shirt, and [go] barefoot. In contrast, the people from La Tortuga use the same trousers but with shirts and tennis shoes, you see?

The ones from La Tortuga wait for the state to give them everything. But not the Mariusans—the ones from Mariusa take from the sea, from the river too, I imagine. From the sea because they live on the coastline where the sea meets the river. They take advantage of their natural environment, they use it for their own benefit, right? And they move around, they are nomads. The people from La Tortuga, on the other hand, don't. The ones on La Tortuga, they stay on La Tortuga. But not the people on the Mariusa coast. If they have to go looking for palm hearts—when it's palm heart season, they go looking for palm hearts. When it's grub season, they go and eat grubs. When it's crab season, you see, they go and eat crabs. They go to the area where the crabs are. And this makes them adapt their habits. We can say that they're not stationary, right? They limit themselves to what the natural environment gives them at that moment.

For example, they preserve their paddles and their canoes, right? [And] the form of the nets they use to catch fish, but that's all. Because they can make a hammock quickly, right? They are capable of making things with what they find in their natural environment. They are capable of making a shanty [*choza*] quickly with what they have in the natural environment. And it's true that the people from La Tortuga aren't capable of making them. And that's why I speak of them as being purer. I try to differentiate them. If you live more in the [lower delta], well, you truly have deeper indigenous roots, and the Mariusan does, it's obvious. And I think that they are the closest that can be seen, what you could have seen a hundred years ago. I imagine that the *indígena* you would have seen a hundred years ago was very similar to these people.

And they're strong *indígenas*. The *indígenas* from Mariusa are strong *indígenas*, with a strong back and musculature. This means that they have paddled a lot. The people from La Tortuga don't look like that. The people from La Tortuga look tubercular [*tuberculosa*], you see, and weak, very weak. And alcohol is killing them, you see. In contrast, the people from Mariusa aren't like that. The people from Mariusa look strong. The women are strong. They're very healthy, very healthy. And that's what I mean. I don't know how an anthropologist would express it, what term you would use, but that is my term. And more or less what I want to get across is that the *indígena* from Mariusa is an *indígena*. The others, we don't know if they are civilized, we don't know if they are *criollos* or *indígenas*. But they don't have roots, they don't have any way of defending themselves within the natural environment. For the Tortugan the natural environment is aggressive, but not for the Mariusan. No, they use the natural environment, and they know how to adapt to that changing natural environment, you see. . . .

The first thing that I came across was that these people were arriving at La Tortuga, and the people from La Tortuga being, quote, "civilized," unquote, had already acquired different customs. They already weren't the same *indígenas*, right? It was as if they had collided, collided within the same indigenous culture—two currents *[afluencias]*, two ways of thinking, right? Let's put it this way: the culture of the Mariusans, right, with the culture of these acculturated *indígenas*, right? And so it happened that the Mariusans found the women from La Tortuga attractive, because they wore dresses that looked more like those worn by civilized people. The women from Mariusa, on the other hand, always had the features of the indigenous Warao—her tight dress, her beaded necklaces. And problems with the women started to arise, you see. That was one of the problems. And the second was that people from La Tortuga didn't want to have the people from Mariusa on their land, constructing cabins, right? And another, to be sure, was that the people from Mariusa were hard workers and the others were not. Because the hardworking people from Mariusa didn't think that the state would give away food, would give them food. And it's true that they didn't like it anyway, right? They don't like the food we eat, right? And they wanted to work, to keep on working, trolling, going after their nets, making their nets, and taking their food out of the river itself. . . .

The truth is that there was a lot of bad feeling among the *indígenas*, and I had to, was obliged to, call the National Guard. And I had at my command *[a mi mandato]* four National Guardsmen. They sent me four National Guardsmen in order to bring the island under control. Because they had started committing acts of violation. Thefts, right? Because the people from La Tortuga were accustomed to being given everything, and they saw that the Mariusans had the fruits of their labor, you see. And so they stole each other's outboard motors, right? There were problems between the women, that the women wanted to steal from each other. They truly wanted to rob each other. It's logical—the people from La Tortuga had more things of our civilization, our civilization, and they wanted to take them, such as manufactured hammocks. The mosquito netting that the Mariusans had were only made of cloth, only of cloth, and in contrast [the ones that the Tortugans] had you could see through, they're manufactured ones. And so I obviously had to call the National Guard by radio. I had a forty-meter radio that I used to communicate with [officials in] Tucupita. And I asked for them and they sent them to me.

And alcohol was another problem. Barely—it would seem impossible—the people from Mariusa don't drink alcohol, you see. That was another problem, because the people from La Tortuga incited the people from Mariusa to drink alcohol. And when they drank alcohol, they were fierce, because the people from Mariusa are fierce *[brava]*, fierce. They're war-like *[guerrera]*, right? A few shots of alcohol in them and they become indomitable *[indominables]*. And they wanted to do whatever they pleased. They went after the women, and they wanted to rape them, just like that. Well, you see, the only way out was to call the police, the military police, and they sent me four military police. I imposed order, I imposed a type of—. Afterward I regretted this because I should have let things evolve by themselves.

In Campins's tale, the gap between the residents of Mariusa and La Tortuga is transformed into that master opposition of modernity: "civilized" versus "uncivilized."[10] The way Campins imagines the Mariusans embodies both sides of the centuries-old stereotype of the savage. His Mariusans fulfill, on the one hand, the image of the natural man. "Pure *indígenas*" live in harmony with nature. By adapting to it perfectly they have rendered nature gentle, a source of comfort. For Jean-Jacques Rousseau, the natural man perfectly embodied the individualism that lay at the core of modern political philosophy, and Campins agrees.[11] He finds the Mariusans hardworking and fiercely independent, relying on no one else for their subsistence and even rejecting civilized foods. Shielded (until recently) from such vices of civilization as alcohol, they are healthy and strong. The Mariusans exist outside of historical time, living today exactly as their ancestors supposedly lived "a hundred years ago." At the same time, however, the uncivilized Mariusan is fierce, warlike, and unable to control his rage. In Campins's narrative, alcohol unlocked the Mariusans' violent nature and prompted them to "do whatever they pleased," including raping women and stealing goods.[12]

Although in Campins's account the Tortugans have lost the ability to harmonize with nature, he implies they haven't adapted successfully to civilization, either. They are doubly displaced. At the same time that they are excluded from the presumably positive dimensions of the noble savage category, Campins suggests that the Tortugans bear only a tangential relationship to the identity categories he invokes—*indígena, criollo*, and civilized. The position of the Mariusans with regard to the civilized-uncivilized distinction is clear, and so is Campins's: he repeatedly speaks for "our civilization." Only one thing seems to link the Tortugans to "pure *indígenas*"—their bodies. Biological difference continues to provide the necessary basis for the racialization process, even though it is not sufficient. The people from La Tortuga retain "the face of an *indígena*, the eyes of an *indígena*, and all of the characteristics of an *indígena*." Here lies a clue to the epistemological status of Campins's account. The young physician constructs himself as an amateur anthropologist and invokes a culturalist logic. He uses a professional discourse in which he lacks authority while acknowledging his interlocutor: "I don't know how an anthropologist would express it, what term you would use, but that is my term."

Campins's representation of conflict on La Tortuga makes use of powerful rhetorical functions. His perception of a cultural chasm provides him with a means of imagining a long-standing, pervasive, explosive, and irresolvable conflict between Mariusans and Tortugans. The narrative neatly erases the roles played by government officials, including bringing the Mariusans to the island, forcing them to stay, and withholding promises and badly needed supplies. It also ignores abusive treatment by *criollos* living in the area, which both Mariusans and Tortugans emphasized in their stories, and the way that priests, physicians, and nurses wielded their power. A language of culture situates the problems solely within the two communities.

The cultural rhetoric that assumes that cultural opposites must "collide" enables Campins to describe events in a way that makes the tension and conflict seem palpable, natural, and inevitable. According to Campins, the envy the Mariusans felt upon seeing the civilized goods possessed by the Tortugans produced a pervasive, inescapable desire to embrace modernity and, thus, inexorable conflict. Campins's description of the Tortugans reflects the common wisdom that *indígenas* who are "acculturated" to *criollo* life become lazy, unhealthy, confused, and socially dislocated. Contact with modernity thus naturally produces cultural pathology for *indígenas*. The sense that contact between culturally distinct communities naturally leads to conflict is a general feature of cultural reasoning.[13]

If difference leads to conflict, then a government official such as Campins has no choice but to invoke the privilege of the state to suppress it. When Campins called in the Guardia Nacional, he placed the power associated with armed soldiers under the "command" of biomedical authority. Campins justifies his actions by describing the "pure *indígena*" as fierce, warlike, and indomitable. Only the power of the state—and of the machine gun—is sufficient to dominate them. This logic provided excellent cover for the threats used to deprive Mariusans of their constitutional right to freedom of transit on La Tortuga and elsewhere. The nation-state's use of force in the cholera epidemic disappears in the image of violent *indígenas*. Campins's narrative and the events it describes recapitulate colonial efforts to preserve the racial economy.[14] It was clear that Campins's job on La Tortuga was not simply to attend to the health of the population but to impede the passage of *indígenas* upriver. The project was militarized and racialized from the start.[15]

A final function of the rhetoric of culture and conflict involves self-representation—that is, the way that Campins places himself within the drama. He plays a number of roles, including those of explorer, physician, magician, and military commander. Confronted by the chaos of the wilderness and the wildness of the "pure *indígenas*," Campins portrays himself as the sole individual capable of controlling violence, disease, death, and disorder. Campins says that he, like heroes in general, faced a challenge that called for inventiveness and willingness to take risks, not a mere capacity to take orders: "Just think, I did everything that I have described to you without the intervention of the state. You could say that I acted alone, and my conscience and my experience told me, 'Do this!' Right, because these weren't policies enacted by the state—they just let you loose there with a load of medicines and that's it!"[16] Campins didn't seem to realize that he *was* the state. The ideological separation of medical and political domains— the modern notion that science and society are autonomous[17]—enabled him to construct the magic he performed as medical, which obscured his position as an employee of a state institution that had accrued special powers in the wake of a "health emergency." Campins shared the stage with other agents of modernity and civilization, including missionaries, nurses, and other physicians, but that fact is never mentioned in his narrative.

STRIVING FOR MODERNITY

The Mariusans and Tortugans I interviewed remembered Ricardo Campins, Gabi Gutiérrez, and others with tremendous fondness, and they lauded their work. These individuals worked extremely long hours and with great dedication to save lives that others seldom thought worthy of protection. Campins and Gutiérrez valued their partnerships with the people from Mariusa and La Tortuga and pointed with affection to a number of friendships that were established during this period. I admire both for the work they did on La Tortuga. The state's principal interest, meanwhile, seems to have been in keeping the Mariusans away from journalists and the residents of Barrancas and Tucupita. Preventing human suffering appears to have been a much lower priority. Campins and Gutiérrez refused to accept this process of dehumanization, and they struggled not only to save lives but also to help people preserve their dignity. That is why I detailed the manner in which racializing discourses came to structure the way that these two newcomers to the region did their work—it helps to demonstrate that the racial economy shaped how even well-trained, dedicated professionals related to their subjects.

Much like the story told by María Vargas, Campins's narrative pits modernity against the premodern and civilization against barbarism. Unlike

Vargas's tale, which is cast as a success story, Campins's story of his journey into darkness and disorder portrays a failure. In contrast to Gutiérrez, who stresses the way that colonial legacies created social and material hierarchies, Campins places the failure of modernity squarely on the shoulders of the *indígenas*. The Mariusans provided Campins with the prototype of the cultural Other, the human being who stands so far beyond the reach of civilization and modernity that he or she cannot assimilate its basic tenets. Although the Tortugans had embraced civilization's material and spiritual manifestations, Campins thought that in their hands the virtues of modernity had turned into vices. He may have been successful in curing their bodies, but he could never transform their minds: "They never understood the origin [of the cholera epidemic]. They will never understand what a virus is, what a bacteria is, what a fungus is. They'll have to study a lot." Campins depicted the cultural gap between *indígenas* and *criollos* as being insurmountable, despite a prolonged process of acculturation: "I think that even the *indígena* who is a physician, Dr. [Vicente Medina], even he must not understand it very well."[18] At the time that Campins made this statement, Medina, "the Warao doctor," was undertaking advanced training in medicine and was serving as a deputy member of Congress. Campins's statement implied that no possible set of circumstances could enable medical modernity to penetrate the *indígenas*' alien culture.

In institutional terms this formula is perfect. Whatever gains are made in improving the health of delta residents are directly attributable to the vision and heroic efforts of *criollo* health professionals. The agency of *indígenas* figures only negatively here, as a force to be overcome. When the discussion shifts to the profound health problems that remain in the delta, the influence of *indígenas* is similarly negative: "their" language and customs impose an insurmountable barrier to civilization and medicine.

The way that Campins positions himself with respect to civilization is much more precarious, complex, and interesting than the orientation of many of his colleagues. Vargas, for example, never seems to waver in her dedication to modern public health practices, remaining steadfast and fully cognizant of what was taking place even in the face of opposition and emergency. Campins, however, seems to embody the opposition between the civilized and the uncivilized. He willingly incorporates magic into his medical practice, extracting screws while administering pills and rehydration solution. Moreover, the uncivilized quality of life on La Tortuga seems to trigger some quiescent barbarism of his own, leading him to drift away from his unquestioned commitment to hygienic practices: "One takes all the precautions at first. But one gets, how can I put it, underdeveloped in the end."

Here we find a second, hidden aspect of Venezuelan modernity: the fear that barbarism might lurk within even the most ardent modernist advances. Julio Salas, recognized as one of the first Venezuelan social scientists, claimed that since the time of independence the civilization of Venezuela has been thwarted by a lingering and internalized barbarism manifested as "retarding forces that promote social decomposition or dissolution."[19] Fascinatingly, in Campins's case this descent into "underdevelopment" came from placing too much faith in modern medicine, which led him to forget "that terrible fear" that he initially experienced. His ambivalent position within civilization assumes visual form when he invites us to picture the site where he perhaps came closest to death: the state-sponsored latrine, which only he used. Ironically, it was the very people who could be effectively civilized—his "uncivilized" or "semi-civilized" subjects—who rescued the physician from this central symbol of modern hygiene.

Campins's account of the Guardia Nacional brings into sharper focus the question of the power exerted by public health authorities. When we reflect on the link between medical and military institutions, other aspects of the Barrancas and La Tortuga stories become much clearer. Recall Ramón Rivera's description of what happened to the terrified Mariusans the moment they arrived in Barrancas: "The National Guardsmen came out of their car. They grabbed us and took us and threw us inside cars and took us away."[20] Vargas made it clear that soldiers were a constant presence at the Eloy Palacios High School, helping to "maintain order" and ensure compliance with medication routines. José Rivera reported that although the Mariusans realized that the promises made regarding supplies were lies, they "couldn't say anything" because there were "lots and lots of soldiers."[21]

Displaying military power strengthened the control of public health authorities over *criollo* residents as well. Vargas made it clear that this support helped her establish control over the powerful fishing industry and local merchants and so gave her an opportunity to transform Barrancas. Soldiers enforced orders by public health officials to confiscate and burn crabs and fish. This type of medical-military might was also apparent when "vaccination campaigns" were undertaken in the delta; physicians openly noted that armed soldiers or police not only prevented trouble but also ensured compliance. The notion that medicine and politics, science and society are separate helps to obscure this connection from view.[22] The power of public health authorities often straddled the line between coercion and hegemony, between the threat of violence and the promise of modernity.[23] The use of military metaphors by public health authorities should not necessarily be read as purely metaphorical.

Campins's narrative of his two-month stay on La Tortuga sharpens our focus on the intricacy of the dance between civilization and barbarism—and the tremendous cost of enabling these categories to retain any semblance of semantic substance and stability. A freshly trained *criollo* physician, newly arrived from the center of Venezuela, would seem to hold modernity comfortably in his grasp, but Campins's narrative implies that modernity can play its civilizing role only when it incorporates elements of barbarism. Here it acquires symbiosis: biomedicine works when it is combined with magic; hygiene can be imposed when its sharp edges have given way to a relaxation of sanitary discipline. Here the modern Latin American subject learns that underneath his (in this case) civilized self lurks a consciousness that is "underdeveloped in the end." It is, ironically, the very fragility of the claim to modernity and civilization that necessitates their violent imposition over racialized subjects.

Campins's experience teaches us that modernity would cease to exist if it succeeded in killing its opponent, the premodern, savage, irrational, traditional community. Without an "Other," modernity has no means of defining, legitimating, and reproducing itself. Campins's narrative also suggests that modernity is most powerful when it is most deeply engaged with its opponent, generating a violence that has great potential for coercion and hegemony. The willingness of the racialized Tortugans to use this logic against their Mariusan cousins bears witness to the puissance of compromised modernity. Perhaps even more important, Campins's narrative reveals that modernity's image as bounded, homogeneous, rational, and ahistorical is no less fallacious and powerful than Campins's claim that the poisoned dogs on La Tortuga died of cholera. The modernity that landed on the island was shot through with institutional resources and interests, racial projects, lies, false promises, and the threat of violence. These modern forces could not have established themselves without a technological base—specifically, without machine guns, IVs, and antibiotics. In Campins's story it was only the sudden appearance of cholera, the quintessence of the premodern, that enabled modernity to be established so visibly, if so ephemerally, on La Tortuga.

9   Culture Equals Cholera
Official Explanations for the Epidemic

No one in Delta Amacuro was prepared for cholera in the opening days of August 1992. Most communities in the fluvial area found themselves in the position of the Mariusans: they didn't know what the disease was, where it came from, how it was transmitted, or what to do about it. In contrast, public health authorities, politicians, and most residents of Tucupita and Barrancas knew that cases were being reported in nearby states and that an epidemic could emerge in Delta Amacuro. Yet almost nothing had been done to enable practitioners to respond swiftly to an outbreak.

Talking and writing about cholera—where it came from, whom it affected, and why it affected them—formed a crucial part of the actions and events that constituted the epidemic. The debate centered on a number of key questions: Where did cholera come from, and how did it get to the delta? How did cholera spread from person to person and place to place? Finally, who was to blame for the high incidence of infection and death in the delta? Laying the blame on "the Warao" and "their culture" could have profound implications for questions of citizenship and civil rights, affecting what sorts of services and legal protections *indígenas* could demand and what they would be likely to gain from pressing those demands. Pinning the responsibility on public institutions could lead to dismissals from influential positions, attacks on the legitimacy of key agencies, disruptions in relations with neighboring states and the national government, and upheavals in the balance of power between political parties and social networks in Delta Amacuro.

Weighing in on these questions was not the prerogative of epidemiologists, physicians, or professionals alone. Shaping perceptions of the disease and its "victims" was a game in which everyone had a stake, including other state institutions and the press.[1] It is emphatically not the case that only *criollos* told "dominant" narratives and *indígenas* their "resistant" counterparts, or that the former were told only on the mainland and the latter in the fluvial area. These explanations circulated widely within the region. Many persons classified as *indígenas* told dominant narratives in the course of explaining why their "less-civilized" neighbors seemed to be more susceptible to cholera, and many *criollos* produced and disseminated the stories that challenged the biomedical underpinnings of accounts advanced by public health officials.

Just three days after the first cases were officially reported, unidentified officials of the Regional Health Service announced that six people had died in the Pedernales area, becoming "victims of cholera after consuming a certain quantity of the crabs that are produced in that region." Although the names of these "victims" were "unknown," they were identified as belonging to "fishermen from the Warao and *criollo* ethnic groups, who in the height of the harvest time for capturing crabs in the Pedernales region and other parts of the lower delta, gather large quantities of these species."[2] An article that appeared in *Notidiario* the next day, based on information provided by Daniel Rodríguez, hedged this assertion regarding the route of transmission of cholera by suggesting that nineteen people had contracted the disease and two had died, "*presumably* due to the ingestion of hairy crabs contaminated by the mortal disease." The epidemiological analysis was more hesitant, but the racialization of cholera became much stronger. All cases were said to have involved *indígenas,* and even the variety of crab was racialized through the assertion that "in their native language it is known as '*motana.'*"[3]

This was a remarkable piece of epidemiological detective work. Although the consumption of crabs formed a good initial hypothesis, it would have been difficult—particularly without visiting the area—to rule out the possibility that travelers from infected areas had contaminated food or drinking water. The rapidity with which this conclusion was reached and presented to the press—as the result of an epidemiological investigation—reflects a racializing logic that was in place long before the epidemic began. Recall that MSAS epidemiologists had asserted that if cholera were to appear in Venezuela, poor and/or *indígena* communities would be responsible. Because of the state's problematic relationship to the national government and the existence of epidemics in other Venezuelan states, discourses of nationalism gained no ground as a tool for representing the disease in Delta Amacuro. The association between cholera and poverty had been occasionally evoked in the delta, especially when patients were classified as *criollos,* but, by and large, the questions of how the epidemic began and how it spread were described in racial terms from the start. Cholera was thus associated with "the favorite dish of the Waraos of that region," to quote the director of the Malariología in Tucupita.[4]

During the following two weeks, crabs became the rhetorical anchor for far-ranging attempts to link cholera to the "customs" and "culture" of *indígenas*. An article in the national newspaper *Ultimas Noticias* stated that crabs were not only "an exquisite dish" but "an aphrodisiac," evoking another image, one of eroticism.[5] Most accounts, however, attributed a religious significance to the crab. An article in *Notidiario* quoted an assertion by "the Warao physician," Vicente Medina, that the gathering of crabs by sons-in-law was the force that lent a "closely unified" character to *indígena* social relations. The collective consumption of crabs and cakes made from moriche palm starch provided not only "camaraderie" but also a crucial context for "the oral transmission of ancient knowledge that constitutes the soul of this seafaring race."[6] Lamenting that this "sacred food" had become the bearer of cholera, Medina suggested that authorities could use the epidemic to "reestablish the confidence of the Warao" by enabling them "to avoid the bad spirits." Medina was the perfect ventriloquist: his account of the origin of cholera was given cultural authenticity as well as scientific authority because he could speak for and about "Warao culture" as an *indígena* at the same time that he could speak in the voice of the physician.

A subsequent article in *Notidiario* illustrated the "traditional" importance of crabs, along with other shellfish and fish, in the diet of the *étnia Warao* by narrating a journey undertaken by "various Warao families" to catch crabs, followed by their consumption in "the annual celebration of the magical liturgical festival known as '*nowara*' in which they celebrate a collective banquet with crabs and *yuruma*, a starch that is extracted from the moriche palm." The article added, "Unfortunately, the crabs had been infected with the *Vibrio cholerae*." The article then moved to the terror that ensued from the death of "one of the principal *wisidatus* of the group, . . . causing panic in the autochthonous collectivity."[7] The source of the epidemic had been pinpointed only two weeks after it started, and it had been presented via the press in the form of a single, easily comprehensible narrative. Epidemiologists generally are hesitant to designate a single, definitive point of origin and means of transmission for epidemics. Epidemiologists are still unsure how the Peruvian epidemic began, and it has been much more thoroughly investigated than the situation in Delta Amacuro.[8] Benavides, Medina, and Rodríguez, on the other hand, apparently drew a definitive epidemiological conclusion.

This narrative constituted a sort of ventriloquism. Nurses and physicians asked patients what they had eaten prior to experiencing cholera symptoms, and crabs appeared on the list. The information that patients offer in clinical encounters is often repeated in a series of subsequent contexts, each with a different setting, audience, and set of rhetorical requirements, which allows medical professionals to control how this information will be used and how it will shape broader perceptions.[9] As information that emerged from initial clinical encounters in the delta was translated by bilingual nurses, relayed to physicians, reported by radio to authorities in Tucupita, used in constructing official stories, and given to the press, crabs were promoted from the status of one item in a list of foods consumed to that of the causal factor in an epidemiological narrative. At the same time, crabs—consumed by nearly everyone in the delta—were racialized and culturalized. They were construed as a facet of the culture of a particular group. Crabs provided a rhetorical glue to join an epidemiological narrative to an anthropological story.

This story was, however, a powerful cultural invention. Although the *noara* is often celebrated by eating crabs in the southeast delta, the feast is virtually unknown in the northwest.[10] I inquired in many communities in the Pedernales area, and in no case did people recall ever having celebrated the *noara* or having eaten crabs as part of a ritual event. Public health authorities and journalists collaborated in taking ethnographic accounts that related to one region, constructing them as the "traditional culture" of another region, and using them to infuse an epidemiological narrative with ethnographic authority. By a cultural logic of synecdoche, one facet of life for some residents of one area of the delta came to stand for activities and ways of thinking that are pervasive and inescapable for an entire racialized population.

Use of the term *noara* helped render the story authentic and authoritative. Officials who make no effort to learn Warao nevertheless generally possess a tiny vocabulary of Warao words and phrases, some of which reflect their particular area of expertise. Slipping one of these into a conversation, report, or statement to the press created the illusion that the official understood how *indígenas* think and feel, speak and act. The use of the word *noara*, which entered this group of catchwords when the article was published, created the impression that the story was based on direct experience of the events in question. Ready acceptance of the story was also fostered by its resonance with other common images of *indígenas*. One widespread image attributed to *indígenas* is a near-pathological tendency to participate in elaborate and even extravagant rituals in which they dance gaily (and perhaps licentiously) even in times of imminent danger. This image invoked the stereotype of *indígenas* as being like animals, unable to develop a sober assessment of their situation.

The crab story was a local transformation of a dominant narrative, which had circulated globally for a year and a half, that blamed ceviche for the Peruvian outbreak. Public health authorities in Delta Amacuro repeated this story, changing details to reflect anthropological narratives of "Warao culture." When "eating blue crabs, . . . one of the most important phases of their ancestral culture[,]" was identified as the source of cholera in the delta, a powerful cultural invention became a credible story that seemed to explain everything.[11]

The crab rhetoric offered a number of benefits to public health institutions. It located cholera far from Tucupita in geographic and cultural terms, thereby mustering the well-established racializing time-space rhetoric to the task of making cholera seem remote for readers in Tucupita. Moreover, it portrayed the epidemic as the unfortunate result of chance: a bacteria had happened to infect a humble creature that lay at the center of a culture. Only elements of the natural and cultural environment of the lower delta figured in this drama—any possible role for government agencies or corporations was conveniently erased. Press releases linked anthropological and medical knowledge, drawing on the lexicons of both. This juxtaposition of scientific authority and cultural authenticity was linked particularly closely in comments offered by Medina. Benavides and Rodríguez became the primary definers of the cholera epidemic. By quoting *indígenas,* either by repeating statements made to these officials or by interviewing cholera refugees in Tucupita, reporters were able to create the impression that they possessed dramatic, first-hand information—without venturing into the delta. The inclusion of photographs of impoverished and diseased *indígena* bodies gave these statements greater authenticity—the persons depicted in the photos seemed to be speaking directly to the reader. Such narrative strategies made these constructions seem like direct reflections of the social world.[12] They imbued quickly concocted stories with the metaphysics of presence and powerful traces of the real.

This initial formulation had, nevertheless, two fatal flaws. First, the claim that crabs were the source of the disease was quickly discredited by the very success of the anti-crab propaganda. The Regional Health Service prohibited the consumption of shellfish and the Guardia Nacional confiscated crabs and fish. A *Notidiario* article quoted *"cacique"* Juan Zambrano as saying that even though they had stopped eating hairy crabs, new cases of cholera were reported.[13] Crabs ordinarily are boiled in the delta, and, since cholera dies quickly at high temperatures, immersion in boiling water removes the danger of infection. Even if some patients did ingest vibrios by eating crabs, this epidemiological story—crabs-equal-cholera—was too simple.

Second, many *indígenas* refuted the validity of the crab stories. Salomón Medina recalled his conversation with the doctor in Nabasanuka.

Salomón Medina, Tucupita, 12 November 1992

We asked ourselves, "How could this have happened?" The *criollos* tell us that "the water is infecting you." The *criollos* say that "the fish are killing you; your food, crabs, is killing you; crabs are angry at you, are hurting you, have killed you; when you eat crabs they kill you."

But we don't believe that. We have eaten them for generations. Ever since I was a small child, ever since as small children we became conscious, we have eaten nothing but crabs. And we didn't die! How could we die from crabs? Crabs won't kill you! Crabs are our food, fish is our food. When we got hungry, we ate them. We ate fish, we cooked them and ate them, and we didn't get sick. Over there [pointing toward Tucupita] they say, "You ate bad fish, those fish that you ate were bad." "No," we responded to them, "no, fish don't cause death." I eat fish. We Warao take our food from the land. We eat palm hearts. And we have eaten them since before there were *criollos*, before we had heard of *criollos*. . . .

That's what I said. The doctor responded, "Is that true?" "It's true." And [the doctor] truly learned from this, he really learned. "Well, then, we can't deny this, it's true."

This passage provides a classic example of reported speech, the invocation of a world brought to life by recounting words spoken within it. Narrators can embed an interpretation of a reported event simply by repeating what was said.[14] Medina portrays two opposed perspectives, those of *criollo* physician and *indígena* patients. He points out that it seems illogical that foods would suddenly become dangerous without any evident reason, but he also places crabs, swamp fish, palm hearts, and grubs at the heart of "Warao" identity and its projected continuity. Although some Mariusans do continue to spend most of the year in the moriche groves and to eat foods derived from the forest, by 1992 many Mariusans spent more time living near the mouth of the Mariusa, where they consumed foods prepared from commercially produced wheat flour, corn flour, rice, and sugar, as well as eating fish and crabs. Simplification and idealization, the erasure of history and heterogeneity, play no less of a role in Medina's than in official accounts, even if the connections he draws between food and identity are more positive than those provided by physicians or the Mariusans' relatives in La Tortuga.

Medina's account differs from official versions in form as well as content. Although his narrative initially places the protagonists in distinct *criollo* and "Warao" camps, the relationship he projects between them is less an insurmountable cultural void than a movement from opposition to synthesis, dialogue, and at least a partial sharing of perspectives. Rather than imagining two homogeneous voices that arose independently of each other, Medina projects a heteroglossia—a complex set of relations between multiple voices that mutually influence one another.[15] It is clear that Medina and others were listening carefully to how physicians explained the epidemic even in the course of constructing alternative accounts, and he gave the doctor credit for the same receptivity.

The crabs-equal-cholera discourse ultimately failed to contain the epidemic in political terms. Some of the very institutional officials who were charged with enforcing it began to deny it. Blanca Cárdenas, then the director of ORAI, loves crabs. She reported, "[*Indígena* residents] would see us there in the [ORAI] pilot center in Arawabisi, right, staying there with them and eating crabs right in front of them."[16] By eating crabs she challenged both key aspects of the epidemiological narrative: the assertion that crabs transmitted cholera, and their racialization as a synecdoche for "Warao culture." Resistance to the initial broadside by public health authorities crossed a supposedly clear-cut racial divide, threatening to reveal that the cultural logic they had employed did not provide a foolproof means of explaining the epidemic or a perfect deus ex machina that could shield state institutions from political scrutiny.

EXPANDING THE CRAB STORY:
FILTH, FOOD, AND SHAMANS

Public health officials realized that they needed a broader, more inclusive, and more complex narrative to successfully juxtapose culture and germs. One strategy maintained the focus on food but widened its scope. Rafael Orihuela, minister of health, laid the groundwork for this expansion by announcing that the high rates of cholera infection were due to "eating habits in the Delta Amacuro."[17] Luís Echezuría, the national epidemiologist, went much further: "The cholera outbreak in Delta Amacuro is the most serious one to emerge in the country by virtue of its sociocultural characteristics, due to the comportment of the *étnia Warao*, who have a nomadic behavior similar to the Yucpa of Zulia state, and who are also characterized by food customs that are difficult to change, such as the ingestion of raw fish and meat."[18] Note the shift here from crabs to "food customs," including methods of preparation, which painted a much more generalized picture of *indígena* culture.

Echezuría's remarks—delivered by one of the most powerful public health officials in the country during a brief visit to the region—did not reflect detailed empirical knowledge of food production, preparation, and consumption. Eating raw meat was deemed to be repulsive in every delta community that I (Charles Briggs) visited. I heard assertions that crabs, particularly the first few harvested at the beginning of the crab season, are sometimes eaten raw, but I have never witnessed anyone eating raw seafood in the delta.

The culturalization of cholera extended beyond "the Warao." Echezuría, quoted in an article in the Caracas newspaper *El Globo,* laid the blame on *indígenas* as a group: "'The *indígenas* have been shown to be the most vulnerable inhabitants of our country to the disease, having been relegated to adverse sanitary conditions in a contaminated natural environment. Moreover,' asserted Echezuría, 'their customs make the work of prevention difficult.'" Echezuría also racialized cholera in Zulia and Delta Amacuro in parallel fashion: "'The situation in Delta Amacuro is similar to what has happened in Zulia, where 80 percent of the cholera cases took place among the Wayú and Parupeno [*sic*] *étnias*. In the delta, 95 percent of the cases are among Warao.'"[19] Daniel Rodríguez accounted for high morbidity and mortality in the delta in similar terms.

Daniel Rodríguez, Tucupita, 14 January 1994

> The Indian is accustomed to living in conditions of very bad environmental hygiene; that's why [there was so much cholera]. We know the situation of these people: they eat on the floor, and they defecate—or, let's say, they don't have a system of defecating discreetly. They do it in the open air. The flies, which land on food, land first on the feces and then on the food and then on the bottle, the pacifier of the child, and then they give it [the child] the bottle.

This statement covers a broad set of material and bodily practices, thereby creating a globalized image of *indígena* domestic space.

Magdalena Benavides also used a common formula of disease transmission, the fecal-oral cycle, in creating a powerful image of hygienic ignorance and resistance.

Magdalena Benavides, Maturín, 31 March 1995

> In the city, well, there are sewage facilities, toilets, etc. But in the delta—they bathe, they go poo-poo, and everything [in the same place]. In the same spot that they contaminate the water, they contaminate the fish, and

this establishes a vicious cycle. And they don't have this habit of washing their hands. They don't want—they don't use toilet paper, nor do they protect their hands, well, [when defecating]. No, no, yes, no—perhaps they don't even—I don't know. I don't even know how they wipe themselves. So there is nothing like, "Look, your fingernails are dirty. Wash them!" No, nothing like that. So then this contamination—anus, hand, mouth— is constant among them. It would be unlikely that an *indígena* would wash his or her hands. First, it's that they eat on the floor.

Using scatological details, Benavides builds an image of people who are not only disgusting but willfully so—they just don't care. The lack of funds to purchase soap or toilet paper and the failure of institutions to provide potable water or to conduct extensive health education programs are washed away by this river of negative images. Journalists reproduced these representations by including photographs of refugees cooking and eating on the ground around open-air fires in articles on cholera (see photograph 21, page 107).

Food preparation and consumption became a key area of surveillance by public health officials. María Vargas (see chapter 6) kept her eye on the *indígenas* living in Barrancas. "I personally went at six in the morning, at twelve o'clock in the day, and at six in the evening to see what they were eating and how they were eating and how they prepared it," she stated. "At that time, I took on the role, I acted as if they were my children. I would scold them and I would make a scene."[20] The precise timing of her visits provides a sense of verisimilitude and makes her observations seem detailed and systematic. This important feature of her narrative is a middle-class projection: members of these households generally prepared two meals a day, mid-morning and mid-afternoon, when sufficient food was available. As Vargas's empirical failing reveals, totalizing images were based less on careful observation than on stereotypes of *indígenas* that circulated widely.

The broader culinary narrative was not only racialized but also gendered, since women did most of the food preparation. Thus the blame for the cholera epidemic was placed especially on *indígena* women. Gender specificity also embraced human reproduction and child survival. Benavides attempted to link not only morbidity and mortality during the epidemic but also infant mortality and poor health conditions in the delta in general to the way that *indígena* mothers view life and death.

Magdalena Benavides, Maturín, 31 March 1995

The Indians—they're people who accept death as a normal, natural event in their lives. And when an Indian dies, it's not anything transcendental. An Indian dies and nothing happens. Or, let's say, there isn't, there isn't this, uh, attachment to life, or anything like that. Or, let's say, this affection for life. Among them, "It's all the same. A child dies and I have another tomorrow and it dies." Okay, maybe it's because it's always been like that—they have their children and they die. Or, let's say, for them death is like, a child is born and it dies. It's all the same. So then this—well, they will think that when a disease comes along that decimates them, it's because one of those evil spirits is getting even with them. They say, "Darn, this spirit is—." Well, okay, in their case we have to teach them to take care of their lives, because they don't love their lives. And I imagine that that must be why they live their lives like that, as if today were their last day.

In the hundreds of interviews that I have conducted during my career, I have never felt such a strong urge to jump to my feet, shout at my interlocutor, burst into tears, and run from the room. I could not believe that she had made this statement, and into a tape recorder at that. But in 2000 a new director of the Regional Health Service provided me with a nearly identical statement. The problem is structural, not individual. Statements such as this one clearly signal the depth of the colonial relationship and the degree to which people internalize racist stereotypes. It recalls the famous quotation from General William C. Westmoreland regarding his Vietnamese adversaries: "Well, the Oriental doesn't put the same high price on life as does the Western. Life is plentiful. Life is cheap in the Orient. And, as the philosophy of the Orient expresses it, life is not important."[21] The promotion of such an image is a tool often used to legitimate state policies that render subaltern lives expendable.

The portraits of "indigenous culture" that replaced the crab story did not focus on food and excretion alone. Recall that Echezuría included "nomadic behavior" as part of the "sociocultural characteristics" that made the epidemic in the delta the most serious in the country. Rodríguez and Benavides juxtaposed crab and nomad tropes to argue that *indígenas* were infected by eating crabs and that they spread the disease through their "migration." After suggesting that *indígenas* underutilized health services because of their greater faith in "shamans," Rodríguez placed this "nomadic" character at the heart of "Warao customs."

Daniel Rodríguez, Tucupita, 14 January 1994

It's also very difficult—even when they want to find us—because their very customs lead them to live in very dispersed, isolated places. They're very dispersed. And they're nomads, too, because they continue moving in keeping with where they find food. And if the fishing is better in a certain place, they look for that place and they leave and settle there. And if that place stops producing, [if] it doesn't have what they're after, they leave—they move to another place. And they keep cutting *[manaca]* palms. They go—if they are planting gardens here, they settle for a little while here, and then they move to another place where they can undertake their activities.

The poetic parallelism in Rodríguez's account—the repetition of phrases that describe movement—creates a sense of ceaseless and random migrations among locations. It implies a logic that reflects only very short-term calculations based on the availability of natural resources. This picture emerged clearly in an article published in a Caracas newspaper, *Ultimas Noticias:* "Hunger and malnutrition are their worst enemies; nevertheless, they swarm *[pululan]* nomadically about the territory in a perpetual search. They fish and then run here and there."[22] The efforts of people to leave an area where cholera was present and medical services were few are extracted from the circumstances of the epidemic and from history itself. The shiftless, chaotic wanderings that these narratives depict become reflections of pervasive, timeless cultural patterns and a life whose terms are dictated by nature.

Here we see a new dimension of the time-space dislocation process. *Indígenas* are displaced from the modern temporal-spatial juncture that is inhabited by public health officials and journalists into a distanced, premodern realm that responds not to historical time but to the seasonal fluctuations of nature. Space is further racialized by imagining modern, *criollo* subjects as occupying fixed points on the mainland and *indígenas* as lacking any stable relationship to space. Rodríguez's reference to fish and *manaca* palms inadvertently draws our attention to the role of capital in shaping this "nomadism." The temporary camps that were established near sites where fish were abundant were generally oriented toward commercial production—the fish were sold in Tucupita or Barrancas—and the *indígena* workers were often in the employ of *criollos*. The factories that processed *manaca* palms paid such a low wage that workers had to travel ever greater distances in order to harvest enough trees—a hundred or more a day—to earn a living wage. Moreover, the state requires *indígenas* to travel frequently to Tucupita in order to obtain bureaucratic documents, paychecks, official permission, and the like, a fact that Rodríguez does not note. A magical sleight of hand rendered the role of the state invisible by converting it into cultural difference.

A "study" conducted by Rodríguez, Benavides, and a colleague, which was concluded some ten days into the epidemic, cited these population movements not only as the primary means by which cholera was spreading through the delta but also as a central facet of Warao culture. The people, said the report, "were trying to escape from the JEBU (spirit) that is causing the disease among the Warao."[23] During her interview, Benavides specified the motive for this nomadism as an irrational fear of death.

Magdalena Benavides, Maturín, 31 March 1995

The most serious problem [during the outbreak] was the problem of the movement of the *indígenas*—that is, those *indígenas* went all over the place. When some *indígenas* died over here, they lost themselves somewhere else, in the areas that had not been infected, and they infected them, the ones who came from here. Or let's say that this movement was what screwed us up, because cases of cholera started to come up all over the place. That was the problem. . . .

You can forget about those communities [if there should be another epidemic]. They're not going to respond because they don't know how to help [cholera patients], they don't know. They forgot about that, they forgot. First, it's that the *indígenas*—they're here in a village and someone dies here and they bury him there and they get lost. They go away from there. Or let's say that memory, they don't have it anymore. At least they aren't seeing that "over there—here, someone died of cholera here." No, they go away from there as if to forget everything, since the spirit is over there. So it's not like us. When my son dies, "Golly, here's my child's picture and my child's car, his toy. I remember him every little while. And, dear God, don't let that other child who I have die, because if this should happen, I don't know how I would face it." No, the *indígenas* don't have that way of thinking.

In the passage quoted earlier Benavides argues that *indígenas* do not love life, that it has no value for "them." Here we see the flip side: the assertion that *indígenas* have such a cultural aversion to death that people flee the place where the death occurred and attempt to erase memory, to wipe the dead from their minds. This feature becomes another means of making a binary contrast between *indígena* and *criollo* cultures. In racializing the production of cultural memory, Benavides excludes *indígenas* from the debates regarding the events that deeply affected their communities by asserting that they are culturally incapable of representing death. The statement repudiates the ethnographic literature, which stresses the centrality of reverence for the dead in delta communities and the wealth of rituals in which memories of *kaidamotuma* (our ancestors) are elaborately enacted.[24]

Benavides's statement also contradicts her interpretation of "Warao" mothers, who seem to care *too little* about the death of their infants. It seems as if Benavides never spent enough time in a delta community to be present when a death occurred. If she had, she would have witnessed the women's *sana*,[25] laments that are sung from the moment people die until after the funeral has ended. *Sana* construct memories that are often remembered—and can be sung word for word—years later. Under the guise of presenting detailed knowledge of *indígena* culture, Benavides imagines opposing and racialized patterns of affective response that produce a vision of a fundamental cultural chasm that obstructs the penetration of modernity into the delta. Her pessimistic projection of the possibility of helping to prevent future cholera outbreaks by teaching *indígenas* about biomedical techniques was presented specifically as a comment on the health education program that Clara and I were attempting to establish for the delta.

Public health rhetoric transformed the Mariusans' response to the epidemic into one of the *causes* that fueled it. Benavides suggested that if the epidemic crossed over into Monagas state, "the movement of the indigenous people" would be to blame.[26] Moreover, the study conducted by Benavides and Rodríguez asserted that this "compulsive exodus" was responsible for impeding the effectiveness of public health measures for controlling cholera.[27]

HEBU VERSUS VIBRIO

Officials also attributed the bodily presence of *indígenas* on urban streets, which Benavides and Rodríguez dubbed an *éxodo compulsivo* (compulsive exodus), to a magico-religious understanding of the world that led them to make unthinking, irrational decisions.[28] Belief in *hebu* was cited over and over as constituting the core of "Warao culture," the basis of *indígenas'* fear of cholera, and one of the central obstacles confronted by public health authorities in general. These assertions by public health authorities and reporters were largely based, however, on an erroneous translation. *Hebu* refers both to spirits that can cause an illness and to particular signs and symptoms associated with a disease. In the early months of the epidemic, vernacular healers openly admitted that they did not know the "origin" *(ahotana)* of cholera; use of the term *hebu* during this period was thus largely confined to physical manifestations of the disease. Choosing to translate *hebu* as "spirit" *(espíritu)* rather than "disease" thus constituted an act of mistranslation that lined up with racist representational practices, efforts to characterize *indígenas* as irrational and foreign. The opposition between science and magic that makes modernity seem real had been reinvented yet again.

As the epidemic wore on into October, *El Diario de Monagas* reported that the problem lay in resistance to institutional medicine.[29] The "shaman" *(piache),* a key symbol of *indígena* culture in the national imagination, served as the principal embodiment of superstition and anti-modernity. Benavides argued, "It was difficult at any given moment to manage the situation . . . because the *indígenas* don't go rapidly to get help when someone is sick. No, they first get treated by their shamans and their ways of curing, and only when they see that the shaman stuff is not working do they go [to the clinic], and by that time nothing can be done."[30]

These narratives turned cholera into a battle between the doctor and the *piache.* Some argued that the ultimate effects of the epidemic might be *positive.* Inadvertently recapitulating the battles between physicians and other practitioners that took place during nineteenth-century epidemics,[31] Cristóbal Bayeh suggested that the terror, the inability of noninstitutional healers to cure patients, the death of numerous healers, and the success of institutional practitioners produced a major step forward in the process of assimilation: "Because their shamans couldn't help anymore—even their shamans died. So, then, in whom should they believe in that moment? They have to believe in the *criollo,* in the physician; this attitude was precisely what led them to have faith that the physician, the government would help them."[32] In this way, cholera stories could have happy endings.

The delta, like the rest of the world, is the home of multiple healing practices. Benavides was a physician and a public health official in the early 1990s, but she was also widely believed to be an active participant in popular vernacular healing practices that evoke the spirit of María Lionza, a mythological *indígena* who is revered as a goddess of the natural world. In centers, or "courts," throughout Venezuela, adepts enter spaces that they believe are filled with the spirits of people who lived in colonial and post-colonial epochs, including *caciques,* physicians, and leaders such as Simón Bolívar. Surrounded by statues, offerings, perfumes, candles, flowers, and incense, adepts become possessed by these spirits—they assume their voices and make dramatic gestures. Followers believe that possession gives them power and the ability to heal the sick.[33] Benavides is said to be a leading practitioner of the Tucupita "court." When she was the director of the Regional Health Service, Father Pablo Romero was called to perform an exorcism to drive evil spirits from the office at Tucupita, whose entrance was graced by a statue of the Virgin of the Valley (photograph 34). Benavides's purported support of such pluralistic healing practices did not preclude *her* from understanding the role of viruses, bacteria, funguses, or other biomedical pathogens or believing in the efficacy of institutional medicine.

How could Benavides combine these forms of therapy without getting branded as intrinsically and irredeemably premodern when racialized sub-

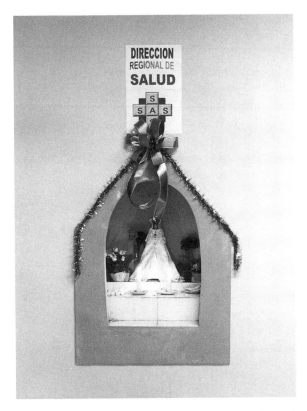

Photograph 34. Shrine to the Virgin of the Valley, located in the vestibule of the headquarters of the Regional Health Service, MSAS, Tucupita. Photograph by Charles L. Briggs.

jects could not? As globalization has led to the growing autonomy of cultural, financial, ethnic, religious, and media domains, social life has become increasingly fragmented.[34] Professionals can occupy complementary roles: a lawyer can also be a churchgoer, sports enthusiast, amateur musician, and so forth.[35] The professional and complementary roles are so compartmentalized, and the complementary roles so privatized, that even obvious contradictions between the two influence neither. In fact, we might see the degree of divergence between the various professional and complementary roles that an individual assumes as functional, creating flexible subjects who can quickly and readily adapt to the shifting demands of the global market.[36] Contradictions thus can be deemed productive for persons granted the status of modern subjects.

Benavides did not seem to be vulnerable to charges of being premodern, irrational, superstitious, or the like. Her complementary roles—political party leader, mariachi singer, and follower of Lionza—were known to virtually all professionals in Tucupita, but they were not seen as contaminating or modifying influences on her professional role. Her purported participation in a religious realm that seemed to contradict her alignment with modernity and science could be construed as a rational response to Venezuela's shifting, often chaotic position in a global world. Indeed, some Venezuelan presidents have been rumored to call upon spirit healers or to participate in the courts of Lionza. Efforts to harness the power of magic constitute a "magic of the state" that is just as apparent in political rituals conducted in Miraflores, the presidential palace, as in Sorte, the magic mountain visited by Lionza.[37]

The situation is very different for racialized subjects, who are defined in opposition to "the national society"—that is, the *criollo* majority. Here the liberty to move among a range of professional and complementary roles was clearly denied. On the one hand, racial gatekeeping mechanisms kept nearly all *indígenas* from entering the professional ranks, except that of teacher in *indígena* communities. An example is provided by Vicente Medina. A graduate of the leading medical school in the country and the recipient of a postdoctoral degree, he held high administrative positions in the regional public health network and served as a deputy congressman. Nevertheless, Ricardo Campins suggested that *indígenas* "will never understand what a virus is, what a bacteria is, what a fungus is. . . . I think that even the *indígena* who is a physician, Dr. [Vicente Medina], even he must not understand it very well." By marking Medina as a racial Other, Campins implies that he could never sufficiently embrace science and modernity to fully gain the status of a professional.

By the same token, racialized subjects are not granted the right to occupy complementary roles, at least in the same way. If an *indígena* went to a nonbiomedical practitioner, she or he was permanently identified with an uncivilized religion and was deemed incapable of entering the modern world. Physicians often warned their patients, "If you go visit that witch, don't ever come back here!" Any dimension of an indigenous life deemed alien to the modern world of the nation-state and global culture can become a sign of that individual's inner essence. An *indígena* could not hold on, however tenuously, to a professional identity were he or she an active participant in the court of María Lionza.

Under globalization, social life is becoming increasingly "deprivatized" as people's lives come under increasing surveillance and regulation by the nation-state and other hegemonic institutions.[38] Several examples point to this phenomenon in the delta. *Indígena* song and dance troupes were often asked to perform aspects of the *nahanamu* for *criollo* audiences, indicating that some of the most private religious activities of the delta had been de-privatized in order to confirm the modernity of the nation-state and its suitability for standing as a liberal, pluralistic, democratic country on a global stage.[39] Missionaries and officials considered the work of indigenous "witches" and "quacks" to be matters for state surveillance and regulation; the regional director of ORAI told me that he planned to standardize the activities of all *indígena* religious practitioners, designating which are appropriate and how they should be performed.[40] Some officials celebrated the demise of the many indigenous practitioners who died during the epidemic and the loss of faith in their curative powers. Finally, Benavides revealed how powerfully social roles had been racialized in the delta when she dismissed *indígena* adults as potential recipients of health care because they combined vernacular and institutional forms of healing.

A META-GEOGRAPHY OF BLAME

Public health officials often cited another factor, the geography of the fluvial region, in their explanations of the epidemic. "The fact that the geography of EDA [Delta Amacuro State] is fragmented *[accidentada]*" limited the very possibility of "governmentality"—the degree to which officials could maintain surveillance and regulate the movement and practices of delta residents.[41] The geographical conditions that formed the basis of this spatial imagining were the region's low population density, the distance between communities, the inaccessible location of some people in the forest, and the fluvial character of the delta itself.[42] By projecting a model of terra firma and a system of roadways as the spatial norm, the geography of the delta was rendered incomprehensible, inaccessible, and foreign.

Spatial divisions for government employees were constructed in terms of administrative boundaries and centers. The seemingly insurmountable distances between health providers were produced, in part, by the failure of these officials to construct an adequate network of clinics in an area of some 40,000 square kilometers. This institutional cartography was naturalized—considered part of the land itself—and this in turn erased the social processes that created it. This image is quite similar to the familiar colonial representation of a "tropical environment" as a natural space that is primitive, alien, and threatening. Assertions that the density of rainfall, seasonal fluctuations, and variations in the depth of the Orinoco made the delta a natural home for cholera characterized the environment as directly propagating disease and inserted a colonial discourse into the arguments of modern officials. Journalists who never left the mainland incorporated this spatial conception into their cholera narratives.

The jump from space to culture was short, as Rodríguez suggests.

Daniel Rodríguez, Tucupita, 14 January 1994

> There are some ["Warao"] for whom it is not so easy to get to a physician, or to reach a nurse, because they live—they don't have an outboard motor, they have to go by paddle. Let's say they have to cross great distances. And in these moments—let's say that there is a whole series of factors that have an influence here: first, they have their healers *[curanderos]*, and then when they [the patients] want to get to a place where they can provide them with medical assistance, they're very far away. So, when they arrive, they arrive in very bad condition, they just can't—. When they are placed in the physician's hands, since it was hard for them to arrive, the physician can't do anything for them [in other words, the patient is too close to death for treatment to be effective].

Here distance is calculated both institutionally and in terms of technology. Locations connected by motorboats seem closer than those linked by paddle-propelled canoes. Rodríguez interweaves the healer trope, creating another length of the familiar rhetorical fabric of "It's not our fault!"

Campins's explanation of why cholera led to such high morbidity in the delta suggested how culture became spatialized and how space became culturalized.

Ricardo Campins, 13 November 1994

> There are many factors that I think are responsible for maintaining—and will keep on maintaining—cholera. Because I imagine—it's been a while since I've been in the delta—but I imagine that they must still be seeing cholera in the delta, even if the health authorities say they aren't. It's that they [the "Warao"] defecate in the river, they eat raw fish, they eat seafood, [they eat] these squid raw. All the fruits of the sea, especially in the outer part of the delta, they eat raw. They defecate in the river, or let's say that they don't have any kind of minimum sanitary norms, right? And evidently due to the geography of the delta, to the way in which it is formed *[está concebido]*, is such as to maintain that disease for years, centuries, you see, because of those same conditions, as much mental as natural. Well, first the mental or psychological ones of the *indígenas*, right, and then the part that has to do with the geography of the delta— these two things become conjoined and they make a spiral. And that is a spiral that will maintain it, right, that will maintain it for a long time.

Beyond the false assumptions regarding the consumption of seafood, this statement reveals how spatial imaginings go beyond the visible features of an area. Here the geography of the delta is conceived as much as a "mental" as a physical phenomenon, one that lies in the interior, at the very essence of things. Cultural practices and space are assimilated to a single "mental" or "psychological" condition that is then converted into a causal factor that produces and sustains the epidemic.

As was true for Conrad's Marlow, the primitivity of the country and of the culture achieves a psychological unity that invades the interior space of all who enter it. As humans fuse with nature, they lose their drive and capacity to control it, a desire that has served as one of the cornerstones of modernity since the seventeenth century.[43] As Sergeant Gilberto Salas, who commanded the Guardia Nacional contingent in Pedernales at the time of the epidemic, put it, "The *indígena* who lives wild *[silvestremente]* on the rivers, the doctor doesn't reach him in time, the teacher doesn't come in time, so he is a man who is living wildly there. He lives in accordance with the natural environment that surrounds him."[44] This fusion of space and culture is projected into the future. The geography prevents teachers and doctors from arriving "in time," and the culture never changes. But the extraction of *indígenas* from history and modernity is a product of the material and discursive strategies of the very institutional actors who are telling the story.[45] For Benavides and Rodríguez, the authority of these spatial and temporal imaginings is enhanced by the scientific language of epidemiology, which takes space, time, population, and microbes as conceptual and empirical foundations. This racialized chronotope, or fusion of notions of space and time, provides a key mode for juxtaposing anthropological, epidemiological, and institutional discourses.[46]

These journeys along the rivers that lead into colonial interiors always end at the same point—Mariusa—which serves as a limiting case of remoteness, primitivism, and cultural conservatism. The desire to dis-locate the "origin" of the epidemic in time and space enabled public health authorities to place Mariusans under guard in Barrancas and to forcibly relocate them to Tortuga. Since one spatializing and racializing logic suggests that *indígena* bodies and minds directly reflect their environment, cholera has become a permanent, invisible, constitutive feature of Mariusan bodies, shaping the way they are perceived and treated to this day. When an outbreak of diarrheal disease was reported in Mariusa in January 1997, the director of the Regional Health Service hoped to dissipate fears of a new epidemic. He told *Notidiario*, "We cannot deny that there was an outbreak of diarrhea in the above-mentioned *indígena* community which alarmed us, given that it happened in the same place that in 1992 cholera made its presence known in Delta Amacuro."[47] Recall that in 1992 public health officials placed the point of origin of the cholera epidemic in Pedernales. The degree to which Mariusans came to embody the quintessence of "Warao culture" and the source of contamination led to a constant rewriting of these narratives.

The comments by Tortugans regarding Mariusans suggest that this colonial language of space, culture, and time had become incorporated into the way people classified as *indígenas* construct one another. Throughout the delta, "the Mariusans" were branded as the human manifestation of cholera's imagined ability to spring up at any point and spread across space. Two of the most prominent *indígena* activists, Graciela Ortega and Feliciano Gómez, identified Mariusa as the origin of the epidemic. Schoolteacher Catalino Pérez of Koboina specified the source of this information: "When the doctor arrived, he told the people about this disease. He himself said that it was from Mariusa. . . . The Mariusans came from over there because they were hungry. The first person got sick there, another got sick, and from there it went to Guayo when they came from Mariusa to the hospital."[48] This epidemiological construction proved to be as infectious as the disease itself.

Points of resistance were apparent. The narrative told to us by Medina in 1994 provides a fascinating counterpoint to the meta-geography of blame. He asserted that when *indígenas* contract a life-threatening illness "they go immediately or try to reach [a clinic]. But, well, there are two things that make them stay away. One is their geographical location, and the other is the mental conception they have."[49] This statement, taken out of context, would seem to place him squarely in the spatial-cultural-causal camp of Campins. But there is an ironic shift in the referent of the third person plural pronoun here, which problematizes "geographical location" and "mental conception." The construction suggests that the public health authorities had placed clinics too far from the areas they needed to serve. The problem comes back to ignorance, but it is official ignorance. Medina implies that health authorities did not know the delta and that they did not take its geographic characteristics into account.

WHERE CULTURE MEETS BIOLOGY

Cultural reasoning emerged toward the end of the nineteenth century as a reaction to evolutionary theory, particularly in opposition to the attempt to explain differences among racial and ethnic groups in physiological terms.[50] This cultural logic adopts a liberal and egalitarian tone, and it seems to project an anti-racist sensibility. It assumes that cultures are equally systematic and complex and that they provide their "bearers" with totally distinct views of the world and ways of behaving. The adherents of cultural evolution claimed that societies could be placed along a continuum from savagery to civilization according to their linguistic, cultural, and technological progress; physiological differences, particularly the size of people's brains, could explain why some populations were more "advanced." Franz Boas and his students argued instead that the differences between societies should be explained by examining each culture on its own terms.[51]

Cultural reasoning was deftly appropriated as a new means of legitimizing racism as biological arguments became less useful: social groups could be separated based on imagined cultural patterns. The differences between the resulting "cultures" were used to justify social inequality and the effects—racism and social conflict—believed to be inevitable when different social groups meet. Etienne Balibar has suggested that biological and cultural explanations of difference operate in what linguists refer to as "complementary distribution"—that they never appear in the same context.[52] A closer look at official explanations of the epidemic suggests, however, that biological reasoning and cultural reasoning can coexist.

Direct references to biological differences between *criollos* and *indígenas* would have contradicted the cultural account of cholera's origin and diminished its effect. Health professionals circumvented this by drawing on the languages of immunology and nutrition. Rodríguez suggested that without medical attention cholera patients "die in less than twenty-four hours—or even less." Then he added, "Well, and given the nutritional status of the *indígenas*, they go even more quickly, of course."[53] Benavides placed nutritional and immunological deficiencies at the heart of the delta's health problems in general, stating that the "common denominator in the entire indigenous area is the problem of diarrhea, diarrhea in times of cholera or when there is no cholera." She continued, "There is a high rate of infant mortality from diarrhea, first, because they are people with very bad nutrition, people with a very, very bad immunological mechanism precisely because of that nutritional deficiency. So they defend themselves very badly from diseases; well, in the face of a problem with diarrhea, after having three or four bowel movements they are already dehydrated."[54]

Given the scientific authority of the discourse and its authors, this formulation circulated widely. The press picked up the story quickly. *Notidiario* stated that *indígenas* "are quite susceptible to any illness, to the extent that even a flu can kill them."[55] Another article suggested that cholera "attacked precisely the poorest sector of the population, the *indígenas*, who are affected seasonally by water-borne diseases, tuberculosis, respiratory diseases, and acute malnutrition, which makes them vulnerable to any contagion, pro-

ducing a high level of mortality."[56] These statements medicalized the political economy of hunger, reducing it to a physiological mechanism, just as
they presented morbidity and morality from all infectious diseases as a question of immunology. Any consideration of inadequacies within the health
care system was erased. The statements pointed to the dearth of detailed information on cholera at the disposal of physicians and public health officials
and revealed their tendency to lump together a wide range of diarrheal diseases. Although susceptibility to dysenteric and other enteric diseases is correlated with malnutrition, leading experts have suggested that this is not
true of cholera.[57] When a racial logic seems to explain everything, gaining
access to up-to-date medical research seems to be unnecessary.

At first glance, tying cholera and other diseases to malnutrition and the
immune system would seem to weaken the force of the cultural argument.
It did, however, help extend culpability from public health to other government institutions; MSAS, after all, could not be blamed for economic conditions. By tying malnutrition to deficient immune systems and the latter
to *indígena* bodies, officials linked the epidemic to biological differences between races.[58] Since "bad nutrition" is related to securing, preparing, and
consuming food, these biological features seemed to be caused by individual and collective choices, a neoliberal explanation par excellence. The adoption of cultural reasoning may subordinate biological rhetorics and place important limits on the ways they can be invoked in the public sphere, but it
does not rule them out. There is hardly a one-way, irreversible historical
passage from biological to cultural reasoning. Balibar's formulation is thus
a bit too simple.[59]

The centuries-old stereotype of *indígenas* as being more susceptible to
disease than Europeans also appeared, supporting a discourse of extinction.
Cárdenas initially believed that the epidemic would lead to the extinction
of the *indígenas*: "I thought that [cholera] was going to finish them off. Really, well, I said, 'If it keeps up like this, the Warao are going to be finished
off.'" Later in the interview she stated, "They laugh at me, because I tell
them: 'I think that the Warao are going to disappear.' . . . I think sometimes
that within a period of five years some will disappear and others will dis-
perse." According to some *criollo* professionals, *indígenas* could not successfully adapt to the modern world, thus their lives were irremediably miserable. Death could therefore be construed as a welcome release. A common
response to reports of high mortality from cholera was, "*Pobrecitos, ya des-
cansaron*" (Poor little things, at least they're out of their misery now). This
rationalization released *criollos,* especially institutional officials, from any
responsibility for these deaths. This attitude was revealed in jokes and off-

hand remarks. Recall the comment by Tomasa Gabaldón, the chief of the nursing office: "Well, I think that the best thing that could happen to them is that they could all die off!"

Such statements, made in voices ranging from lamentation to gruesome irony, were uttered off the record by, and for, individuals who shared a common racial identity and, in general, worked for the same institution. In fact, it is impossible to grasp the full complexity of the relationship between biological and cultural reasoning without considering how private commentary seeps into the public arena.[60] When Venezuelan officials publicly alluded to deficient immune systems and the greater susceptibility of *indígenas* to disease and death, they were operating within a framework that had been partly shaped by behind-closed-doors comments. These comments were made in much more overtly biological and racist terms than were public statements. Clara's account of such conversations in MSAS offices during the early days of the outbreak provides a case in point. The dynamic and complementary relationship between biological and cultural reasoning was more apparent in private discourse. Jokes and off-hand remarks made in casual conversations and in meetings between officials in a broad range of institutions during the epidemic characterized the outbreak as proving the biological preeminence of *criollos*. Much like the exchange of sexist jokes among men, these private exchanges enhanced social bonds between officials and confirmed their social superiority. Individuals who found such remarks shocking repeated them in other contexts, expressing their sense of outrage. As a result, these words were in general circulation alongside other representations of the epidemic. These private remarks created powerful connections between biological and cultural explanations that were carried over into the public sphere. Such hybridity should not surprise us. Notions of creolization, *mestizaje*, and Indianness brought cultural and biological constructions of difference in twentieth-century Latin America together in complex and shifting ways.[61]

Science studies specialist Bruno Latour has commented on the miraculous power that the concept of the microbe has to enable practitioners to connect the most heterogeneous sets of phenomena.[62] By joining microbiological definitions of the epidemic to cultural reasoning, officials could juxtapose imaginings of food, fiestas, dirty habits, nomadism, spirits, and shamans in such a way that they not only seemed to go together seamlessly but also explained why so many people were getting infected and dying. Official narratives construed *indígena* culture as *sui generis*—existing apart from political economy, history, modernity, and the cultural norms of "the national society." Cultural reasoning was cast as a form of scientific knowledge produced by anthropological study of "the Warao." Curiapo physician Manuel Mato suggested that his statements were based not only on his work as a physician with *indígena* patients but also on extensive conversations with Caracas anthropologist Leonora Vásquez, who had worked for decades in the delta and knew Warao well. Rodríguez specified that culture, not class, was the source of the cholera problem: "They are—the question of hygiene, hygienic habits, that they don't have because of their very cultural level—more than anything else, I think that it's because of their cultural level. Because it's not so much the lack of resources, because there are people who have few resources and there are people who have better hygienic habits, and even though they don't have many resources, these people, of course, don't get cholera."

The division between the "two cultures" of Delta Amacuro was represented as an impenetrable barrier for *indígenas*, one that made it impossible for an *indígena* to become a *criollo* or to understand *"criollo* culture." Nevertheless, physicians and public health practitioners seemed to take it for granted that their gaze could comprehend *indígena* culture even when the depth of their experience in the delta was minimal. Physicians would never suggest that *criollos* who lack medical training could accurately characterize biomedical knowledge, yet they felt perfectly capable of comprehending the specialized beliefs and practices utilized by "shamans."

This "millenarian culture" was portrayed as being stubbornly resistant to change, even in the face of new knowledge or life-threatening circumstances. As Rodríguez put it, "They can try to make me change a custom—I, who knows how things are—and they want me to change them, and often I don't want to change them. So how will it be with them, who have patterns with deep roots, more difficult, right?" Here he assumes the voice of a member of the *criollo* population, one of the people whose health-related behaviors physicians want to change. "Know[ing] how things are" refers to awareness of causal connections that are deduced on the basis of at least some grasp of scientific reasoning. "The Warao," who relied on "their beliefs" and who inferred that cholera was caused by "spirits" rather than by bacteria, lacked an epistemology that would enable "them" to produce or even receive new knowledge. Physicians and public health practitioners often cited the problem of language, referring not to their failure to learn Warao but to the seemingly illogical characteristics of the language and the limited command of Spanish evident in many communities. Similarly overlooking the failure of the state to provide adequate schools, these professionals sidestepped blame for ineffective institutional efforts and their failure to improve health conditions by citing low levels of literacy as the cause.

Benavides suggested what would be needed to truly change Warao culture: "It is a very complex problem, the one with the *indígenas;* darn, to get them to put a few ideas into their heads. But you have to begin, and you have to begin with the little children who are in the schools, with these new generations, because the old folks, damn! Like the proverb says, 'An old parrot can't learn to talk.'" Here we see the flip side of the "bad mother" stereotype cited earlier. Benavides racializes *indígenas* differentially according to age: although adults are beyond the pale of modernity, sanitary citizenship, and "the national society," young children are still potentially valuable subjects.

Constructions of age and family dehumanized adult *indígenas.* Recall Vargas's assertion regarding the *indígenas* living in Barrancas: "I acted as if they were my children. I would scold them and I would make a scene." Here she infantilizes her *indígena* patients within a racial patriarchy. The state had such an abiding interest in the welfare of *indígena* children that it could exercise the right to break the hold of Warao culture over the early socialization process, potentially resulting in what has been referred to as ethnocide. Adults could be construed as threats to the survival of their children, giving the state the right to usurp the parental role. This purported obligation of the state to protect the lives of racialized children sometimes led to the criminalization of *indígenas* for infanticide.[63] It is, of course, bitterly ironic that the obligation of the state to protect the lives of *indígena* children did not seem to entail any serious effort to reduce the unconscionable rates of infant mortality.

10 Challenging the Logic of Culture
Resisting Official Explanations for the Epidemic

Official narratives of crabs, *hebu* spirits, unsanitary habits, geographic isolation, immunological deficiency, and extinction were repeated by physicians, visiting epidemiologists, and just about everyone else. These dominant narratives—particularly the crab story—were sometimes turned on their head by activists, opposition politicians, and delta residents. Two obvious differences separated the alternative narratives from those told by government officials. First, thanks to the government's failure to launch a serious health education program, the disease generally arrived before the word *cholera* or any information on what it was or how to prevent and treat it. Second, delta residents immediately linked the disease to broad-based critiques of social inequality, exploitation, and the growing effects of globalization.

Feliciano Gómez of Nabasanuka has long been one of the most consistent and articulate critics of the Venezuelan government. Educated by the Capuchin missionaries, he initially trained for the priesthood. After leaving the seminary, Gómez became a teacher. He wrote several short bilingual readers and a substantive textbook on Warao narrative.[1] His efforts to oppose ecological destruction and labor exploitation by owners of palm hearts factories and to organize delta communities brought him great visibility—and triggered frequent attempts to discredit him. He served as president of the Unión de Comunidades Indígenas Warao (Union of Warao Communities). Gómez was in his mid-forties when we interviewed him in 1995. His face was often lit by passion and his penetrating gaze matched his measured, confident tone. He assessed the factors responsible for the virulence of the cholera epidemic.

Feliciano Gómez, Nabasanuka, 8 July 1995

The people suffered a lot, and many Warao died. This is true—many, many Warao died. I think that the Warao, I don't know, didn't have time, let's say, to prevent it—well, cholera just came. "To prevent cholera, you need to do this"—and it wasn't done. When it had begun, when the Warao were dying, that's when it happened, when many Warao were already dying, that's when they came to correct [*corregir*] the Warao, and the Warao began to boil water. The Warao never boil water. Until that date they had never boiled water. They drank water straight from the river. And when cholera came, it was then they began to boil water. And, yes, we were scared, because lots of people died, to be sure, children and adults. More than anything, this was probably because the government didn't take preventive measures. Before it arrived, cholera was in Colombia. "Okay, we're going to tell the Warao that cholera might come here. We're going to have meetings with the people in order to advise everyone about everything you need to know so that cholera won't come." I think that in this way cholera wouldn't have killed so many Warao.

Gómez largely accepts official cholera narratives. He racializes the disease as a Warao problem, and he constructs the disease as a question of specialists imparting biomedical knowledge to change the behavior of laypersons. He departs from official accounts when he explains why cholera killed so many, implying that just as the power to prevent cholera lay with the government, so did the blame. "Warao culture" has no part in Gomez's narrative; at the same time, "the Warao" seem to have little agency.

In the course of my interview with him, Vicente Medina placed the assertion regarding crabs and culture that he gave to reporters in August 1992 in a very different light.

Vicente Medina, Caracas, 13 December 1994

No one in the Ministry of Health, let's put it this way, either on the state or national level, understands the customs or the indigenous worldview or their conception of health and disease. And [physicians] try to give their treatments in a very mechanical fashion. . . . This is disastrous, because that's some of what lies behind the ignorance of our leading [public health] figures. If you know how this disease attacks and if you know what the people eat, then you should have an idea as to how these people could become infected. Then, since the people [meaning public health authorities] didn't know, or if they had known that all of the crabs could become infected and the people were going to eat them in huge quantities during a certain period, if they had realized this, they would have acted before that period arrived. Or at least they would have been alert during that period in order to see if this was going to occur or not, right? But our authorities weren't familiar with these Warao customs. . . .

On the one hand we have the intellectual understandings of researchers regarding the Warao, with all the studies by Wilbert, Dieter Heinen,

Bernarda Escalante.[2] These constitute a way of understanding the Warao world. So we have one sector that is the human masses, the suffering human masses in which there are diseases. We have a material sector [the health infrastructure] and a source of information. There are people who are directly interested in how we should proceed. I see that the conditions are available to make a good start or to begin again in the direction of a new approach. That's why I say that this is the moment to truly work in accord with existing conditions, you see. So I believe that along with all of these researchers, anthropologists, linguists, missionaries, and in my case, being a Warao who is a physician, there are people in education, such as the example of a Warao who just received a bachelor's degree, she graduated a short time ago, a teacher who is the mother of a family, a teacher in Arawaimuhu—let's say that all of this means that we can reach some kind of agreement, right, and coordinate a bit and come up with [better health] policies.

Although ignorance and culture are central tropes here, Medina places the ignorance in the minds of public health officials, characterizing it as the failure to learn the "customs" of the population they serve. This lack of knowledge leads to a epidemiological blunder: the failure to foresee the risk of a massive epidemic during the crab-harvesting season. Because cultural reasoning has been used in very problematic ways by these professionals and those in other institutions, granting epistemological and political privilege to the "intellectual understandings" of *indígena* culture produced by anthropologists—myself included—would seem to be no less dangerous than accepting the authority of public health officials and practitioners.

Medina's acknowledgment of the authority of "anthropologists, linguists, [and] missionaries" may be partially tied to the interview setting (I was trained in anthropology and linguistics), but his public statements suggest that the cultural formulations of these professionals have affected his perspective. In proposing that a new program for reconfiguring health care and education be developed, Medina seems to suggest that Warao professionals join these students of culture as key participants. Those who lack such credentials form part of the "human masses" that *receive* information. Cultural reasoning enables Medina to juxtapose the language of public health, a muted ethnic nationalism, and the rough and tumble of party politics in complex ways. He seems to want to extend the penetration of cultural reasoning into public health rather than give more authority to community leaders and social movements in representing *indígena* perspectives and interests. The racialization of *indígenas* as bearers of a homogeneous and totally distinct culture remains intact, even if its status as a causal factor in explaining the epidemic is challenged.

THE SALE OF "WARAO CULTURE" IN CARACAS

The sudden death of Mariusa's leader, principal *wisidatu*, and seven other persons in August of 1992 left the survivors terrorized and confused as they immediately turned to the task of trying to explain what the disease could be, where it had come from, and why it was killing people. The first focus of the narratives that sought to address these questions was patriarchy, particularly the struggle between Santiago Rivera and Manuel Torres for political control of the Mariusa community. These narratives were partisan accounts that incorporated patriarchal ideologies; for example, María Rivera's narrative of her brother's death lauds Rivera's heroism, casts Torres as a treacherous villain, and blames her niece for running away from an arranged marriage with the much older Torres.

Manuel Torres had a twofold motivation for finding an alternative explanation for cholera. He needed to make sense of the disease, and he needed to defend himself against charges of being a coward and having murdered his old rival. Torres is a remarkable and enigmatic person. His manner is quite unlike that of Santiago Rivera, who spoke rapidly and often conveyed a sense of being constantly worried about what he could immediately do to ensure the survival of all Mariusans. Torres usually articulates his words slowly and assuredly. He addresses many people in the delta as *mauka* (my son) or *maukwatida* (my daughter). We are close, and I am one of his "sons." He decided in 1989 that I should learn *hoa* curing. This pursuit had certainly not been on my research agenda, since I had been critical of the tremendous preoccupation of North American and European ethnographers with "shamanism." I was, however, very interested in learning more about how people cope with such difficult health conditions. Furthermore, Torres was not an easy person to refuse.[3]

Tall and distinguished, with silver hair and handsome features, Torres is recognized as one of the most skilled healers of *hoa* sickness in the delta. He is also a *wisidatu*, but he is not as widely recognized for his skill in this area. This grandfatherly figure is widely feared because he has a reputation for being quick to anger and for using *hoa* vindictively. I heard more sorcery accusations against Torres than anyone else. Small wonder that people pointed to him when a strange disease began to take lives in Mariusa.

I spoke with Torres about the epidemic and Santiago Rivera's death in November 1992. Having heard that I was in Tucupita, he made the journey from Barrancas and found me in the Hotel Delta. Torres connected the beginning of the epidemic to a command performance by residents of the Arawabisi and Winikina areas that took place in Caracas in July 1992, just before cholera began to kill Mariusans. The performance was part of the Diálogo Intercultural (Intercultural Encounter), which was a component of the Columbian Quincentennial and the fifty-fifth anniversary celebration of the Guardia Nacional.[4] In addition to the performances, the dancers participated in a series of well-publicized events held in conjunction with the anniversary celebration, including visits to the National Congress, the birthplace of Simón Bolívar, and the presidential palace, where participants were received by President Pérez. Uncharacteristically, Torres spoke rapidly, anxiously, and quite unpoetically. He seemed to be searching desperately for meaning amid chaos.

Manuel Torres, Tucupita, 13 November 1992

Our ancestral sprits *[kanobo]* must have come from far away. The ones who brought this thing were *hebu* practitioners. They brought it. When the *hebu* heard what was going on they rose up in anger. And then his younger brother rose up to try and control the *hebu*. . . .

The people from Arawabisi tried to control the *hebu*. The people from Winikina and the people from Arawabisi danced in Caracas.

I asked what the dancers had taken as offerings for the spirits.

Those people didn't have any moriche palm starch, no moriche palm starch. Since they danced at night, [the spirits] inflicted the curse of the old people. But that's just gossip. That's why, damn it, our children [the spirits] kept hearing, kept hearing the music, kept hearing the music, and it hurt them. . . .

They found some food, but there was no moriche palm starch, just a little wheat flour, and they got mad! Bam! Bam! Bam! Then they did the same over there. Then they came back through [the communities along] the other side of the river. [It was] the spell of the Caribs. . . .

We haven't heard what the ancestral spirits are saying yet, but it's said that they have wings, wings. After the guy came back after having called [the spirits], he had *wings* inside of him. It's said you could hear the wings beating inside him. And [the spirit] lodged itself inside of him and he died, because it was sucking up the water, sucking up the water just like that! "Bad things are going to happen to you folks, really bad things!"

I asked whether the sickness could be cured.

Huh! You can't cure the sickness of the Caribs, the true sickness of the Caribs. There are just too many cases to cure. Even if you speak the name of the disease, you can't cure it. And as for me, my children are buried here. That's why I don't have any children left. They all died.

Torres makes imaginative links between the broad outlines of the past and the most concrete events of the day, and between a particular death from a new disease and the day-to-day health conditions that plagued his community, all the while admitting that he was just thrashing around blindly. He is, of course, trying to get himself off the hook. It was bad enough to be accused by most of the members of his community of having killed a man who was not only an old rival but also the community's most important leader. Earlier Torres had asserted that people from all over the delta were suffering from cholera, and he stressed the physicians' amazing success in treating cholera patients. Both of these observations would seem to remove the blame from his shoulders: even a practitioner of his stature could not harm people in a number of communities simultaneously, and a *criollo* doctor would never be able to cure *hoa*.

In linking the epidemic to a dance performance in Caracas, Torres distanced himself more systematically from the *ahotana* (origins) of the epidemic and placed the blame on residents of Arawabisi and Winikina. Since *indígenas* and *criollos* alike blamed the Mariusans for starting the epidemic, Torres was attempting to get his community off the hot seat as well as defend himself. Here he adapts a familiar rhetoric to a most unfamiliar set of circumstances. *Nahanamu* ritual cycles are held when the *hebu* spirits tell the *wisidatu* in a dream that they are hungry for moriche palm starch. The dancing does not begin until the *nahanamu*, the huge receptacle that holds the collective cache of palm starch, has been filled. Then the *hebu* spirits can be summoned. If people get sick in the weeks or months after a *nahanamu* is held, some ritual infraction is generally thought to be the cause. The *wisidatu* may be blamed for having failed to follow proper procedures, or menstruating women may be accused of entering the dance platform.

In the eyes of many people in the delta, the folks from Arawabisi and Winikina made a serious mistake by performing in Caracas. The troupe included a *wisidatu*, who took his *hebu* rattle and the *isimoi*, a single-reed instrument.[5] When the spirits heard their sacred music they came looking for the palm flour. Yet they were never called—their names were not uttered by the *wisidatu*. In their attempt to re-create the ritual, the troupe used wheat flour instead of the real stuff. All in all, the spirits' feelings got hurt, and they got mad. The *wisidatu* died shortly after returning from Caracas. This kind of performance had long been criticized in delta communities as cultural theft, and many delta residents believed that performers were just asking for a wave of illness and death. When people started dying from cholera, these criticisms spread rapidly through the delta.

The leader of Danzas Wirinoko, the troupe that performed in Caracas, is Ramón Gómez. A tenacious and savvy advocate for Warao political rights,

Gómez has long served as a cultural broker. Thoroughly bilingual, he walks a political tightrope. He is one of the boldest critics of violations of the human, labor, and political rights of delta residents; at the same time, he is affiliated with the COPEI (Christian Democratic) Party and was for many years employed as a community worker by ORAI. Gómez is short, gaunt, and extremely animated, and his passion emerges as readily in relating a humorous incident as in articulating another incident of social injustice. He was some sixty-five years of age when I interviewed him in June 1993.

Gómez proudly related the way that he and other performers had staged a small takeover of the government's agenda during their visit to the Congress, delivering their own addresses to legislators and reporters regarding indigenous land struggles and protesting a proposed constitutional amendment that would have eroded indigenous rights.[6] I asked about the accusations that *hebu* had sent cholera to the delta in retribution for Danzas Wirinoko's performances in Caracas.

Ramón Gómez, Arawabisi Akoho, 16 June 1993

That's true! That's why we can't use the sacred rattle anymore—without providing palm starch. We'll dance again next time, but first we'll provide palm starch in order to make the *hebu* content. We'll call the *hebu* and place them in the palm starch. But we won't call them in Caracas—we won't call them there. Before we leave, we'll provide palm starch here. And then we'll dance *nahanamu*, with the rattle. It won't be dangerous, because we'll gather palm starch, we'll gather palm starch for a *nahanamu*, we'll give it to the *kanobo arima* [grandfather, or chief *hebu*]. . . . [The *wisidatu*] will ask, "If we go [to Caracas] again, should the people dance [the *nahanamu*]?" That's what he will say. "Can the people dance in Caracas?" And he will tell the *hebu*, "Now we have amassed palm starch for you, so don't get angry!" . . . I'm not afraid, the *hebu* won't be angry, because he'll talk to them. . . . [He'll say,] "Now we're going to hoe palm starch, so don't get angry." He'll tell them while we're still here. The *wisidatu* will tell . . . the father of the *kanobo*, "We're telling you, we're going to offer you tobacco." The grandfather *hebu* will smoke. We're going to go dance, we're going to play the *isimoi*, we're going to play the *isimoi* [in Caracas]. They won't get angry.

Gómez went on to report that they had already tried out this new procedure and that it apparently had worked. The performance, which took place outside the delta, had not led to any retaliation by the *hebu*.

Gómez also blamed the Guardia Nacional for demanding that the delta troupe perform "the *nahanamu* dance."[7] Here his narrative embraced the broader historical context in which the epidemic took place, a dimension that was conspicuously absent in official accounts. The Guardia Nacional had been severely criticized for failing to protect Venezuela's southern border from the illegal influx of Brazilian *garimperos* (gold miners) that had decimated Yanomami people through disease, mercury contamination, and repeated massacres. The Guardia Nacional had been frequently criticized for mistreating *indígenas,* including conducting vaginal searches as a form of sexualized racial violence, and it had also been accused of massacring poor Venezuelans in both urban and rural communities in the wake of the 1989 uprising.[8] The Diálogo Intercultural seems to have been designed to counter these accusations by exhibiting "the close ties which exist" between the Guardia Nacional and "our principal settlers of the national border."[9] The event also seems to have been calculated to counter widespread protests that marked *indígena* responses to the Quincentennial. This debate provided Torres with a basis for defending himself against charges of having killed Rivera, though in the end the narrative failed, as Torres himself admitted: "But that's just gossip."

Torres used the power of narrative to explore a range of possible explanations for the epidemic. He also related a story about young Mariusans who had refused to share a large cache of crabs with a *wisidatu* from Winikina. In retaliation, the *wisidatu* sent *hebu* against them. Torres also spoke about a *wisidatu* who failed to care properly for the stones that embody ancestral spirits, which had been entrusted to him, thereby bringing the spirits' wrath down upon the entire area. None of these familiar modes of explanation could adequately account for the scope and ineffability of the crisis. The Warao language contains an elaborate system for assessing the evidence that lies behind a particular statement, and Torres set aside his usual airy confidence by inserting into his narrative the formula that indicates the lowest level of confidence in the information that is being conveyed. He asserted, *"Marioso kokotuka iabanae!"* (I have abandoned all of my gods!). Feeling impotent as a healer and believing health conditions in Mariusa to be impossible, Torres moved to Barrancas in an attempt to escape from the sudden inflation in the economy of death.

Torres's account provides us with important clues as to how people were coping during the early days of the epidemic. While some individuals, such as María Rivera, minutely examined the details of daily life, others looked at how officials of the nation-state and entrepreneurs who claimed to speak for "Venezuela" affected the residents of delta communities. This direction ultimately came to dominate the ways in which delta residents conceptualized and attempted to explain cholera.

REJECTING *VIBRIO CHOLERAE*

Attempts to look in other directions to explain the epidemic often involved imaginative leaps to transnational trade, international conflicts, and genocidal plots undertaken by the nation-state. Many of these narratives can thus be characterized as conspiracy theories, juxtapositions of fact and fantasy that attempt to make sense of dizzying arrays of detail and hidden causal connections. The conspiracy theories provided resources for challenging official narratives, going beyond biomedical and cultural explanations, and imagining ways of coping with the epidemic. Official statements regarding cholera were often treated as a smokescreen. For those who accepted this version of events, the problem was not how to explain cholera but how to expose why the government was talking about the disease in the first place. Others accepted the idea that *indígenas* were dying at the same time that they asserted that the epidemic was not caused by *Vibrio cholerae*.

One of these alternative narratives circulated in Mariusa—and in different versions throughout much of the delta—after residents returned there in early 1993. In October 1994 a young man named Leonard López, who described himself as a biologist, was living in the Bustamante fishing camp in Mariusa. He explained his presence there as part of an attempt to secure funding for small-scale development projects. About the same age as Jacobo Bustamante, López is a tanned, slender, and robust man. He spoke with great conviction and a liberal use of scientific terms, but he engendered a feeling of distrust, at least on my part. López offered an alternative theory of the origin of the epidemic.

Leonard López, Mariusa Akoho, 8 October 1994

> For me, it was some substance that was in the water, as much in the area of Winikina as here in Mariusa, Macareo, and Pedernales. Because they took samples of it and it turned out to be an unknown substance. And I even had problems with the Guardia Nacional on account of the samples and such—"No, it's just not possible, guy." Who was I to take this on if it had already been diagnosed as cholera? That's as far as I got with my investigation. . . .
>
> People said that that it was crabs—that was one hypothesis. [People became infected] by consuming crabs here in this area. But crabs go around the Caribbean, and they didn't report any cases of cholera there, not even one. And many of these crabs go even farther than the Caribbean. But no, they didn't report any cases of cholera. Or maybe it was something fictitious or something to stop up a leak [*para tapar un hueco*], something that truly—. We really don't know what happened there.

I asked if he thought that something had been spread in this area on purpose.

> It could have been due to the ship traffic, some sort of a spill of a liquid from one of those boats. If we look into it, they inspect the areas where there are rivers. They inspect ships, the port captain inspects them. But when these boats enter Venezuela they don't have a technician from the Ministry of Health who inspects these ships, what the ship is carrying, what it dumps into the river. And this could be one case out of many. . . .
>
> Yes, there are thousands and thousands of details and, if we organize them, we can find a way out of these cases of the famous cholera. Okay, let's say that this year it was cholera. So then why wasn't there any last year, if ever since they have existed the Warao have eaten crabs? There are things, questions that remain clouded, if we just take a little bit of time to see what's going on there. This was a singular and specific moment—why didn't cholera continue? They took preventative measures only at that precise time, and it disappeared. Let's reflect a little bit, and if we reflect, we're going to see that this supposed cholera truly never existed. Because some plants when the tide came up were left with strange residues, which weren't oil or gasoline or any kind of fuel. It was a chemical product that entered as a kind of foam. But nobody talked about that. We don't know what happened there.

At this point Jacobo Bustamante cut in to suggest that he knew conclusively that the account was correct because "the Warao themselves know this, they know that it wasn't the supposed cholera but that it was a ship that spread this chemical in the entire area and contaminated it." López later recounted a meeting with Magdalena Benavides in which she confiscated all his samples and threatened to jail him unless he stopped looking into the source of the epidemic.

López and Bustamante present a classic conspiracy theory, combining an abundance of readily observable details with secret knowledge of nefarious linkages. The result is a hypercoherent explanation that yields only one conclusion.[10] They suggest that international shipping in and out of Venezuelan waters was not sufficiently supervised by government institutions, which led to illegal spills and dumps. By taking samples López sought to out-scientize public health officials, suggesting than any serious investigation of the matter would show that the cholera theory was not supported by the evidence. Bustamante, who lacks scientific training but has intimate contact with Mariusans, incorporates voices of "the Warao themselves" as his evidence. The two men argued that officials used journalistic narratives regarding the presence of cholera in Latin America to concoct their story, one that covered up a case of illegal dumping.

Why would a commercial fisherman and a self-styled biologist want to deny the existence of *Vibrio cholerae?* Perhaps an element of economic self-interest was at work. The epidemic threatened the economic well-being of the Bustamante family and other small commercial fishermen. It initially deprived them of their labor source, forcing them to cut back operations drastically between August and December 1992. The sale of fish was prohibited during the early months of the epidemic. Sales were later resumed, but the catch was stringently inspected. The consumption of fish fell. Antonio Bustamante marketed his fish in many Venezuelan states, and consumers were unlikely to buy fish caught in a region that bore the stigma of cholera, particularly after epidemiologists cited the consumption of fish as a key route of transmission. If it could be established that the epidemic was caused by a one-time industrial accident, more economic losses could be avoided. López's angry assertions regarding a conspiracy by the Guardia Nacional and MSAS to thwart his investigations suggest that he was aware of the power of public health authorities to produce cholera narratives.

The conspiracy in this case was limited to covering up an accidental spill. Some activists, including José Guevara, the enigmatic commander of the Escuela Forestal of San Félix, suggested that public health officials played a key role in *causing* the epidemic.

José Guevara, Tekoboroho, 22 October 1994

They situated the sites in which they inspect the vessels that go upriver toward the basic industries in this region right here, precisely at the mouth of the river. That's where they placed the checkpoints, the sanitary sites, and that's where they discovered that some ships had cholera. But they didn't take the necessary precautions with those ships. "They have cholera, we're going to subject them to quarantine right here," in the same place. They didn't take into account that those ships had to be opened up on the high seas. That's where all the waste that those ships threw out started to fall into the water. And you can see the results. The crabs, which are the ones that go along eating everything that reaches the edge of the beach, were the first things to blow when cholera first came. Then the catfish were the second to produce massive death here—the catfish and the crabs; and other fish took charge of spreading it farther upriver. . . .

I am going to tell you honestly, I am not a scientist and I don't know anything about medicine, nor do I know about—, but my own natural instinct has enabled me to calculate precisely how cholera arrived. You saw—and I said it in the office of the national attorney general—that it isn't the case that cholera was born. Cholera was planted *[sembrado]* here by the ships that take products to the basic industries—that they detected cholera and then they were anchored on the edge of the shore, submitting them to quarantine in an area that was not appropriate for this purpose.

Guevara not only accepts the epidemiological assessment that the outbreak was caused by cholera but also develops this argument precisely on the basis of public health procedures for cholera control.[11] Recall that the most common narrative regarding how cholera reached South America, as widely reported in the press, pictured a commercial vessel from Asia anchored off the Peruvian coast discharging its ballast into coastal waters. Indeed, press reports noted that MSAS was checking ships entering Venezuelan ports and controlling the release of ballast and garbage.[12] Guevara presupposes that public health authorities, knowing that the coastal waters of the delta are estuarial, also knew that any discharge released there would spread along the coast and a few kilometers upstream into nearby rivers. His account suggests that cholera cases were reported on large commercial vessels that transport the steel, aluminum, and other products produced by industries just upriver on the Orinoco in Ciudad Guayana (see map 2, page 13). Guevara argues that detaining these vessels on the delta coast violated the very rationale for a cholera quarantine: preventing transmission of the disease. He then incorporates MSAS's own prime suspect for transmission of the disease in the delta: crabs, catfish, and other aquatic species.

Unlike López, Guevara admits that he lacks scientific or medical authority. He dialogically engages MSAS's own discourse by suggesting that public health officials caused the outbreak in the delta. He thus shifts the attribution of agency away from *Vibrio cholerae* and "Warao culture." Guevara stops short of explicitly accusing MSAS, and he does not advance any sort of claim regarding the intended targets of the infection or why officials would want to create an epidemic. As we will see, many accounts of the epidemic went much further in terms of attributions of agency and intention. They become outright charges of genocide.

CHOLERA AND THE NEW WORLD ORDER

Officials in Caracas characterized the Latin American cholera epidemic as part of the seventh global pandemic. The clinical and epidemiological training that Benavides and Rodríguez received was shaped by international standards for diagnosis and treatment. Health officials considered themselves to be bearers of modernity and modern hygiene. Nevertheless, official accounts of the epidemic in Venezuela were *localized*, focused on what officials perceived to be particular features of the "local" culture and the geography of the delta. Their narratives seldom explored broader connections.

Paradoxically, many "locals," some of whom had never left the region, traveled much further in their attempts to explain the epidemic. From the start Mariusans drew on a wide conception of social and political-economic relations in trying to make sense of the disease. Most residents asserted that the first case was a *criollo* fisherman who lived in a neighboring state, thereby placing the "origin" of the epidemic within the context of the commercial exploitation of delta resources for a market that exists beyond it.

Hénaro Romero took the story into the murky waters of international relations. Romero is a *wisidatu* in Huanakasi, a small community of some fifty residents on the edge of the Siawani River, which proceeds from nearby Nabasanuka to the sea. He was about sixty years of age when I interviewed him. Tall and slender, with graying hair, Romero has a serious, distinguished look. He told me that like all the residents of Huanakasi, he became ill with cholera and was treated at the clinic in Nabasanuka. He described the "origin" of cholera in the following terms.

Hénaro Romero, Huanakasi, 17 October 1994

This is a *criollo* disease. That is its origin. The *criollos* made it, and its owners are the people from Trinidad. That's what we heard. It's said that they brought more and more and more and more crabs from there [in Mariusa]. But then: What happened? The owners of the crabs, it's said, didn't want to go get them—it appears that they hadn't been paid. Okay, fine! So right then they started putting poison [in the water], for the crabs. They kept on making poison. Then the black people [Trinidadians] left. So [the Mariusans] in turn went and got crabs and they ate them, see? But they had become bad. Maybe that's why they made [the poison]. That's how it happened. And that's how the disease began. . . .

It came from Mariusa. And after it came from there, life was awful. The people from Winikina first brought it. Before they brought it here, they went to get crabs. They went to the mouth of the Mariusa River to get crabs. Having gone there, they got crabs and took the guts of the crab. They gathered moriche fruit, they mixed it with the guts of the crabs, and they ate it. Then their stomachs started hurting. That's how the disease began, that's exactly the way it started, right there.

I asked whether the crabs had been cooked or eaten raw.

They didn't cook them. They didn't cook them, they ate them just like that, without cooking them. They ate some in their canoe, they ate them in the canoe with moriche fruit, with the pulp of the moriche fruit. That's why the disease began. If they had cooked them, things would have been fine. . . . Since they were hungry in the canoe, that's why things turned out badly. When they arrived they were gravely ill, so they went immediately to the hospital. Since they brought the disease from over there, that's why it infected all the people from around here. If they had gone instead to Tucupita, then we wouldn't have it around here. But since they came here, this disease, cholera, arrived. That's how it happened, that's why there is death here. And many children died from that disease. How many people must have died around here! A great many, with that disease. It's a different sort of disease. It makes your stomach hurt, your whole body gets sick, you get fever, and that's how so many people died. Our children have died. Three of my own children died.

The points of convergence between Romero's narrative and those told by public health officials are as fascinating as the points of divergence. Romero heard official accounts of the epidemic in Nabasanuka during trips to take his relatives to the clinic and his own stay as a patient, and he subsequently heard other narratives as they circulated around the delta. Like many officials, he places the origin of the epidemic in Mariusa, and the consumption of crabs provides the mode of infection and transmission. In response to my question he adds an episode to his narrative that relates that the Winikinans ate some crabs raw, and he states that the outbreak would never have occurred if the crabs had been cooked. Although Romero says that it is not the Mariusans but people from adjacent Winikina who are responsible for spreading cholera to his community, crab-consuming Warao bodies continue to be the mode of transmission. Romero's narrative thus incorporates clinicians' readings of epidemiological information.

There are two crucial differences between Romero's story and official accounts. First, Romero places the epidemic in the context of transnational commerce, albeit on a very small scale. For years Trinidadians arrived illegally in small fishing boats every few days to purchase crabs from Mariusans. Santiago Rivera constantly fought to raise the meager sum paid for each gunnysack of crabs. On several occasions when the Trinidadians refused to increase the amount they paid, I heard Rivera threaten them with a strike. Romero's story suggests that he made good on this threat, and that the Trinidadians retaliated by poisoning the crabs. From that point on the epidemic proceeds according to the epidemiological narratives of cholera transmission.

Although Romero's narrative is set in Mariusa, it is deeply enmeshed in shared knowledge of the broader political and historical context. Everyone in the delta knew in the mid-1990s that a great deal of illegal trade with Trinidad and Guyana traversed the delta, and most people knew that cocaine constituted part of the contraband. A subject that was sensitive for the nation-state and delta residents alike was the way that Trinidadian fishermen often dropped their nets in Venezuelan waters. This is not to say that relations between delta residents and Trinidadians were hostile. *Indígenas* often traveled to Trinidad to trade, and these long-standing exchanges produced positive and poignant memories for each side.[13] At the same time, myths told in Warao construct Trinidadians, like *criollos,* as belonging to a class of humans distinct from *indígenas.*[14]

Despite the Trinidadian involvement, Romero's narrative places the "origin" of the epidemic within the delta. Some stories, told almost from the start, placed the "origin" of the outbreak far beyond Venezuela. In January and February 1991, the United States, Great Britain, and other nations bombed Iraq and Kuwait and attacked Iraqi ground forces. News of the war reached delta communities via *Notidiario* and Radio Tucupita; individuals who lacked access to media reports learned through word of mouth. Unbeknownst to me, I was placed at the center of the conflict in the geopolitical imaginings of many delta residents. The U.S. government was seen as Iraq's central adversary, and many people assumed that, because it was centrally involved, it was also defending its own territory against a foreign invasion. Accordingly, all persons who could fight, myself included, were thought to have taken up arms. Indeed, my friends referred to the U.S. government as *Dokomuru aidamotuma*—Charles's leaders. After the conflict ended, teacher Feliciano Gómez was asked to write a letter to me, as I was told over and over, "to see if you were still alive." The missive never reached me. When I did not respond, the rumor that I had died in the war traveled around the delta. I had to convince quite a number of friends that I was still alive when I went to Tucupita in November 1992.

In 1992 friends from Guayo reported an imagined link between the two cases of widespread death, telling me that the "origin" of the epidemic lay in the war. I did not record the narrative at that time, but Ramón Gómez offered a version of this story during a visit to our house in Tucupita on Venezuelan Independence Day. His niece had been incarcerated, and he was seeking her release. He had come to us for help. Carmen Chávez (Gómez's wife), Clara, and I were seated with Gómez on the back patio when he spontaneously began to talk about the "origin" of the cholera epidemic.

Ramón Gómez, Tucupita, 5 July 1994

I'm going to tell the story of the origin of cholera [*hebu sabana nakakitane*], the origin of cholera, the disease that is called cholera in Spanish. Five hundred years ago, five hundred years ago the Spaniards arrived—

Christopher Columbus saw this land five hundred years ago. For five hundred years now our ancestors, our great-grandfathers, have eaten crabs just like us. They ate red crabs and blue crabs, and they ate all kinds of fish. And more and more and more years have gone by until just two years ago. And then when the river had reached its high point, we heard that a war was going on.

It was the Americans, with Iraq. They fought and fought, and they dropped their fire into the water—that's what we call it. In Warao we call it that, in Spanish they're called "bombs." They dropped them on the ground and they dropped in the water and then dropped them in the water. They have some sort of poison in them that affects the fish, the water, and the crabs. And crabs come from the sea, from the sea when their season arrives. From the time that they fought one year passed, and that water came from over there, very slowly. [The poison] dispersed in the water and came slowly. And that poison made the fish turn bad. Now you can no longer eat them or you get diarrhea. Since the crabs also live in the ocean, they also got the poison. It doesn't kill them, but the crabs come to where the people live. When they catch fish and they eat them, they get diarrhea and vomit; and when they eat crabs the same thing happens. They get diarrhea and vomit and their soft bodies become rigid. It's just as if they were poisoned. They get really sick.

So the Warao people think, "*Criollo* doctors say that crabs are to blame for this cholera." But we Warao say, "Crabs don't have cholera." We think that the water is to blame. The people who were fighting dropped an element that made the water bad, and it spread throughout the oceans. It's because they dropped bombs, they dropped bombs from the sky on ships. . . . What sort of disease did the bombs produce there in the water, in the ocean? A gas or a microbe that somehow infected the water and, by infecting the water, also infected the fish and infected the crabs. And so, for us Warao, this cholera didn't come on its own.

Gómez's narrative is immersed in broad historical and political contexts in a number of ways. He assesses the amount of time that *indígenas* had been eating crabs by referring to Columbus's arrival in the Americas. In this way he projects five hundred years of geographically and culturally continuous Warao existence in the delta at the same time that he constructs the epidemic as a decisive historical break. He explains the temporal gap between the end of the ground war in the Persian Gulf in February 1991 and the beginning of the epidemic eighteen months later by describing the gradual spreading of the poison through the oceans.[15]

Here is another example of local-global paradox. *Indígenas* who live in "remote" communities are supposed to be quintessential locals, people whose experience is limited by history and geography to a "traditional" knowledge that does not incorporate new information or global perspectives. In contrast, public health officials are trained in a field that lays claim to scientific, universal knowledge that is not tied to any local place, and, it is assumed, they develop global perspectives. When Gómez criticizes "*criollo* doctors," however, he implies that their crab theory is too local, restricted, and reductionist. Gómez, who divides his time between Arawabisi and Tucupita, follows the news in print and on television while he is in town. Many delta residents are similarly aware of the ways that transnational capital and the international use of political and military power shape contemporary experience, even in Delta Amacuro. In Gómez's narrative a postcolonial critique merges with a critique of the effects of globalization on people who usually do not have the opportunity to influence the transnational flow of capital, goods, and technology or political-cum-military power.

As the leader of the dance troupe that had performed in Caracas just before the epidemic began, Gómez had been personally implicated in many cholera stories. Moreover, he knew that I am a citizen of the country that dropped most of the bombs that, he asserted, caused the epidemic. Yet Gómez certainly did not produce the Gulf War story himself—I heard many versions. Such narratives explicitly challenge the hegemony of "localized" accounts and provide spaces where people can develop critical perspectives on the forces that shape their everyday lives.

Official narratives medicalized the epidemic in the sense that the deaths were framed as questions of knowledge legitimately produced and circulated by professionals in medicine and public health. From the start, however, popular discourses about cholera sought to explain the epidemic in historical and political terms. The "smokescreen" reaction radically de-medicalized cholera as lacking any pathogenic basis whatsoever. As the epidemic wore on, activists in Tucupita and delta residents turned increasingly to efforts to link epidemiological explanations to the historical and political circumstances of everyday life. In 1992 activists were concerned with questions of land rights, economic exploitation, political representation, and human rights. Cholera rarely figured on the agenda of organizing efforts or marches protesting the Columbian Quincentennial. This is not to say that activists did not participate in the circulation of cholera narratives or that questions of land expropriation did not shape them.

Esteban Castro makes a meager living through subsistence farming and small jobs related to research and political projects. Conversant in Warao, he collects files, briefcases, and boxes of reports and newspaper clippings on delta communities. He has reportedly authored a number of manuscripts, none of which have been submitted for publication. He is tall, bearded, and sunburned, and his unkempt hair, beard, and old soiled clothes seem to reflect more closely his self-identification as a *campesino* or peasant agriculturalist than the well-groomed appearance of other patrons in the library or the office of Hector Romero, a socialist lawyer-cum-sociologist, which we both frequent. His animated face and eyes burn passionately, and he gestures dramatically as he provides accounts of injustices committed against *indígenas*.

Castro's narrative directly connects cholera with the land issue. Not one to present information in such formal events as interviews, he nearly shouted his theory of the epidemic one night at eleven o'clock in the street in front of our house, as a party that Clara and I had given was breaking up. He directly attacked epidemiological narratives that attributed agency to *Vibrio cholerae* and blamed "Warao culture." He asserted that the epidemic was a master plan developed by government institutions and their staffs who wished to get rid of "the Warao" once and for all so that they could enjoy free access to the land and natural resources of the delta. Six months later, while we were having lunch, Castro specified that the causal agent for the epidemic was a "superbacteria" that had been developed by the U.S. military for use in the Persian Gulf War. Remaining mute about his sources, he concluded that Venezuelan government officials had obtained quantities of this bacteria and had spread them at strategic points in the delta. We heard this narrative repeated by people in Tucupita and in the delta.

CHOLERA AND VERNACULAR HEALING

Vernacular healers, particularly *wisidatus*, came to play an increasingly important role in the process of rendering the epidemic comprehensible in historical, political, and social terms in the fluvial area. To be sure, the early days of the epidemic dealt a powerful blow to the prestige of noninstitutional medicine in the delta. Healers were unable to treat patients, and they admitted ignorance of the new disease.[16] They were also quick to admit that institutional practitioners enjoyed remarkable success. A substantial proportion of the noninstitutional healers died in the epidemic. Nearly all the *wisidatus* who are recognized as powerful through their abilities to "own" sacred ancestral stones and other ritual objects, hold *nahanamu*, and cure patients are senior men holding other positions of authority. Since the epidemic threatened the legitimacy of vernacular medical knowledge and, to an extent, patriarchy, leaders sought to reestablish their authority, particularly after the terror began to subside and many of the people who had fled the delta returned home.

Fernando Rivera was one of the most prominent *wisidatus* in the Mariusan community for years. Until 1992 he was second in prestige to Claudio Martín, who was the "owner" of the ancestral stones. When cholera killed Martín, Rivera inherited them. Rivera lived to the age of about seventy, a remarkable accomplishment. He died in 1999, probably of tuberculosis. Until the time of his death he was animated by a bravado that sometimes bordered on braggadocio. During week-long *nahanamu* celebrations he worked virtually all day, played the *isimoi,* danced all night, and held lengthy dialogues with *hebu* spirits while ingesting massive amounts of tobacco. His words were uttered with force, conviction, and often great volume, and his gestures bordered on the theatrical. Rivera and his family spent most of their time in Nabaribuhu in the moriche groves, rejecting the life of wage labor and store-bought foods adopted by people living in the company of fishermen on the coast.

As the economic crisis worsened, more and more people rejoined Rivera in the forest. Globalization, it seemed, was driving Mariusans back into what was commonly considered the epitome of the premodern world. Nabaribuhu was not a refuge from cholera, however, and several people died. Rivera himself got "a little sick" with the disease and was treated in Nabasanuka. He, too, fled the area when the epidemic hit, but he spent most of that time near the mouth of the Winikina River—a site that enabled him to live within the forest as well as be much closer to the clinic at Nabasanuka.

I first returned to Mariusa after the epidemic in June 1993; this was Clara's first visit. We called a community meeting with Rivera and other Mariusan medical practitioners to make arrangements for building an infirmary and bringing a nurse to work in Mariusa. Fisherman Antonio Bustamante loaned us his house, the largest (if the most odiferous) in the community. When Rivera arrived he took me to the back of the house and proudly whispered that he had dreamed of cholera and wished to recount his dream. I grabbed my tape recorder, and we hid behind a huge box of rusting metal filled with ice and fish.

Fernando Rivera, mouth of the Mariusa River, 19 June 1993

I'm going to tell you about my dream. This disease began when the sun arose and began to shine in the sky. The house of this *hebu,* "Poison," is there [points toward Trinidad]. This poison that comes from up there is just like the *hebu's* poison, and that's what started it. That's how my dream goes. That "Poison" is a *hebu,* cholera. Its poison arose in order to exterminate the Warao, to finish off all the Warao. My dream is really powerful, and that's what I dreamt! Not every *wisidatu* will recount his dreams!

I asked how this *hebu* had arisen.

> This cholera's food is grease. Cholera's food is grease—it's like a hard ball of grease. When you eat it you vomit. When you eat it you get diarrhea. That's what I dreamt, that's my dream.

I then asked what had made the *hebu* mad.

> This *hebu*'s name is "Poison" *[Veneno]!* This poison is like the *criollo*'s poison. That's its work [killing Warao]. It's mute, it can't talk. It's a *hebu* that can't talk, can't talk, nor can it respond. It's silent. That *hebu*, Poison, rose up in order to finish off the Warao, to kill the Warao. That *hebu*, who lives up there, rose up to kill all the Warao. That *hebu* that had never existed before rose up, the one that is the master *[arotu]* of the end of the earth, where the earth ends far away, at the end of all the mountains, it is in charge there. . . . That *hebu* rose up with all of its power so that it could finish us off, so that not even one of us would be left. That's what happened *[saa]*. But now medicines appeared and people were cured, that's what I dreamt.
>   The *hebu* took its gun, bang!—it shot me. But I didn't die! It ran through the corridor up there [in the sky], stopped, and fired at me with its shotgun. It hit me, slam! But I still didn't die! I grabbed it—bam!— the master itself. I killed my prey, the master of the *hebu*, their leader died. And then I also destroyed all their boats in my dream. That's my dream. Um hum, I'm strong, ha ha ha. What I am telling you is the absolute truth.

It is clear that the cholera stories told in June 1993 by men in Mariusa and other parts of the delta had changed radically from the previous year. From fragmented adumbrations of a range of possible scenarios, which were often marked as unverifiable gossip, healers had moved to dreams that purported to reveal the invisible dimensions of the disease, objectify it, and locate its "master" or "leader." Rivera reveals the name of the *hebu*, "Poison," thus suggesting that he can now control it. For vernacular healers in the delta, healer's dreams are regarded as the most definitive form of evidence, far more powerful and reliable than what is seen or heard. Instead of punctuating his narrative with "I don't know," Rivera uses evidentials, grammatical forms that mark the nature and strength of the evidence that lies behind a statement, such as *saa*. To impress me further, Rivera makes the authority of his narrative—and thus of himself as narrator and *wisidatu*— evident: "My dream is really powerful," and "What I am telling you is the absolute truth."

Rivera places cholera in a very prominent place in the ontological realm of *hebu*. The narrative of the "origin" of the Sun is one of the most powerful narratives that informs vernacular healing practices.[17] Some of the most potent forces dwell where the Sun rises, and the *arotu* (master) of the cholera *hebu* is none other than the *arotu* of that realm. Rivera provides a nifty rationalization for his inability, and that of other *wisidatus,* to communicate with the cholera *hebu:* they are mute and, as he explained later, deaf as well since they have no ears. The word he uses, *dibumoni,* creates a double entendre: it refers to *dibu* (speech) that has become defective, unintelligible. *Dibumoni* is often used to refer to the English language, and its use here thus links the epidemic to Trinidadians as well (an allusion that Rivera clarifies later by referring to the *hebu* as *mekoro,* or "blacks"). Having learned the identity of the pathogens, he determines their goal—to exterminate all "the Warao." Although the *hebu* also try to kill him, Rivera constructs himself as being such a powerful healer that he is not harmed by their bullets and is able to kill the "master," destroy the *hebu's* means of transportation, and send the remainder of the *hebu* away. He thus claims to have rid the area of cholera.

Ah ha, you might say, *indígenas* really do believe that cholera is produced by spirits, as many public health authorities and clinicians suggest, and they thus rely on medical beliefs that are incompatible with medicine and accordingly resist "modern" health care.

Since Rivera is an elderly *wisidatu* who lives in the moriche groves near the coast in the most "culturally conservative" area (as anthropologists and Tucupita residents often put it), his narrative would be a good candidate for this reading. But Rivera's story resists appropriation by dominant narratives. Cholera is not constructed as a "traditional Warao" *hebu* but as a "new" disease that is associated with *criollos* and Trinidadians. It is modeled on the poisons used by *criollos,* and its secret name is in Spanish, not Warao. Moreover, by dreaming of medicines, Rivera indirectly incorporates biomedical therapies into vernacular medical practices. The dream thus ratifies the status of institutionally based treatments as the cure for cholera, and it follows on the heels of Rivera's sojourn as a cholera patient in the Nabasanuka clinic. Believing in vernacular disease etiologies and receiving treatment from vernacular healers did not preclude *indígenas* from seeking institutional health care or following through with treatment, and it did not undermine the success of biomedical treatment.[18]

Rivera's narrative clearly racializes cholera, pitting all *criollos* and Trinidadians against all Warao. He is aware of assertions that *criollos* want to get rid of *indígenas* and that the former believe that cholera just might accomplish this. Diego Rivera, the *wisidatu* of La Tortuga, reported a dream in which Trinidadians sent two *wisidatu* who were half wild pig *(vaquiro)* and half human to kill all the Mariusans to take their lands. A number of accounts suggested that *criollos* had, through their own vernacular practitioners, ordered *"criollo hebu"* to come and kill all Warao so that they could have the entire delta to themselves. People often described Caracas as the place of "origin" of cholera, strongly implying that officials of the national government had started the epidemic and were attempting to exterminate *indígenas*. Most of the dream-based narratives amount to charges of genocide.

Most surviving healers moved from confusion to a recovery of knowledge and authority, but a few practitioners claimed that they had dealt successfully with cholera right from the start. We came upon one case in España, a community located along the Winikina River. The chief *wisidatu* was Raúl Leoni. Sixty-eight years of age at the time, thin and frail, Leoni was unable to walk without assistance, and he wrestled with symptoms of dementia. Nevertheless, he was tremendously engaged with questions of healing, and he demonstrated a dramatic flair and more than a touch of braggadocio, much like Rivera. Unlike Rivera, however, he had a strong sense of humor, and he enjoyed making fun of himself and others. The two men's lives had been quite different as well. Missionaries had not made more than occasional visits to Mariusa, but they have had a strong presence in the Winikina area since the early part of the twentieth century, and Leoni was taken as a child to a mission boarding school in the delta. "Interned" by the Capuchins, he escaped.

Leoni was one of the first residents of España to contract cholera. After he was treated in Nabasanuka he was able to combine what he had learned at the clinic with his own training as a *wisidatu* to develop ways of treating cholera. He dreamed the name of the cholera *hebu* and the song he needed to send them away. Accompanying himself with his rattle, which provides voices of the spirits, he sang the cholera music for us. Leoni noted that he used these songs both in treating his grandson and in the course of a *nahanamu* ritual that he held to rid the community of cholera. In his dream he learned that he was indirectly responsible for bringing cholera into his community because he had insulted *criollo* politicians when they came to campaign in Winikina. In retaliation, they sent the disease. Cholera was, once again, the vengeance that the nation-state exacted on *indígenas* who dared to resist it. Leoni claimed the capacity to identify state violence, render it impotent, and return it to its source: his song sent cholera back to Caracas. Although cholera is often imagined as a racialized form of violence, in his song Leoni ordered the cholera *hebu* to leave *criollos* in peace as well. Leoni, along with his son and grandson, who are local officials, made sure that España residents drank only potable water, washed their hands, and cleaned food containers well.

We discovered a remarkably successful integration of institutional and vernacular healing in Wakuhana, which is quite close to the large coastal settlement of Cangrejito. In November 1994, with the help of Tirso Gómez, I extended our survey of health conditions to the community. We were astounded to find that the Wakuhanans had been unaffected by recent outbreaks of measles, whooping cough, and chicken pox, that they had had only one cholera case, and that the community was, according to *wisidatu* Eulalio Torres and other residents, free from other diarrheal diseases. Amazed, we ask Torres why Wakuhana did not suffer from the diseases that had taken many lives nearby. Torres said that one person had shown symptoms of cholera. They took him to the hospital in Curiapo, and Torres listened carefully to the doctor's instructions. Upon returning to Wakuhana he announced that every drop of water destined for consumption in the community would, henceforth, be boiled, that no one would travel to adjacent communities, thereby avoiding the risk of becoming infected and bringing the disease home, and that a *nahanamu* would be held to send away the *hebu* causing cholera. These three steps were performed, the community continued to boil drinking water, and health conditions improved considerably. Wakuhana's experience provides a model for generating the sort of integration of medical perspectives that could save lives elsewhere.

CONTROLLING INEQUITY

Ghosts—cholera narratives are full of them. Every attempt to narrate cholera—to explain what it is, where it came from, and why it was killing *indígenas* in the delta—had to contend with a powerful relationship between the hypervisible and the invisible. People with cholera were highly visible. They were easily spotted and, horrible to apprehend once dehydration was severe, frequently photographed. At the same time, the pathogen that sickened and killed so many in such rapid succession was invisible, unlike an atomic bomb, a tidal wave, or an earthquake. In this sense public health officials, cholera patients, *wisidatu*, and reporters were faced with the same epistemological dilemma. Since the cholera epidemic brought questions of social inequality right out into the open, those who controlled social memory of the epidemic would shape the ideologies and practices that regulate daily life and death in the delta—and social inequality as well—for years to come.

Clara and I heard many more variants of the narratives recounted here. We should not, however, conclude that some sort of postmodern epistemological democracy emerged in which each narrative circulated without constraint through social space. Nothing could be further from the truth. If we take as measures of authority those narratives that were published and broadcast, figured in health education programs, were embedded in official statements, and shaped how government resources were deployed in the delta, it is clear that some narratives fared much better than others. Even though dominant narratives were not monolithic—individuals connected with oppositional parties and some journalists presented quite different variants that often portrayed public health authorities as villains or incompetents rather than heroes—they too racialized the disease and historical agency. Accounts that linked the epidemic to the Persian Gulf War, transnational capital flows, or command performances of sacred dances or that described heroic attempts by *indígenas* to save their communities from cholera seldom appeared in the press or prompted government investigations.

We might conclude that official narratives were more widely disseminated because they emerged from specialized training in medicine and public health and were in accordance with international standards and a global conversation between scientists and health professionals. The other set of narratives, in contrast, reflected local cultural norms such as beliefs in *hebu* and magical practices, and many presented conspiracy theories that reflected fleeting local conditions, or perceptions of them. A rather substantial amount of scientific evidence confirmed the status of *Vibrio cholerae* as the pathogen, and public health authorities enjoyed exclusive access to laboratories that could detect it.

Perhaps the cachet of the official narratives lay in the way cholera was medicalized, which invested authority solely in the discourses, epistemologies, and technologies controlled by public health authorities and, to a lesser extent, by physicians. This was true—in a way. The narratives told by public health officials and physicians were medicalized, but only very imperfectly, and they were also shot through with popular conceptions of geography, ecology, hydrology, culture, psychology, social relations, sexuality, nutrition, demography, religion, education, language, history, and race, creating bizarre and somewhat surreal juxtapositions of disparate discourses. Perhaps all of the physicians that I encountered knew their basic microbiology, physiology, and pharmacology, and all the public health specialists knew their epidemiology and biostatistics. Nevertheless, they spoke about matters, such as culture, that lay beyond their specialized training. When they turned to these areas, health professionals drew on rough-and-ready amalgamations of what they gleaned from specialists in other disciplines and popular discourses. Laypersons generated statements about medicine and public health in the same way.

This is not to say that no one should venture an opinion about areas in which they lack specialized, scientific training. Yet by framing their statements as authoritative descriptions, Benavides, Rodríguez, Vargas, and others gave the impression that their statements were based upon specialized, circumscribed scientific knowledge—the sort of understanding that nonspecialists lack. The sense that these statements reflected self-contained, coherent medical and/or public health knowledge is thus an illusion, one based on the speakers' institutional and occupational status and the infusion of public health and medical jargon in their statements. Not only were these narratives epistemologically quite heterogeneous, microbiological and clinical knowledge was no more central than the other sorts of information they incorporated. The illusion of homogeneity, empirical validity, and scientific sophistication imbued these accounts with authority and augmented their social, political, and medical impact. As they came together repeatedly in official narratives, public health and racial discourses came to be more than simply juxtaposed. The scientific and social realms, which are supposed to be kept separate, became hybridized.[19] As they provided rationales for medical profiling, public health and medical knowledge became racialized at the same time that medical meanings more deeply and pervasively shaped the construction of racial categories.

Moreover, statements and decisions by public health officials in the delta were based on relatively little empirical information. Benavides, Rodríguez, Vargas, and Orihuela all made statements regarding *indígena* culture, diet, and sanitary practices even though none of them had conducted in-depth research in this area. Recall that Benavides and Rodríguez's "study" of population movements and religious and medical beliefs, which purportedly demonstrated their role in transmitting cholera, was completed in only ten days at a time when Benavides and Rodríguez were primarily concerned with vast logistical problems. One would suspect that the requirements for validity and reliability of investigations in these areas were somewhat lower than those required for microbiological or clinical work. The real point, however, is not whether official imaginings of culture, history, language, and sanitary practices were scientific. The point is that what was paraded as empirical information about local populations and geographic spaces was not, by and large, either empirical or local. This "information" was drawn from stereotypes, encountered all over the world, that circulated, in general, through anecdotes recounted by *criollo* professionals who had worked in Delta Amacuro.[20]

Claims for the modernity and scientific authority of official narratives should be considered critically, despite Rodríguez's reassuring assertion that the epidemic was being studied "by way of all of the angles of the scientific vision."[21] For example, a great deal had been learned about the way that *Vibrio cholerae* can attach themselves to algae, assume a passive state (and thus become quite difficult to detect using standard laboratory techniques), and then, when the temperature and salinity are suitable, become active again.[22] Further ecological research could have provided valuable information about how cholera was being transmitted and how to predict and prevent future outbreaks, but it does not appear that work along these lines was executed. None of the public health officials or physicians that we interviewed knew very much about recent work on the ecology, microbiology, or immunology of cholera.

The emphasis on controlling the movement of delta residents, particularly the quarantine of Mariusans, ran counter to modern scientific guidelines, including those issued by PAHO and WHO. Like the distribution of Bactron to keep people from fleeing to the mainland, some of the decisions that were made by public health authorities reflected not science but the political constraints under which they were operating. These statements contained a great deal more than science, and the scientific perspective they reflected was not the only one available. The power of the narrative sprang more from the position of the speaker or writer and the status of their account (as journalism, official report, rumor, personal statement, and so on) than from the content.

The cholera narratives provide invaluable insight into how denigrating stereotypes can be reconstituted, blended, and placed on the science shelf of the discursive supermarket. Faced with a potential institutional catastrophe, public health officials first searched common imaginings of a racialized population for one or more elements that resonated with the specific features of the case at hand. Since seafood and specifically ceviche had provided leitmotifs for the Peruvian epidemic, Venezuelan officials seized on crabs as a logical villain, and they were immediately served up to journalists and politicians. The specialized discourse had to be modified to fit the target culture, so crabs and fish were, in official narratives, always eaten raw. The rhetoric of culture thus played a crucial role in giving the heterogeneous discourses of public health officials the ring of truth.

Next, synecdoche was employed to strengthen the narrative: officials declared that all "Warao" ate crabs at that time of the year. This generated an empirical problem because crabs had been prohibited. Many people had stopped eating them (even cooked), and delta residents were still getting sick. The solution was found in the scientific rhetoric of culture, which generally asserts that a culture is systematic, complex, and integrated. If an individual or a community can be said to possess one element of a cultural complex, they can be considered its members; if one element is criticized or doesn't support the official explanation, there are others that can serve. Thus the crab story was expanded to incorporate other areas of "the culture," augmenting explanatory resources and opening up escape routes for possible retreat from future empirical problems. Crabs were depicted as part of a ritual that involved migration, social organization, and vernacular curing practices. The story was expanded to include not only food procurement, preparation, and consumption but also religion, sanitary practices, child-rearing, nomadism—and on and on. Cultural reasoning even embraced two of the formulations it was meant to displace: environmental and physiological (read: racial) determinism.[23] If an individual, or a community, can be said to possess one aspect of a cultural complex, he or she has it all. If one element is criticized or doesn't support the official explanation, there are others that will serve.

Finally, stereotype was transformed into cultural truth in two steps. In the first step, cultural patterns were contrasted element by element with the cultural patterns of *criollos*, "the national society." This promoted the sense that *indígena* culture had developed independently from and shared no features with its *criollo* counterpart. Each individual in Delta Amacuro was determined to have a single, bounded identity as *either* "Warao" or *criollo*. No one—neither "Warao" who had lived for years in Tucupita or Barrancas nor *criollos* who were born and raised in predominantly *indígena* areas of the delta—could have composite identities or even any in-depth knowledge of the "other culture." Bilingualism was conveniently overlooked. In the second step the culture of the Other was deemed to be ahistorical and static, in contrast to the *criollo* culture, which was seen as constantly changing and adapting. Once an *indígena*, always an *indígena*, as Benavides claimed. *Voilà!* Culture had been objectified and constructed as an agent, making "them" do the things that caused the crisis and rendering "them" unable to let "us"—those who knew exactly what was happening and could have stopped the epidemic if "their" culture hadn't gotten in the way— help.[24]

All of the needed oppositions were in place: us versus them, science versus magic, civilized versus uncivilized, modern versus premodern. The liberal veneer of cultural reasoning suggests that the opposition between "us" and "them" simply defines a local cultural economy as separate but equal. What seem to be balanced oppositions are generally a cover for asymmetrical relationships, where one group is constructed as the complete version and the other is a partial and defective copy.[25] Franz Fanon, a physician and critic of colonialism, pointed out long ago that the categories "white people" and "people of color" stand in this sort of asymmetrical relationship: whiteness is the unmarked, natural, fundamental category that defines what is universal and expected; "nonwhite" defines what is derivative, pathological, or incomplete.[26]

The category of *indígena* that emerged from official cholera narratives—like other racialized discourses in Delta Amacuro—followed this pattern to the letter. "Warao culture" added up to a thoroughgoing lack of all the essential characteristics of bourgeois *criollos*, who were modern, rational, strong, independent, intelligent, and hygienic. It was, in short, a classically Orientalist construction, the specific features of which were mapped to fit the specific contours of the problem at hand—a cholera epidemic.[27] The tellers were "complex subjects," while the objects of their description were only partial and fragmentary subjects, lacking such purportedly universal and necessary attributes as rationality, history, awareness of causation, and agency.[28] Individuals racialized as members of "the national society" confirmed their status as modern subjects by accruing complementary roles, even as adepts in spirit possession; in contrast, those cast as *indígenas* were cast out of modernity when they created hybrid selves. As incomplete subjects, *indígenas* were incomplete citizens, people with distinct and incompatible political norms and values. The protests that emerged in 1992 were thus dismissed because incomplete subjects could not legitimately demand the same rights and legal protections as complex subjects—members of "the national society." Casting *indígenas* as unsanitary subjects enabled *criollo* sanitary citizens to use cholera narratives to exclude *indígenas* from full participation in social and political life.

The dominant cholera narratives created global and local subjects. Public health professionals had a global vision: they were able to take modern information from the metropolis and use it to infuse modernity and rationality into a backward world. *Indígenas*, on the other hand, became classic locals, people incapable of either seeing beyond their immediate circumstances or incorporating knowledge that came from beyond the boundaries of their parish (from laboratories, international organizations, trade organizations, and universities, for example). The local politicians criticized by Rodríguez, the local doctors who were modernized by Vargas, and local *crio-*

llos in general formed an intermediate category. Most were too provincial to be bearers of civilized, metropolitan knowledge and too accustomed to local, backward conditions to want to change them. But they at least had the *potential* to change: it was Vargas's assertion that cholera provided just the right stimulus.

Public health officials are hardly alone in creating local subjects. The role of anthropologists has been to discover, describe, and compare various types of locals.[29] Nevertheless, in Delta Amacuro, it was public health officials—the supposedly global subjects—who localized the epidemic. In contrast, many of the quintessential locals—the members of an "uncivilized" population—sought to make the most global connections they could imagine, linking cholera to global capitalism, global warfare, the degradation of the global environment, the marketing of local culture in national (or nationalistic) arenas, and the transnational politics of race. The officials abstracted cholera from time as radically as they extracted it from space (at least any conception of space that extended beyond the delta), imagining unchanging, inherent properties of the environment and millenarian beliefs and cultural patterns. The locals, however, tied cholera to the social, political-economic, and environmental parameters of the historical moment in which the epidemic occurred. How ironic.[30]

It would certainly be easy to disqualify some narratives as conspiracy theories based on ludicrous assumptions. Many of the stories that challenged official accounts did exhibit features that characterize such accounts. Conspiracy theories centrally involve a theory of power, and they tell how an individual or group seized power illicitly (such as the use of genocide in taking away *indígena* lands). Stories that resist official versions often treat events as signs of hidden meanings. The usual traffic of ocean-going vessels becomes a clue for understanding mysterious illnesses and revealing government secrets. Not satisfied with normal boundaries between categories, domains of analysis (such as medical versus economic), or conventional types of meaning and methods of decoding them, conspiracy theories engage in a constant play between the hyperreal (such as visually compelling cholera symptoms) and that which can only be imagined (scientists creating a superbacteria). They form hybrid mixtures of what we might refer to as the metaphysics of presence and absence.[31] The narrators of alternative cholera stories, including self-styled biologists, activists, and vernacular healers, were the perfect middlemen between visible and invisible realms.

Conspiracy theories have recently become a focus of researchers in cultural studies because they depict a world that seems to be entirely illusory and question the validity of common representations.[32] They attempt to dismantle the rational, taken-for-granted world and show it to be unreal and irrational. Conspiracy theories take normal bureaucratic, political, and physical rules and show that they are incapable of making sense of the visible world. This interpretive strategy seemingly offered a way to explain why the colossal promises frequently made by politicians and bureaucrats seldom produced any tangible benefits, at least for their ostensible beneficiaries. Cholera conspiracy narratives were called upon to explain the experience of racialized subjects with bureaucratic rules that had special modes of implementation for *indígenas*. These rules always seemed to allow officials to avoid providing promised papers or resources and to then blame the failure on the client. Many of these conspiracy theories challenged the ideological basis of medical profiling. Although they generally failed to challenge the racialization of the epidemic—the idea that *Vibrio cholerae* and *indígenas* were intimately connected—these narratives attempted to unravel the cultural and geographic logics that linked race and bacteria in official accounts. Medical profiling was variously reinterpreted as negligence, institutional indifference, exploitation, and genocide.

Conspiracy theories always involve a curious leap of imagination that takes narrators and audiences beyond the realm of the rational.[33] Such logical jumps emerge in many narratives: Trinidadian wrath over a crab workers' strike produces a delta-wide epidemic; the U.S. military sells Venezuela its new superbacteria; cholera begins as collateral damage from Persian Gulf War bombs. But the official narratives that these stories challenged also involved striking leaps of faith: religious rituals produce cholera epidemics; antibiotic-saturated *indígena* bodies are a threat to *criollo* populations. The use of cultural reasoning also involved tremendous leaps of faith: religious and dietary practices were ascribed to an entire population and then transformed into modes of bacterial transmission, even when literature on the role of water-borne transmission in Latin America was readily available. Indeed, one might say that modernity itself is built on a fundamental leap of the imagination, one that converts egalitarian promises into schemes of social inequality that revolve around the restriction of access to modern knowledge and that then evaluate individuals in terms of how well they have internalized the unavailable information.

Fredric Jameson suggests that conspiracy theories provide a particularly appropriate narrative form for use in an era "whose abominations are heightened by their concealment and their bureaucratic impersonality."[34]

He suggests that they perform a sort of "cognitive mapping" of the totality of contemporary social life, an effort to see how one's local experience fits into the global system of late capitalism. Jameson could have been thinking about the delta. Official narratives attempted to confine people's vision to what took place after the first case of cholera was reported, making it difficult to look beyond the rivers and coast that limit the geography of the delta. The conspiracy theories sought to connect transnational corporations, policies of the nation-state, and the mechanisms for legitimating and extending a racial economy that had cost numerous lives.

Politically progressive critics who might be attracted to the oppositional politics that sometimes emerge in conspiracy theories generally distance themselves from such accounts because they are flawed by their reliance on questionable sources and by an analytic fixation on individuals and cabals rather than institutional, systemic, or structural factors. These critics argue that these shortcomings render them ineffective in confronting the real causes of oppression. Academics generally focus on debunking conspiracy theories rather than on exploring the social and cultural contexts in which they arise and the theories of power and political subjectivity they present.[35] A major problem with such critiques is that they simply presuppose that conspiracy theorists enjoy equal access to the sites where knowledge and authority are produced and circulated and the cognitive and material practices entailed. For racialized and impoverished subjects who are largely denied the rights of citizenship, challenging the structures of authority and the limits of discourse and perception constitutes a very real act of resisting the racial economy and the institutional and political-economic mechanisms that produce it.

Critiques that dismissed the alternative stories that arose during the epidemic failed to appreciate these stories' role in helping delta residents look beyond the disempowering rhetorics that pinned the blame for the epidemic on their beliefs and behaviors. These critiques failed to grasp how these stories revealed the logical leaps that provided the basis for official narratives. By refusing to listen to alternative narratives, progressive critics limited the power of their own analyses and helped to silence those people who knew racism intimately and could penetrate its institutional mechanisms.

I am not arguing that the narratives I present in this chapter are right and official narratives wrong—that would be a great conceit indeed. It would also thwart my efforts to extend the circulation of the cholera narratives that we heard and to show how intimately these very different sorts of stories are in dialogue with one another. It would limit my efforts to explore the social and cultural settings in which the cholera narratives arose, the material interests they served and helped shape, and the complex political subjectivities they constructed for all parties. The alternative narratives undermined the assignment of individuals, populations, places, and subjectivity to local or global categories and demonstrated the imaginary and destructive character of this process. These stories and epistemological issues continue to be, for some narrators, matters of life and death.

11 Local Numbers and Global Power
The Role of Statistics

There is one area of institutional effort that seems to be maximally apolitical, authoritative, and safe: the collection and dissemination of health statistics. Yet these numbers play a central role in shaping how infectious diseases are perceived as global, national, or regional phenomena and in stratifying the position of nation-states in terms of the health of their populations. Here we have a global discourse par excellence, one that is produced by rural clinics, urban hospitals, and other "local" institutions and transmitted through global hierarchies to WHO, whose jurisdiction is the entire world.

After it was founded in 1945, WHO became the global clearinghouse for annual reports and official health statistics as well as information regarding health-related laws and regulations. Statistics are circulated worldwide in the *Weekly Epidemiological Record (WER)* and other publications. The WHO constitution grants nation-states the authority to collect these statistics, a stipulation made more explicit in 1951:

> For the application of these Regulations, each State recognizes the right of the Organization to communicate directly with the health administration of its territory or territories. Any notification or information sent by the Organization to the health administration shall be considered as having been sent to the State, and any notification or information sent by the health administration to the Organization shall be considered as having been sent by the State.[1]

The legitimacy attached to the regulations developed by WHO, PAHO, and Pan-American and international health conferences was greatly augmented when these regulations were adopted as national law or incorporated into the rules and regulations of nation-states. Venezuela ratified the

1905 Washington Sanitary Convention in 1907, and the Pan American Heath Code of 1924 and the Additional Protocol of 1927 were directly incorporated in 1933 into the legislation that shaped MSAS.[2] Venezuelan President Rómulo Gallegos signed the WHO constitution into law in 1948. Its assertion that "the enjoyment of the highest standard of health is one of the fundamental rights of all human beings without regard to race, religion, political ideology, or economic social condition" must have appealed to the populist rhetoric of Gallegos's Partido Acción Democrática.[3]

These national laws and regulations shaped the bureaucratic structures that produce medical statistics. A flow chart published by the MSAS (figure 1, page 24) distinguishes four institutional levels: (1) hospitals and clinics, referred to as *puestos centinelas* (sentry posts), a category that also includes "community officials, neighborhood organizations, undertakers, teachers, pharmacists, and churches"; (2) the district epidemiologist; (3) the regional epidemiologist; and (4) the Departamento de Vigilancia Epidemiológica (Department of Epidemiological Surveillance) of the División de Enfermedades Transmisibles (Division of Communicable Diseases).[4] These offices are connected to the Servicio de Laboratorio (Laboratory Service). The information that must be submitted by the institutions in the first tier is progressively amalgamated by the district, regional, and national epidemiological offices. The national office creates both state-by-state and national summaries that are published in its *Boletín Epidemiológico Semanal*.

This process creates a flow of statistics from the "sentry posts" at the bottom to the national offices at the top, and then on to the international organizations, PAHO and WHO. Ideally, each statistic should be what Bruno Latour refers to as an "immutable mobile," an entity that can move between bureaucratic and other contexts without a change of meaning.[5] In order for this system to work, cases must be defined in accordance with a stable and universal code. The *International Classification of Diseases (ICD)*, first devised in the nineteenth century and periodically revised, attempts to impose a single classificatory schema on clinicians and statisticians around the world.[6] WHO controls the compilation of statistics and the amalgamation of statistics into broader and broader summaries. WHO also decides which composite data and technical analyses will move back down the hierarchy. The statistical compilations, guidelines, manuals, epidemiological bulletins, and other texts move in this direction. In general, however, physical texts, be they faxes or copies of weekly epidemiological reports, move only one node in either direction. For example, district and regional epidemiologists seldom receive epidemiological bulletins published by PAHO or WHO; instead, the national epidemiologist sends them MSAS's own reports and publications. WHO and PAHO technical manuals are translated and adapted in Caracas before being distributed to regional offices. In theory, the policies that determine what is counted and how it is passed along are shaped by globally distributed manuals (including the *ICD*), issues of *WER*, and international officials stationed in member countries.

The transnational replication of institutions and procedures for compiling medical statistics creates tremendous authority as well as colossal risks for international and national institutions. Once they accept international agreements regarding infectious diseases, nation-states are committed to providing international officials with the materials used to create precisely the sorts of national images that their governments most want to avoid. This process accords great powers of surveillance and regulation to WHO and PAHO, and nation-states secure the right to exercise control over the production of health statistics within their borders. It is nearly impossible for outsiders—individuals, communities, nongovernmental organizations, or other government agencies—to produce independent epidemiological evidence that could be used to challenge official representations. Some numbers never seem to burst out of their local starting gates, and others get disqualified before they can finish the race. When opposing discourses arise, they are by definition unofficial or even illegitimate.[7]

Since the production and dissemination of epidemiological statistics quintessentially embodies the workings of public health institutions and their specialized authority, tracing this process provides a privileged perspective on globalization and its effects. Whether you define the concept in terms of global "flows," processes of inclusion or exclusion, or the restructuring of national institutions in keeping with transnational dictates, the branches of public health agencies that keep statistics were globalized long ago.

CONSTRUCTING OFFICIAL STATISTICS IN DELTA AMACURO

Any depiction of international epidemiologists and public health officials as hegemonic bureaucrats who coolly survey a transnational terrain over which they have firm command would certainly infuriate the people who occupy these positions—or simply make them laugh. Public health institutions are generally subordinated to other government agencies, and they often get the short end of the budgetary stick. The opening days of the Latin American epidemic placed these institutions in a tremendously vulnerable position, and this exposure—and the strategies they used to deal with it—were especially apparent in how epidemiological statistics were collected.

Articles appeared on the front pages of local and national newspapers when rumors of the epidemic began to circulate in Tucupita, yet international awareness of the epidemic was virtually blocked by official statistics for Delta Amacuro: 735 cases and 9 deaths were reported for 1992, and 88 cases and 3 deaths for 1993.[8] The national epidemiologist could thus report to PAHO that in 1992 there were only 2,842 cases of cholera and 68 deaths in all of Venezuela.[9] Peru, Ecuador, Brazil, and Bolivia were reporting many more cases, so Venezuela received relatively little attention in the international press. As I have noted previously, Clara and I estimated that roughly 500 people died from cholera in Delta Amacuro in 1992 and 1993.

How were the official statistics compiled? The *prefecto*, or magistrate, for Pedernales, Horacio Rondón, provided an insider's account of how deaths in delta communities were converted into vital statistics. When he took the job, Rondón found that the previous magistrate had reported mortality statistics only rarely, even when they took place in town. Realizing that the deaths of *indígenas* "almost never get recorded," Rondón asked the *comisarios*, the leaders of larger *indígena* communities, to come by his office when they came to Pedernales and orally relay information on births and deaths. But even this attempt by a conscientious official did not yield more accurate statistics on cholera morbidity. Rondón was not allowed to make diagnoses like a physician. He recorded either *vómito y diarrea* (vomit and diarrhea) or *fiebre* (fever) as the cause of death. He concluded, "I couldn't put down, just imagine, that it was cholera, because I didn't know if it was cholera, and probably the *indígena* doesn't know that it was cholera either." Even when people died in communities that had *comisarios* (and many do not), and the *comisario* had the means of getting to Pedernales, cholera deaths remained invisible.

The underreporting hardly stopped there. During his interview Rodríguez showed me two sets of statistics. One, posted on the wall across from his desk, listed both "confirmed" and "suspected" cases; the other, a typescript, contained only "confirmed" cases. Rodríguez permitted me to photocopy the latter document, but I was not allowed to copy the more inclusive set. He explained the two sets of statistics as follows. At first he counted every case and death that clinicians attributed to cholera and sent the totals by fax to the national epidemiologist, Luís Echezuría. When these figures had surpassed the totals for Sucre state and nearly equaled those for Zulia, "the ministry told us, well, that they had to be run through the laboratory, with positive results. Okay, we started doing it the way they wanted. And from that moment on, we have been working on that basis."

No laboratory in the state was equipped to process cholera samples at the beginning of the epidemic. Rodríguez thus had to rely on taxis that connect

Tucupita to nearby cities. Even after the laboratory was installed, only a relatively small number of the patients treated at rural clinics were tested. Recall that Ricardo Campins stated, "I didn't take any stool samples because
we didn't have the specimen tubes, the special specimen tubes that [the Ministry of] Health was giving out. They never came during the month that I
was on La Tortuga. During the first month and a half of cholera I never saw
a specimen tube. I only saw them at the very end."

In any case, treating scores of gravely ill patients and attempting to halt
routes of transmission left clinicians little time to worry about rectal swabs.
How many people died from cholera in 1992 and 1993 in Delta Amacuro
state? The total, as stated by Rodríguez, was twelve, but the other document
on his wall listed sixty-three. During his interview Rodríguez shuffled between "positive" and "suspected" cases: "Because there are other deaths in
which, well, in which it was unfortunately not possible to take samples due
to the remoteness of the areas. . . . And epidemiologically one could say that
it was cholera." Adopting MSAS's laboratory-confirmation criterion created a wide gap between the perspectives of epidemiologists and clinicians.
Physicians could contribute only indirectly to cholera statistics by sending
samples to the laboratory. Their assessments did not, in the end, constitute
knowledge of cholera, as Campins noted: "The [regional] epidemiologist can
be watching an *indígena* die of profuse diarrhea and he will say that it's not
cholera until he sees a positive result from a specimen tube." MSAS laboratories became an obligatory passage point for statistics. No quantity of diarrhea or vomit and no death could be counted as an official case unless
cholera's fecal trace passed through one of these labs. Remarkably, personnel and equipment housed in a corner of the Luís Razetti Hospital shaped
what everyone else in the region—and from there to Geneva—could learn
about the epidemic.

As science studies specialists Geoffrey Bowker and Susan Leigh Star suggest, institutions need to forget, to erase information that is deemed irrel-
evant or potentially damaging, as much as they need to remember. At the
same time that some means of preserving information as long-term memory may be officially sanctioned (such as the statistics for "positive" cases
sent to Caracas), institutions have a "complex ecology of memory practices"
that shape how different types of information will be retained, if at all.[10]
That clinicians often resist their obligations to spend time filling out epidemiological forms, such as death certificates, thus may reflect not only their
reluctance to take time away from saving lives but also their recognition
that the forms of knowledge they control most directly are placed on a lower
rung in these institutional memory practices—although much higher than

those associated with nurses or laypeople. Campins was not complaining that he had to fill the specimen tubes but rather that he had none to fill—and that his clinical judgment did not, as it were, count. At the same time that this policy greatly multiplied MSAS statistical and representational control, it divided professionals within the institution: the clinical gaze was subordinated to microbiology and epidemiology.[11]

The low statistical counts also created a cavernous gap between epidemiological and popular discourses. As delta residents spoke with people from other communities, accounts of who had become ill and who had died circulated widely. Reports broadcast by Radio Tucupita and published in *Notidiario* and Caracas newspapers also provided a sense of the scale of the epidemic. On 16 September, *Notidiario* reported that MSAS had tallied 1,138 cases and 25 deaths.[12] On 12 November an article titled "Cholera Decimates the Warao" quoted the anti-cholera committees of various delta communities as saying that the tally had reached 5,000 cases, resulting in some 300 deaths.[13] Because the state had been able to render a ludicrous count into statistics that were deemed to be authoritative in Caracas, Washington, and Geneva, people's appreciation of the power of the state grew.

No one seemed more aware of this enigma than the political activists fighting discrimination in Delta Amacuro. Activist Graciela Ortega, in her fifties in 1992, was educated in English in Guyana. Possessed of an aristocratic air and a splendid sense of humor, she enjoyed conversing with me on the streets of Tucupita, winding back and forth between English, Spanish, and Warao. This scene inevitably drew a group of onlookers, who were amused by the linguistic acrobatics of the *indígena* and the gringo. A skilled negotiator, she later served as the first *indígena* director of ORAI. Suggesting that "at least six hundred, eight hundred, one thousand Warao died" from cholera, Ortega argued that MSAS epidemiologists required laboratory confirmation "because none of them wanted to tell the people the truth, they wanted to say that the government is doing a good job." Lacking their own epidemiological infrastructure, activists could not effectively challenge the official statistics or the political authority that lay behind them.

AND THE NUMBERS MARCHED ON

Statistics were transferred by radio once a week from rural clinics to the office of the regional epidemiologist, where the number of "suspected" and laboratory-confirmed cases and deaths and the number of patients hospitalized were tabulated. Rodríguez then faxed the total of "confirmed" cases to the national epidemiologist each week. He also presented cumulative totals of "positive" cases broken down by department (the major political division within the state), age, sex, and race. Although distinguishing *criollo* from "Warao" would seem to violate the official, race-blind policies that guide MSAS procedures nationally, it was a natural distinction in Delta Amacuro.

The weekly statistics from Tucupita arrived at MSAS's Department of Epidemiological Surveillance in Caracas. The weekly totals for the entire country were transmitted to Venezuela's PAHO representative in Caracas, and this official faxed the figures to Washington. In Washington the numbers went personally to Claudio Silva, a Brazilian epidemiologist who worked at the time in PAHO headquarters. Of medium build and with slightly graying hair, Silva has a youthful and informal manner, and he is equally at home in English, Spanish, and Portuguese. Silva put the numbers into a database that included cases, number of persons hospitalized, and deaths by country and province. Specifying regions within nation-states was important, Silva told me, because this procedure enabled PAHO to warn neighboring countries when cholera approached an international border. Statistics were published in the *Epidemiological Bulletin* and occasional reports titled *Cholera Situation in the Americas* and were sent to WHO's Global Task Force on Cholera Control and to organizations that participated in an inter-institutional coalition set up by PAHO that included the CDC, UNICEF, Care, the U.S. Army, USAID, the European Economic Community, and other institutions.

Epidemiologists at PAHO and WHO suspected that some nation-states were not fully complying with their obligation to report cholera cases. WHO linked underreporting to "fear that restrictions may be imposed on exports and on travel by their citizens, or that tourism may be affected."[14] Feliciana García, the head of WHO's Global Task Force on Cholera Control, pointed to the organization's reliance on offering carrots to countries suspected of withholding information in the absence of any available sticks. García is a young, attractive, and self-confident Spanish physician who was trained in Paris. She moves fluently in and out of English, Spanish, French, and Italian. She was the highest public health official in the world specifically charged with overseeing cholera prevention and treatment. Clara and I interviewed her in WHO's Geneva headquarters.

Feliciana García, Geneva, 5 January 1995

It is very sad but very true. The worldwide mentality regarding cholera is to blame, because it prompts a panic about being censured rather than having the opposite effect. Because when we make cholera an obligatorily reported disease, it's precisely to help countries combat cholera, to mobilize resources, to avoid unjustified control measures, to distribute medications. Yes, it's necessary, but notification is achieving the opposite effect in that some countries hide their cases out of fear of reprisals. . . .

When cholera arrived in Africa for the first time, when a country was characterized by a pandemic, it was a country that did not report cholera cases. It hid them for many weeks. This was tremendously important, because they should have taken measures to stop the infection, and they didn't take them because the country didn't want to provide notification that they had cholera conditions. To be sure, when they finally declared that they had a cholera epidemic it was because it had become impossible to hide it. So, then, from that point cholera overran the entire continent.

García's perspective was shared by Silva: "The argument that we at PAHO use with all countries, not just on that occasion [in 1991], but today in the face of any problem, is that you can't hide this type of situation generally. It's very difficult to hide situations of outbreaks of communicable diseases, not just because of their magnitude, but due to the gravity of the problem. It's something that becomes public knowledge."[15] Events in Delta Amacuro both confirm and qualify such statements. It was indeed difficult to keep powerful images of dehydrated cholera patients out of the newspapers and away from television cameras. Nevertheless, WHO and PAHO constitutions and practices granted nation-states so much power over the reporting of epidemiological statistics that it was easy to provide numbers that shielded countries from international scrutiny, even when "public knowledge" clearly contradicted them.

The underreporting problem was closely tied by officials to a second issue, that of "case definitions," meaning what counts as a case of cholera. In its guidelines WHO invokes the authority of the International Health Regulations to argue that "standard definitions should be used and certain information should be included in reports from all levels of the health system": "When cholera is newly suspected in an area, the International Health Regulations require that the diagnosis should be confirmed by laboratory investigations as soon as possible. Once the presence of cholera has been confirmed in an area, it is not necessary to confirm all subsequent cases. Neither the treatment nor the notification of suspected cases of cholera requires laboratory confirmation of the presence of *Vibrio cholerae* o1."[16]

Clinical knowledge does not provide a sufficient basis for confirming that a cholera epidemic has begun, so knowledge produced in the laboratory is epistemologically privileged when an outbreak is suspected. During an epidemic, however, microbiology takes a back seat to clinical epidemiology, weighing in periodically to reconfirm the authority of clinicians. Once cases have disappeared or the results of laboratory tests are predominantly negative, microbiology again becomes privileged.

In Venezuela, MSAS recontextualized WHO and PAHO guidelines: "It is not always possible to examine stool specimens for all suspected cases, especially when the outbreak is large and prolonged. Just as laboratory diagnosis is essential in order to establish the nature of the outbreak in an endemic zone and the presence of the disease in a recently infected area, it can be necessary to restrict laboratory examinations to representative samples for logistical reasons."[17]

Although WHO and MSAS guidelines both stated that laboratory identification of *Vibrio cholerae* was crucial at the outset of an outbreak and of lesser importance as it progressed, the grammatical framing of the MSAS statement opened the door to explicitly political considerations. By suggesting that laboratory analysis *"no siempre es posible"* (is not always possible) and that taking representative samples *"puede ser necesario"* (can be necessary), the Department of Epidemiological Surveillance reserved the right to require laboratory confirmation. MSAS distinguished "suspected" from "confirmed" cases, but WHO stated clearly that once the presence of *Vibrio cholerae* had been confirmed, "it is not necessary to make a distinction between suspect and confirmed cases; all should be reported as cholera."[18]

These guidelines provided MSAS with tremendous flexibility and impressive control over the representation of cholera. The distinction between "suspected" and "confirmed" cases, which was published months before cholera was reported in Venezuela, provided a ready means of creating two scientific and systematic methods of producing statistics. If the counts were too high for official comfort, the number of suspected cases could be relegated to the status of an official secret—that is, circulated only among MSAS officials, while the total for confirmed cases could be given to PAHO and WHO.

PAHO and WHO knew that countries were underreporting during the epidemic, but it wasn't until after the epidemic that the problem with case definitions was revealed. Dr. John Schwartz, a U.S.-based epidemiologist who was involved in PAHO's cholera efforts from the outset, described how officials learned of the problem. Schwartz is a bearded, strong, friendly fellow. Although he had been up all night with a new baby when we visited him in 1998, he patiently detailed PAHO's efforts to compile and disseminate accurate cholera statistics. He stated that although case definitions were "a big problem from the very beginning," the scope of the problem did not become apparent until 1993, when a questionnaire was sent out to individual countries that asked how they had compiled their statistics. PAHO discovered that Peru had counted all cases of acute watery diarrhea in persons five years of age and older as cholera, whereas some other countries had reported only confirmed cases. At that point the Communicable Diseases Program "tried to clarify in greater detail each country's definitions, how they were utilizing their definitions." Schwartz said that they "also tried to create a standardized format for reporting" and added that some countries accepted the standardized case definitions while others did not.[19]

Some PAHO and WHO officials complained about the production of epidemiological procedures, but they overlooked the way in which their institutions helped to create the problems. International guidelines set up an epistemological hierarchy that privileged microbiological above clinical knowledge, at least during certain phases of epidemics, and institutional structures granted nation-states complete authority over the statistics that public health organizations produced. Bypassing nongovernmental organizations, community groups, social movements, activists, and other parties strengthened the power of nation-states over the representation of cholera by giving health ministries a freer hand to do as they pleased with statistics as well as prevention and treatment efforts. The problems were not simply products of political pressure or individual misjudgment.

THE STATISTICAL IMAGINATION

What can we learn from statistical imaginings of the epidemic? European countries collected statistics in the eighteenth century, but these numbers were mainly kept behind locked doors. In the following century the circulation of statistics in printed form became a preoccupation. New numbers created new political technologies for classifying and enumerating people, a new "style of reasoning," and a statistical and probabilistic view of society that identified "normal" and "deviant" characteristics and populations.[20] Another view suggests that the growing administrative use of statistics derived more from disputes among bureaucracies, government regulators, and skeptical publics. Their use initially was a sign of weakness, not strength. Many bureaucrats actively resisted the growing ascendancy of quantification.[21]

Scientific writers use numbers, maps, charts, and diagrams to stratify their texts, creating layers of auto-referentiality by rhetorically bringing the referent of the work into the text itself.[22] Authors thereby attempt to shape how their findings are interpreted and how they will be recontextualized in future writings as "facts"; how often a scientific text is cited and how it is portrayed is where the scientific action lies. Since statistics seem to be so decontextualized—to exist apart from the institutional contexts in which they were created and the textual setting in which they are being presented—they are ready-made for circulation in future texts and contexts. This illusion of decontextualization is not simply an epistemological question; it is deeply embedded in the power of international regulatory organizations and nation-states to monopolize the production of statistics and to control the sites and technologies needed to produce them. In a study of the role of WHO and the *International Classification of Diseases,* Bowker and Star argue that disease categories and the statistics they produce are not immutable but rather are closely tied to the heterogeneous administrative contexts in which they are produced and circulated.[23] Nevertheless, these procedures cover up the traces of the contradictions between these multiple contexts and contrasting political and administrative demands; the decontextualized character of statistics is thus a carefully orchestrated effect.

Although the use of quantification in medicine and public health is often seen as a model of the power of statistics to enhance disciplinary authority, the struggle between clinical judgment and statistics in medicine is acute. Medicine and public health enjoy considerable prestige, but they also bear a substantial weight of public scrutiny, governmental supervision and regulation, and political intervention.[24] Cholera epidemics in the United States during the first half of the nineteenth century heightened popular mistrust of the medical profession and exacerbated discontent with its attempt to monopolize curing. John Snow's famous study of water-borne transmission in the London epidemic of 1854 and Robert Koch's discovery of *Vibrio cholerae* in 1883–1884 helped public health officials confront institutional challenges and gain authority.[25]

Epidemiologists would have us believe that medical statistics are politically neutral reflections of disease distribution because they use scientific, standardized procedures and case definitions. In their eyes politicians and panicky publics react irrationally, and, as a result, epidemiologists are pressured to underreport statistics, adopt case definitions that make national statistics incomparable, and use ineffective measures such as quarantines, travel restrictions, and embargoes. To counter this pressure officials at PAHO, WHO, the CDC, and other leading institutions strive valiantly to thwart the politicization of cholera by promoting scientific knowledge about disease as the sole guide for representations and concrete action.

This perspective fails precisely because it rests on a number of fundamental misunderstandings of the nature and effects of epidemiological statistics. Social statistics are never just about the objects they purport to measure; they constitute powerful imaginings of society and our place within it.[26] Bowker and Star argue that bureaucratic practices and larger questions of state formation, international relations, and, starting in the second half of the twentieth century, multinational corporations are built into the way epidemiological statistics are produced and read.[27] Accordingly, politicians and publics will always read cholera statistics as potent social and political forces. Such readings are neither irrational nor misinformed: statistics are not neutral numbers but rather are closely tied to schemes of social classification and governance.

Statistics are also closely tied to the institutional circumstances in which they travel. The authority of a set of numbers is related to the prestige of the agency with which they are identified. Tremendous cachet was attached to PAHO and WHO cholera statistics even though these institutions did not produce the numbers, were often skeptical of the numbers they received, and were largely powerless to end underreporting. Numbers produced by organizations not connected to the nation-state were not likely to be taken seriously, and statistics proposed by individuals who were not physicians or epidemiologists seldom even made it into the press.

The way statistics are produced, circulated, and reported is profoundly affected by institutional threats, whether existing or potential. This process is strikingly apparent in the way that Echezuría, clearly under pressure from the minister of health and the president, forced Rodríguez to include only confirmed cases, thereby hiding the extent of the epidemic in Delta Amacuro from international scrutiny. The production, aggregation, circulation, and interpretation of statistics was at each and every point embedded in these sorts of complex institutional and political relations. To pretend that underreporting was an aberration or that cholera statistics were ideally apolitical would simply be an invitation to reproduce the conditions that rendered these numbers problematic.

Statistics are powerful and dangerous. The way that numbers can cover their tracks, their histories, and their political economies of production, and the way that they can be inserted into almost any new context—their purported status as immutable mobiles—weaken institutional control over their circulation. PAHO and WHO were relatively powerless to challenge numbers that they doubted or even to perceive just how far the numbers departed from standard case definitions. Numbers travel longer and farther than their producers anticipate or desire; clearly, they can be used for purposes that are deemed inflammatory or illegitimate.

Let us not forget that these statistics referred to people who were sick and dying from cholera. We must reverse the abstracting and dehumanizing work done by numbers. Ever since efforts to control nineteenth-century cholera epidemics helped to create the category of the sanitary citizen, the disease has provided a key means of assessing the hygiene—or, modernity—of individuals and populations. The irrepressible social meanings of cholera statistics center on charged assessments of social worth, and, given the way that the disease has represented social inequality for nearly two centuries, comparisons between individuals, classes, communities, races, nations, and continents usually follow. When the disease is afoot, cholera statistics inevitably become contested sites that provide opportunities for exposing *and* legitimating gaps between the rich and the poor. In today's world it would be irresponsible not to add that international institutions—including not just PAHO and WHO but the World Bank, the International Monetary Fund, trade blocs, and others—play a role no less important in this regard than that of the national institutions they regulate.

12 Sanitation and Global Citizenship

International Institutions and the Latin American Epidemic

Will the real global cholera expert please stand up?

Quite a number of institutional players represented themselves as the bearers of perspectives that would modernize backward Tucupita and Barrancas. Ironically, the modernity they proclaimed bore a strong resemblance to precisely the perspectives that international experts on cholera described as outmoded and ineffectual. These experts were employed by the leading international public health institutions and constituted the epitome of authority. They decided how cholera was defined, prevented, and treated worldwide, and they not only shaped the institutions that had access to cutting-edge technologies and epistemologies for studying cholera in the lab and in the field but also set the standards for international reference laboratories. They determined which practices constituted modern modes of preventing and treating cholera and which practices should be thrown into the dustbin of public health history. They constructed global narratives of cholera, including accounts of where cholera was, whom it was infecting, and why.

The first cases of cholera in Latin America in the twentieth century appeared in Peru in January 1991, and in a little over eleven months, cholera had surfaced in most countries in the region. Cholera had not posed a problem in the Americas since the International Sanitary Bureau was conceived in 1902. International cooperation in the form of sanitary conferences had led to the formulation of agreements aimed at controlling cholera, yellow fever, plague, and smallpox.[1] Although officials were aware that endemic cholera had existed along the Texas and Louisiana coast of the United States starting in the 1970s, this fact failed to generate much concern.[2] Cholera did become a significant preoccupation in the 1970s, when the disease was widely reported in Africa. When it was speculated that it likely would be transmitted

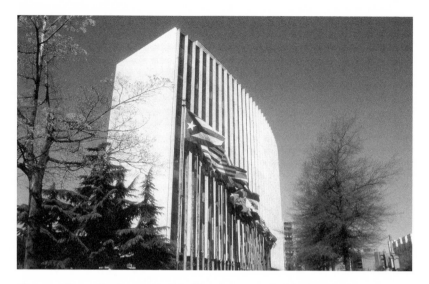

Photograph 35. Headquarters of the Pan American Health Organization, Washington, D.C. Photograph by Armando Waak, courtesy of the Pan American Health Organization.

to Brazil from former Portuguese colonies such as Mozambique, Brazil constructed cholera beds, trained medical personnel, and stockpiled medicines. Mysteriously, the disease never came. Cholera then disappeared from the agenda. Public health authorities seemed to think that the region was somehow immune from the disease. I was told that PAHO officials discarded copies of WHO cholera guidelines.

Nearly all of the PAHO officials with whom I spoke dated the end of this idyll to one moment of shock on 5 February 1991.[3] Dr. Richard Huntington tells the story well. Before being appointed director of PAHO's Disease Prevention and Control program, Huntington had worked in Kenya, Thailand, and Central America for the CDC. He is a tall, dark-haired man in his fifties, and his manner combines a strong sense of cordiality, gentility, and professionalism, as well as a touch of formality. The interview was conducted at the headquarters of PAHO (photograph 35).

Richard Huntington, Washington, D.C., 13 April 1999

It was quite remarkable when we met with the minister of Peru, Dr. Carlos Vidal. I remember very clearly our meeting . . . with [PAHO director] Dr. Guerra de Macedo in his office, in which Dr. Vidal told us that there were cholera cases in Peru, and we were all just stunned. What do we do? You know the response was very quick, but we had not been thinking about cholera for twenty years, or at least certainly the last ten years, after the threat from Africa, or the example of Africa, sort of disappeared from the mind. Cholera didn't seem to be a threat for the Americas. Looking back on it—of course, hindsight is twenty-twenty—we realized that was foolish. But it's hard to sustain a state of preparedness for ten or twenty years when the disease doesn't come. It came with a vengeance. . . .

We sort of said, "Well, what do we need to do?" And, actually, Dr. Guerra de Macedo, since I was head of epidemiology at that point, turned to me and said, "Well, you will lead the thing until I gather, you know, all the people I can lay my hands on," basically. And so, "Okay," you know, "what do we do?" We sort of laid down a plan of attack initially focusing on, of course, collecting as much information as we could in what areas of responsibility people had, and we developed it from there.

Peruvian public health officials had suspected that the disease might be cholera, but Vidal left for Washington before he knew for sure. He received confirmation there and informed PAHO director Dr. Caryle Guerra de Macedo. The famed meeting lasted less than an hour.[4] This must have been a worst-case scenario for an international public health organization: your job is to guard the hemisphere's health, and the minister of health of a member country announces that one of the most dreaded epidemic diseases is afoot.

Another of the participants at the meeting was Claudio Silva, a Brazilian epidemiologist who then worked in PAHO's Health and Human Development and Health Situation Analysis programs. Silva was right in the middle of PAHO's cholera program, visiting Latin American countries and compiling the statistics sent from PAHO offices in member countries. Clara and I met with him in his office in November 1999. I asked him what the participants did after leaving the meeting.

Claudio Silva, Washington, D.C., 8 November 1999

Well, I think that the first was to study, to read up on cholera in all of its many dimensions. Because really, even though we had at some point seen what cholera was, we had to review all its dimensions—those having to do with clinical diagnosis, those having to do with treatment, chemoprophylaxis, the *vibrio*'s resistance to the antibiotics that are used, its relationship to the major modes of transmission in terms of water, goods, person-to-person—all of the dimensions we needed to be able to talk about some mechanism of control, some form of control, right? And the aspect of social communication was very serious. It was a situation that we knew would generate panic among the population, and for that reason we would have to think about how to teach the population, how to inform it in such a way that the situation could be kept under control.

Medical education revolves around building a close relationship between text-based knowledge and clinical experience. Reading a section on cholera in a textbook or reference manual in medical school and having detailed knowledge of the disease are, to be sure, very different. In the interview Silva said that his crash course on cholera did not end after he had scoured all the materials at PAHO: he left for Peru in the second week of the epidemic "in order to continue learning alongside them as well as to assist in coordinating the [international] aid." PAHO officials had little idea of what was coming, as Silva noted: "I don't think that anyone, not anyone, suspected that [cholera] was going to have this kind of dissemination in the country"—let alone in the region as a whole.

The circulation of information about cholera was a central concern from the start. Whereas Huntington stressed PAHO's communication with member countries, Silva emphasized the transmission of information to the public and suggested that fear of cholera was itself a threat to public health. PAHO sought to shape how the epidemic would be reported by the press by issuing reports and giving press briefings. Guidelines published in the *Epidemiological Bulletin* outlined how national public health officials should control the flow of information.

WHO UNDER FIRE

WHO's response to cholera, like that of Venezuelan public health agencies, was deeply embedded in how the disease threatened WHO's institutional legitimacy. During roughly the first two decades following its founding in 1946, WHO, a specialized agency within the United Nations, was a model of institutional stability. It pursued a medicalized, disease-oriented agenda that focused on uncontroversial efforts to provide member countries with technical advice.[5] Hesitant forays into controversial issues such as family planning and health insurance brought harsh criticism—particularly from the United States—and WHO retreated into safer areas.

WHO's agenda changed as former colonies became sovereign nations and members pushed the agency to be more responsive to the needs of their citizens. In the 1970s a new director general, Halfdan Mahler, charted a much more activist course, one that focused on health rights and social inequality. Two controversies provide striking examples. First, in a response to corporate marketing strategies that contributed to infant mortality in poor areas, UNICEF, other multilateral organizations, and some countries pushed

WHO to adopt an international code that set standards for marketing breast milk substitutes. Second, WHO started an Action Programme on Essential Drugs that attempted to facilitate access to medicines in developing countries. In both cases WHO clashed with transnational companies that were based in industrialized nations.[6] Despite criticism from wealthier nations and intense lobbying from the transnationals, the World Health Assembly (WHO's governing body) passed both issues.

In the 1980s globalization and neoconservative politics challenged this activist agenda in powerful ways. Inaugurated in 1975 by Mahler, the "Health for All by the Year 2000" campaign spotlighted the links between poverty, disease, and health and reshaped discourses of international health around the world.[7] But an international restructuring of capital and power turned the slogan into bitter medicine.[8] The anti-internationalist politics of the Reagan administration, coupled with anger over the agenda of WHO and other UN agencies, led the United States to withhold its contributions to WHO and to the United Nations as a whole. This policy was strongly influenced by strategies produced in conservative think tanks. For example, the Heritage Foundation published a short book by John Starrels that attacked "Health for All" as part of a call for a "new International Economic Order" bent on regulating transnational corporations, redistributing wealth between the northern and southern hemispheres, and launching a campaign against free markets.[9]

Neoconservatives criticized WHO for becoming "politicized." This strategy presupposed the medicalization of health and the restriction of public health to narrowly scientistic questions, weakening awareness of the fact that the distribution of health and disease is always a question of politics and economics. At the same time, it covered its own tracks, making it harder to focus on the corporate and political agenda that lay behind attempts to make WHO apolitical. In the face of the budgetary crisis that resulted from the withholding of dues and the inability of poor member nations to make their contributions, WHO turned increasingly to extrabudgetary reliance on special funding from governments, nongovernmental organizations, and multilateral organizations. In turn, WHO accepted much greater external control, particularly by donors. As leading industrialized countries once again became dominant, WHO moved back to a more conservative agenda.[10]

Enter the Latin American cholera epidemic. Huntington, Silva, and others with whom I spoke did not think that PAHO had been attacked or even strongly criticized for how it handled the epidemic, despite its lack of preparedness. Indeed, the opening chapter of PAHO's recent institutional history focuses on the epidemic, describing it as having "exemplified the quintessential institutional story of PAHO in action."[11] It was WHO, which had worked actively on cholera for may years, that took a major political hit for its response to the Latin American epidemic.

The 4 December 1994 production of CBS News's *60 Minutes* focused on WHO's opposition to the use of cholera vaccine in Peru and Rwanda. Co-host Lesley Stahl opened the segment with the following statement:

> When Swedish scientists came up with a safe, proven oral vaccine against cholera, the deadly diarrheal disease that Third World countries live in fear of, the United States Army bought $4 million worth of it to inoculate American troops in the Persian Gulf. But when the Gulf War ended abruptly, the Army found itself with a large surplus, which it offered to donate to countries like Peru, where, in 1991, an epidemic struck 300,000 people. But before the Army could ship the vaccine, which protects against cholera for three years, the United Nations' World Health Organization threw a monkey wrench into the works. Why? That's what we set out to discover.[12]

Producer Howard Rosenberg pitted Colonel Jerry Sadoff, the chief of infectious diseases at the Walter Reed Research Institute in Washington, D.C., against Paul Thomas, the director of WHO's Programme for Control of Diarrhoeal Diseases.[13] In the segment Stahl took viewers on a tour of Lima. Shots of poor houses, piles of garbage, dirty rivers, and disheveled children provided visual images that directly equated cholera and "Third World countries" in an affectively charged way. No Peruvian public health officials appeared. Peruvians (and Rwandans) were cast as pathetic figures waiting for assistance from the north, lacking professional or critical voices. CBS accused WHO of opposing use of the vaccine "to protect their own bureaucratic turf," of being "stuck in some sort of time warp," and of pushing "a political agenda" that was aimed at getting "the politicians to clean up the water."[14] These claims were expressed by Stahl and Colonel Sadoff. WHO, which is charged with determining what counts as modern practices and condemning outmoded responses, was itself portrayed as premodern and anti-scientific.

CBS News did not mention that two doses of the oral vaccine must be administered, preferably a week apart, or that it takes some time to build immunity. Thomas told me, when we spoke in Geneva in January 1995, that CBS had refused to broadcast a brief rejoinder. In the end, WHO was cast in the role of the baby-killer, an ironic replay in reverse of the infant-formula controversy of the 1970s. The epidemiological profile of the Peruvian epidemic—the fact that children under five did not figure prominently in terms of mortality or morbidity—was not mentioned. WHO's public information packet (contained in the "Cholera Information Kit") states that "even in the midst of a cholera outbreak, more children die from *other* causes of diarrhoea. *Approximately 120 persons died from cholera in the first three weeks of the outbreak in Peru. However, it is estimated that during the same period ten to twenty times more Peruvian children—and almost 200,000 globally—died from diarrhoea due to other causes. These children have been given little attention in the press.*"[15] This point received little attention in the *60 Minutes* program.

A leading U.S. Army public health physician charged that WHO was rejecting biomedicine in favor of politics. CBS seemed to ask why the politicized, indifferent, and antiquated WHO remained in control when U.S. capital, technology, and goodwill could do the job better. The program presented the convenient notion that biomedicine can take care of cholera without having to worry about economic inequalities or structural adjustment, as if cholera vaccine could also inoculate the poor against these factors. The program caused quite a stir in the United States, catalyzing another anti–United Nations, anti-WHO salvo. It led people of a variety of political persuasions to believe that WHO was coldly and bureaucratically turning its back on poor children. Thomas told me that criticism coming from the United States following the program was so strong that it threatened WHO's precarious funding.[16]

PLACING CHOLERA IN SPACE AND TIME

Among its many functions, WHO coordinates the collection and circulation of epidemiological statistics worldwide. A special section at the end of each weekly issue of the *Weekly Epidemiological Record (WER)* lists national totals for obligatorily reported diseases: cholera, plague, and yellow fever. How a nation-state registers in these pages is often a matter of intense official anxiety, given that this information is disseminated to every nation-state; these numbers are also incorporated into press accounts, official decisions regarding health-related trade and travel restrictions, and warnings offered by embassies, consulates, and travel agents to tourists. WHO's Global Task Force on Cholera Control bears the responsibility for weaving together myriad cholera stories into weekly announcements of statistics, periodic articles in *WER*, annual summaries of information on cholera, manuals destined for use by public health authorities worldwide, and other materials. The way WHO characterized the Latin American epidemic was thus crucial. What epidemiologists in Geneva, Dhaka, Washington, and Atlanta said affected how journalists and public health officials in Venezuela portrayed cholera and attempted to control it. In turn, how officials in Venezuela portrayed cholera shaped what the most powerful health officials in the world said about the disease.

WHO's first mention of the Latin American cholera epidemic appeared on 8 February 1991. After stating that the Peruvian Ministry of Health had reported "an outbreak of cholera" that began on 31 January, the statement concludes: "This is the first time that cholera has been reported in South America during the current pandemic which started in 1961."[17] This brief report provides a sense of the scope, speed, and power of the circulation of epidemiological statistics: just over a week after the epidemic was believed to have begun, its existence was officially noted in *WER*. The Peruvian experience had been located within global cholera narratives. One week later another brief note placed the number of cases at 7,089 and deaths at 49; this article specifies the "causative agent" as "*Vibrio cholerae* 01 biotype El Tor, serotype Inaba."[18] The epistemological authority of microbiology had already been incorporated within authoritative representations of the epidemic.

A more in-depth analysis of the epidemic appeared on 1 March 1991. It begins with a "Brief Historical Review" of cholera.

> Cholera is one of mankind's oldest diseases. During the nineteenth century it reached Europe for the first time and caused six major pandemics, earning its reputation as a killer disease. After the sixth pandemic, cholera returned to Asia, its region of origin.
> The seventh pandemic began in 1961 when *Vibrio cholerae*, biotype El Tor, spread outside its endemic area in the Celebes (Sulawesi), in Indonesia, probably because of increased population movements.[19]

This passage illustrates the powerful influence of a chronotope.[20] Medical topographies of disease have played a key role in epidemiology ever since the rise of medical geography, or geographical epidemiology, in the late eighteenth century,[21] and contemporary epidemiologists continue to describe the distribution of diseases in terms of categories of person, place, and time.[22] Epidemiological discourse structures time in narrative frames that impose Aristotelian qualities of beginning, middle, and end onto diseases.[23] The centrality of etiological reasoning in epidemiology, as frequently expressed in "causal webs" or "assemblages," provides a narrative device for connecting social, biological, and spatial elements and ordering them in temporal sequences and interpretive frameworks. In these frameworks space is divided primarily into regions—for example, Africa, the Americas, Asia, and Europe—and countries. Time is organized in chronological terms vis-à-vis the Christian calendar; years form the basic units, and months are used to describe the spread of cholera within regions. Precise dates generally refer to discur-

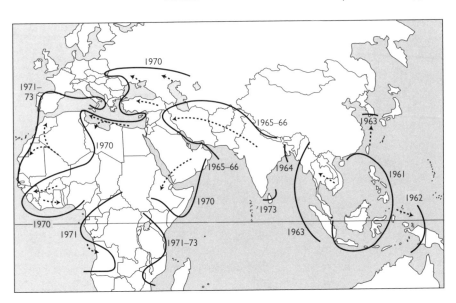

Map 3. Global spread of cholera, 1961–1973, based on map from the *Weekly Epidemiological Record* 66, no. 9 (1991): 61. Courtesy of the World Health Organization.

sive and institutional events, particularly the announcement of diagnoses or laboratory results, their transmission to PAHO and WHO, and earlier mentions in epidemiological publications. By March 1991 a medical topography had linked Peru to nineteenth-century Europe and to Asia, past and present, as well. Even before we get to Peru, the Latin American outbreak is situated within a master narrative that purports to track the "spread" of cholera through vast stretches of space and time.

The cholera chronotope was calibrated in terms of seven "pandemics" and major events within them, providing a schema for organizing cholera stories and weaving them into larger narratives. The opening sentence of "Cholera in 1991," an annual summary of WHO cholera epidemiology, places the Latin American epidemic in a vast chronotopic framework: "In 1991, the pandemic of cholera El Tor, which started in 1961 in the Celebes (Sulawesi), in Indonesia, finally completed its encirclement of the globe."[24] Modes of representation such as maps and tables interact with the text in fascinating ways. The following maps are based on those that appeared in WHO's annual summaries on cholera for 1991 and 1992.[25] One map (map 3) provides a chronotopic representation of the seventh pandemic in visual form. The arrows trace the "movement" of cholera across vast stretches of time and space. Two other maps (maps 4 and 5) are of tremendous social and political-economic significance. Map 4 divides countries into three categories: (1) "Already infected in 1990" (shaded), (2) "newly infected or re-infected" (dark cross-hatching), and (3) "imported cases" (a single black dot). The map also includes an implicit fourth category, countries not reporting any cases (depicted in white). Map 5 uses shading and ranges of statistics to map Latin American countries in terms of their location in the geography of cholera; black marks the epicenter in Peru.

Tables provide more detailed information. Here the story is told by specifying the number of reported cholera cases and deaths as divided by region and country. One of the richest tabular representations appears in WHO's annual summary for 1992.[26] In table 1 we see the story of the first two years of the Latin American epidemic as told by the date on which the first case was reported and by a comparison of morbidity and mortality in 1991 and 1992. This table presents the data in such a way as to facilitate nation-by-nation comparisons regarding (1) the temporal sequence in which countries entered into cholera topography, (2) the number of cases and deaths in each, and (3) the way these statistics changed during the second year of the epidemic. Statistics get connected to nation-states, which in turn are placed in categories of cholera morbidity and laid out in powerful visual representations. To be sure, WHO and PAHO consistently and vigorously oppose quarantines, trade embargoes, and other sanctions against countries reporting cholera cases. Nevertheless, the statistics that they are required to compile and the documents that they disseminate play a key role in shaping international images of countries and their populations in terms of infectious diseases. Particularly when reported by the media and used by individual nation-states, these epidemiological statistics help project medical profiling on a global scale.

These time-space connections were perhaps nowhere as naturalized and powerful as in references to places of origin. The association of cholera with Asia, particularly the Indian subcontinent, was formerly reflected in the designation of the disease as "Asiatic cholera" or "Indian cholera."[27] The British used cholera in their assertion that they had the right and duty to maintain colonial dominance over India. The disease became so connected to India that other countries blamed the British for bringing cholera from India to Europe; it was so deeply embedded in colonial discourses that it was used to criticize British imperialism.[28] When WHO cast Peru as the origin of cholera in Latin America, it applied the imprimatur of the highest public health institution in the world to such modes of imagination.

WHO is surrounded by political, scientific, and institutional controversies,

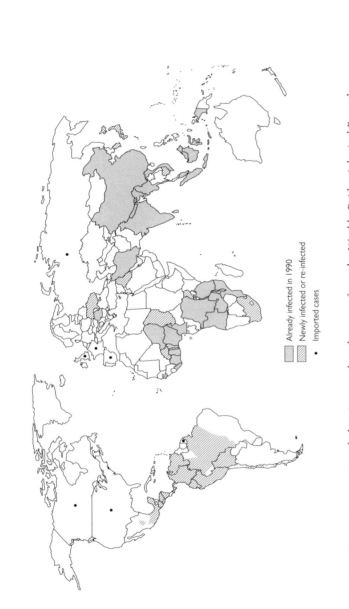

Map 4. Countries reporting cholera in 1991, based on map from the *Weekly Epidemiological Record 34,* no. 21 (August 1992). Courtesy of the World Health Organization.

Already infected in 1990

Newly infected or re-infected

• Imported cases

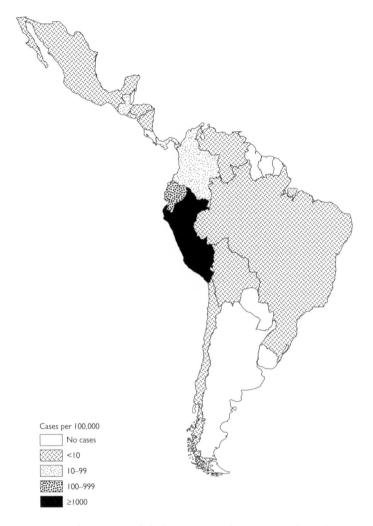

Cases per 100,000

	No cases
	<10
	10–99
	100–999
	≥1000

Map 5. Incidence rates of cholera in Central America and South America, 1991, based on map from the *Weekly Epidemiological Record* 67, no. 34 (1992): 255. Courtesy of the World Health Organization.

Table 1. Cholera in the Americas, 1991–1992

Date of First Report [d/m/y]	Country	Cumulative Cases		Cumulative Deaths	
		1991	1992	1991	1992
23/01/91	Peru	322,562	212,642	2,909	727
01/03/91	Ecuador	46,320	31,870	697	208
10/03/91	Colombia	11,979	15,129	207	158
08/04/91	United States of America	26	102	—	1
09/04/91	Brazil	1,567	30,309	26	363
12/04/91	Chile	41	73	2	1
13/06/91	Mexico	2,690	8,162	34	99
24/07/91	Guatemala	3,674	15,395	50	207
19/08/91	El Salvador	947	8,106	34	45
26/08/91	Bolivia	206	22,260	12	383
10/09/91	Panama	1,178	2,416	29	49
13/10/91	Honduras	11	384	—	17
12/11/91	Nicaragua	1	3,067	—	46
29/11/91	Venezuela	15	2,842	2	68
14/12/91	French Guiana	1	16	—	1
03/01/92	Costa Rica	—	12	—	—
09/01/92	Belize	—	159	—	4
05/02/92	Argentina	—	553	—	15
06/03/92	Suriname	—	12	—	1
03/06/92	Canada	2	4	—	—
05/11/92	Guyana	—	576	—	8
	TOTAL	391,220	354,089	4,002	2,401

SOURCE: Data drawn from World Health Organization, "Cholera in the Americas, 1991–1992/ Le choléra dans les Amériques, 1991–1992," *Weekly Epidemiological Record* 68, no. 21 (21 May 1993): 149–155, table 2. Courtesy of the World Health Organization.

and the accounts in *WER* are written in such a way as to steer clear of these disputes. They are published anonymously, thereby enabling officials to speak with an authoritative institutional voice. Careful scrutiny suggests, however, that even this most seemingly homogeneous, self-contained, epidemiological mode of representation is heteroglossic—that is, it incorporates a number of different vocabularies and voices.[29]

WER reports often accord agency to cholera. Although the bacteria is capable of relatively little movement, being transmitted through the movement of water, food, and people, individual human beings rarely stand as agents in these narratives. The most frequent grammatical objects in these constructions are geographic entities. The phrase "cholera invaded West Africa" is typical. This metaphorical attribution of agency to *Vibrio cholerae*, which was also apparent in the way that public health authorities narrated the epidemic in the delta, enjoys a truly global distribution. *WER* accounts of cholera are also double-voiced: they are tied into multiple discourses simultaneously through their vocabularies.[30] These documents were written by and for specialists—primarily physicians and public health officials— and they draw on the lexicons associated with epidemiology, microbiology, ecology, clinical medicine, and public health. We thus read about serogroups, biotypes, ribotypes, and serotypes of cholera, each with its respective name and/or number, as well as fecal coliforms, ORT (oral rehydration therapy), chemoprophylaxis, morbidity and mortality, attack rates, excreta disposal, and the like. The use of these terms enhances the discursive authority of epidemiological texts and accords to specialists rights over the production and reception of the cholera discourse. Few references are made to non-specialists or to other types of texts. Such esoterica help to construct the epidemiological gaze, which is capable of perceiving microbiological and clinical objects that would escape the layperson's eye.

Nevertheless, cholera texts are connected intertextually to popular vocabularies and perspectives. For example, the frequent use of verbs associated with war casts cholera in the metaphorical guise of a hostile army: "In 1970 cholera invaded West Africa which, apart from an outbreak in 1868 in the Senegambia region and another poorly reported incident in 1893, had always remained free from the disease."[31] *WER*'s first extended discussion of the Latin American epidemic begins its assessment of "the current epidemic in Peru" by noting the bacteria's previous munificence: "Only one region of the world, South America, had been spared by cholera during this pandemic."[32] In these reports cholera also *strikes,* and epidemics *gather strength.* Nouns drawn from the same lexicon are often incorporated into verb phrases: "Cholera also made many raids into the industrialized countries during the 1970s."[33] The use of *raids* is interesting since it seems to present cholera cases in industrialized countries as the result of sporadic foreign invasions rather than a lingering presence, thereby helping to reproduce a hiatus between "First" and "Third" worlds. The term *surveillance* is used frequently in cholera narratives.[34] Military metaphors may make the use of direct military and police force in supposedly consent-based health measures seem more legitimate, natural, and invisible.[35]

More than simply adding rhetorical pizzazz to technical reports, heteroglossic features enable these texts to project an authoritative, self-contained, and auto-referential image *and* to remain open to penetration by other kinds of lexicons and discourses. The analysis of the epidemic that appeared on 1 March 1991 in *WER* links epidemiology with popular fear by stating that cholera is "earning its reputation as a killer disease" in nineteenth-century epidemics.[36] Given the fascination with and fear of infectious diseases projected by the popular media, this infusion of popular images helped shape the political economy of epidemiological discourse.

Chronotopes in WHO publications cast geographic regions and nation-states as natural units of disease transmission, surveillance, and containment. Texts, tables, and maps compare regions and countries in ways that create hierarchies of success and failure in combating cholera, and annual summaries provide powerful points of comparison. National pride is particularly on the line with regard to case-fatality rates;[37] countries that reported that less than 1 percent of cholera patients had died could claim victory on behalf of their public health systems.[38] "Cholera in 1992" calls the difference between the Latin American average of 1 percent and Africa's 11.7 percent "striking."[39]

Interestingly, WHO maps commonly include the following statement: "The designations employed and the presentation of material on this map do not imply the expression of any opinion whatsoever on the part of the World Health Organization concerning the legal status of any country, territory, city, or area or of its authorities, or concerning the delimitation of its frontiers or boundaries." WHO seems to recognize the tremendous power of *WER* to shape international and national agendas. Indeed, if the emergence of International Health Regulations, the *International Classification of Diseases,* and WHO itself was connected to the formation of and transformations in nation-states and international relations, such disclaimers would seem to be oriented more toward preserving the illusions that medicine and politics are unrelated and that epidemiological statistics can be read apolitically than toward preventing the politicization of numbers and institutions that are shaped exclusively by medical knowledge.[40] The structure of *WER* accounts invited readers to connect statistics regarding "a killer disease" with particular nation-states. Such distinctions as "free from the disease," "imported," "newly infected or re-infected," and "already infected in 1990" imposed spatial and temporal projections that were far from neutral or politically inconsequential. Just as individuals and social communities are assigned the status of either sanitary citizens or unsanitary subjects, countries face the prospect of being thrust into the category of unsanitary states. Map 4 uses seemingly objective and politically neutral numbers in placing some countries in white areas, signaling their status as sanitary states; for others, the darkness of the shading indicates the degree to which they have been thrust into the realm of the unsanitary state.

INTERNATIONAL EXPERTS ON EPIDEMIOLOGY

Starting in February 1991, accounts of the Latin American epidemic were published in leading scientific journals, including *The Lancet, Science, American Journal of Tropical Medicine and Hygiene, Journal of Infectious Diseases,* and *Journal of the American Medical Association.* Many of these works were more open than the cautious *WER* to the infusion of popular discourses. The organizing principle behind many of these international narratives was precisely the same one that structured accounts of cholera in Venezuela—social inequality. Leading cholera expert Robert Tauxe put the case succinctly: "Cholera is a disease of poverty."[41] Imagining social inequality and converting it into a nexus of causal factors in the transmission of cholera played a central role in publications that crucially shaped how the epidemic was perceived by public health officials, journalists, politicians, publics, and even patients worldwide.

The opening lines of "Cholera in the Nineties," which appeared in *CDC Briefs,* characterize the epidemic in unequivocal terms:

> When one thinks of cholera, images of pre-twentieth-century sanitation come to mind . . . sewage in the streets, children suffering miserably. Does this sound like a plague from long ago?
>
> Not so. After an absence of nearly a century, epidemic cholera has reappeared in the Americas. Hundreds of thousands of cases of cholera have been reported in the past year in many South American countries. The death toll is estimated to be around 4,000, but officials have concluded that the numbers would have been much higher if modern treatment had not been available.[42]

The article calls up the historical imaginings of poverty, filth, suffering, and backwardness with which cholera is associated and then connects them to contemporary Latin America. These powerful images are juxtaposed with the concept of "modern treatment," placing the epidemic into a dramatic and perilous confrontation between modernity and its opposite.

This process of disconnecting Latin America from the modern world is also apparent in the way many leading international cholera experts represented the epidemic. Tauxe is the chief of one of the branches of the CDC's National Center for Infectious Diseases and a faculty member at the Rollins School of Public Health and the Department of Biology of Emory University. The author of more than 150 journal articles and book chapters, he is one of the leading experts on cholera worldwide and the co-author of a chapter on the Latin American epidemic that appears in an influential reference work on the disease.[43] Tauxe provided this description of the epidemic: "The explosive spread of cholera in Peru and other countries occurred in large, poor urban populations. Millions of people in the urban slums of Latin America lack safe piped water and sewage disposal. They live crowded together, in primitive circumstances, eating 'fast food' from street vendors and storing their drinking water in whatever buckets can be found."[44] This statement brings together two of the most prevalent themes in the international epidemiological literature on the Latin American epidemic: the failure of nation-states to provide such crucial sanitary services as potable water and sewage, and the poverty of the citizens themselves.

PAHO cited work by Tauxe and the CDC when it identified deficiencies in municipal water systems as the major means of transmission of the disease in two Peruvian cities. It went on to state that "this water quality situation is representative of many countries of Latin America and the Caribbean."[45] What was the source of the problem? PAHO suggested that the Peruvian state was both too organized and too disorganized, suffering from "excessive governmental centralization" and a failure to plan and control such processes as urban growth, which had taken place "in a disorganized fashion."[46] Authorities were criticized for being unconcerned with water-quality surveillance and for failing to correct problems when they were noted.

Critical epidemiologists, who systematically explore links between health and political economy, criticized perspectives that blamed the epidemic on the behavior of individuals, emphasizing structural factors. Ecuadorian epidemiologist Jaime Breilh analyzed municipal data in showing how conditions fostered by macroeconomic deterioration correlated with cholera morbidity.[47] Norman Gall suggests that the epidemic must be placed in the context of macroeconomic changes in Latin America during the 1970s and 1980s. In the case of Peru, he cites population increase, rapid urbanization, hyperinflation, the effects of neoliberal economics on health infrastructures and real wages, and a dramatic rise in malaria, dengue, yellow fever, leprosy, and tuberculosis. He thus places cholera within "the polarization of health," a growing medical gap between rich and poor. Nevertheless, he seems to undercut his argument by concluding with respect to "Third World countries" that "their fate is in their own hands."[48]

Similarly, causal factors were sometimes placed in a timeless world of tradition rather than in history, as Tauxe and Paul Blake have suggested: "As in the time of the Incas, raw sewage is used to irrigate and fertilize fruits and vegetables that are often eaten without cooking."[49] Similarly, Tauxe wrote that the lack of modern hygiene left populations "at risk for ancient scourges."[50] Writers such as Richard Guerrant stressed that Europe and the United States embraced the sanitary reform movement—a major point of entry into modernity—in the nineteenth century, thereby rendering them immune from a cholera epidemic in this era: "It was the fear of cholera that drove the sanitary revolution with improved sewage disposal and water supplies in Western Europe and in the United States in the last century. . . . We can only hope that the fear of cholera in the Western Hemisphere can drive a similar sanitary revolution in the 1990s."[51] Here we find a classic modernist narrative, a tale of a decisive rupture that separates premodern and modern worlds. The sanitary revolution becomes the quintessential means of separating sanitary from unsanitary states. It seems to apply to both halves of the nation-state equation, separating states that do not invest in sanitary infrastructures from those that brought their revolutions to successful conclusions, and nations (meaning peoples) that failed to embrace hygiene from those that internalized modern hygiene and medicine.

These statements oversimplify the story in two significant ways. First, sanitation was often rendered as a question of "investment"; recall the title of the World Bank's World Development Report for 1993: "Investing in Health." PAHO stated that unless Latin American governments made "sufficient investment in environmental health," cholera and other diseases would continue into the distant future.[52] PAHO noted that it had raised "over US $21 million from the international community" to invest in Latin American health, while it estimated that it would take over $21 billion over ten years "to correct deficiencies and return the Americas to a situation in which it is no longer susceptible to epidemic cholera."[53] PAHO suggested that the choices were stark: "The countries of the Region have little choice: either they make the necessary investments in environmental health interventions, including pollution control, or they pay the consequences in terms of economic loss as well as suffering, disease, and death."[54]

The notion that Latin American governments could freely choose whether to spend public funds in this fashion was largely illusory when international lending agencies were pressing them to reduce public expenditures. In suggesting that these expenses were "beyond the means of some Latin American countries," Tauxe and Blake seemed to recognize that these exhortations were unrealistic. By placing such tremendous burdens on the shoulders of the same Latin American governments that they accused of negligence, incompetence, and inefficiency, authors and international agencies created pessimistic projections that failed to identify the roots of sanitary and health problems. Indeed, the word *investment* constituted a misleading metaphor that created the impression that Latin American governments had simply made the wrong decisions. PAHO's assertion that "all of this could have been avoided with timely investments in water and sanitation infrastructures" made about as much sense as blaming the homeless for failing to help themselves by investing in the stock market.

A second oversimplification was encapsulated in recurrent invocations of John Snow's 1854 demonstration in London, which identified the role of environmental contamination in creating cholera epidemics and "prompted the improvement of sanitation services to prevent the spread of the disease."[55] Snow's success story was used as a compelling model of how modernity could be achieved: scientists would generate authoritative knowledge that public health officials would use to enlighten the press, politicians, and public, thereby catalyzing the modernization of institutions, infrastructures, and behavior. Like public health officials in Delta Amacuro, international authorities suggested that the fear inspired by cholera was the catalyst that sparked sanitary revolutions.[56] (It was precisely this imagining of the relationship between biomedicine and politics that fueled María Vargas's identity as a crusader for hygiene and modernity.) Since the science was theoretically accessible to everyone, international epidemiologists concluded that the problem in Latin America must be either the failure of public health officials there to disseminate this knowledge or the inability or unwillingness of politicians and citizens to embrace it. By bringing the nineteenth-century discovery of *Vibrio cholerae* into the story, relations were created among microbiological, statistical, ecological, clinical, and demographic understandings that were used to project a model of how decisions should be made, with scientists directing politicians and the public.

Such stories of the authority of epidemiology and public health rest, historians tell us, on an invented history. Sanitary reforms in Europe and the United States were carried out despite acrimonious debate between proponents of various theories of cholera and other infectious diseases. The arguments continued long after Filippo Pacini had identified *Vibrio cholerae* in 1854 and Robert Koch's work in 1883–1884 on the bacteria had gained acceptance.[57] Cholera epidemics were probably more of a distraction from than a stimulus to sanitary reform, and few institutional responses to epidemics had any lasting impact.[58] Nineteenth-century sanitary reforms resulted from economic changes and the growth of state regulation of the lives of the poor. Moreover, suggestions that this revolution had not yet come to Latin America erased the importance of sanitary reform movements in Latin America, which began in the eighteenth century.[59] In reality, Venezuelan Arnoldo Gabaldón, who was trained in Germany and the United States as well as in Venezuela, established in 1936 the Escuela de Malaria (the Malarial School) in Aragua state, which trained generations of sanitarians from all over Latin America and beyond. He certainly would be shocked to learn that the sanitary revolution that he started, which changed the face of Venezuelan towns and cities, had been erased from the record. García Márquez's protagonist Juvenal Urbino would be shocked to learn that he had not brought modernity and hygiene to Colombia after all!

Discourses of poverty played no less central a role in the accounts of the epidemic offered by international epidemiologists than in those presented by their Venezuelan counterparts. PAHO linked the poverty-cholera connection to its own institutional history: "The epidemic drove home, in alarming terms, the truth of PAHO's basic message—without socioeconomic development there can be no health and, without health, social and economic progress will grind to a halt."[60] PAHO also suggested in 1991 that health improvements "have not been distributed equitably throughout the entire population"[61] and that "the most important factor relating to cholera deaths has been access to and use of health services."[62]

Note the double-voiced character of the statement regarding accessibility. While "access to" health services points to broader issues of social inequality, "use of" places the burden on patients and their communities, thereby moving PAHO's conclusions in the direction of rhetorics that individualize and blame. PAHO later repeated the same statement with a coda, suggesting that the problem revolved around certain cholera victims: those "usually not seeking care or arriving late at health facilities."[63] This statement paralleled assertions made later in Delta Amacuro state regarding *indígenas'* purported rejection of institutional care in favor of "shamans." Even though PAHO did characterize the problem as one of "structural poverty," which countered rhetorics that blamed cholera on the individuals it infected,[64] in 1994 it stated that although "cholera was a disease almost exclusively of the poor, . . . those with some resources quickly learned how to decontaminate their water or obtain clean water, and cholera became a disease of those without means and knowledge."[65] As did Venezuelan accounts, PAHO individualized and reduced poverty and cholera, at least in part, to questions of knowledge and behavior.

Practices relating to water and food, attendance at fiestas, the failure of health education programs, and the nefarious figure of the street vendor had central roles in the accounts of international epidemiologists, just as they did in accounts offered by Venezuelan officials. Epidemiologists cited the "health-related behaviors" of communities in which cases were concentrated. Failure to boil drinking water was emphasized, along with such practices as storing water in open-mouthed vessels, washing one's hands in drinking water, and making contact with water while scooping it out.[66] The failure to wash one's hands with soap prior to handling food or water was often cited. PAHO pointed to the importance of "traditional and local food customs" and envisioned the epidemic as an opportunity for changing them.[67]

Tauxe and Blake brought together a number of tropes: "The food habits of the population may also put some Latin American populations at increased risk for cholera. Fish and shellfish are often consumed raw or nearly so, often as ceviche, a dish of raw fish and shellfish with variable exposure to lemon juice. Street vendors sell home-prepared foods and beverages held for many hours at warm ambient temperatures."[68] In these accounts, practices that placed populations at risk seemed to emerge from tradition and culture, not from the global economic constraints faced by people suffering from poverty and malnutrition. Given PAHO's status as the preeminent public health institution in the western hemisphere, and given the dissemination of its reports to all its member countries, the appearance of these tropes in subsequent statements by Venezuelan officials and the press is far from surprising.

A study conducted by CDC and Peruvian researchers and published in the prestigious British journal *The Lancet* blamed attendance at fiestas for increasing consumption of contaminated food and drink.[69] Statements regarding fiestas, such as this one from PAHO, contained messages regarding class and race: "Cases proliferated in the poor neighborhoods of Guayaquil, and by the end of March, following festivities that brought rural inhabitants to the city, there began to be reports of cases in various parts of El Guayas Province."[70] Accounts told by officials in Tucupita were reminiscent of a PAHO report that placed new outbreaks "mainly in some of the provinces in the mountains" in Ecuador in October 1991: "The latter [outbreak] has been attributed to religious ceremonies among the indigenous populations living in Cotopaxi and Tungurahua provinces. The preparation and consumption of food during funeral services of cholera cases in these communities also were found to be associated with the occurrence of cases."[71] Street vendors of food and drink were identified as purveyors of cholera in PAHO accounts as well: "Many operate as itinerant peddlers, including thousands of street vendors who sell food under unhygienic conditions and without any type of sanitary control."[72] Selling "a variety of traditional foods" on the street was identified as a longstanding "traditional practice in Latin America."[73] At the same time, the proliferation of street vendors and customers who sought quick, cheap meals close to their work sites were tied to modern labor practices. Street sales were thus placed both in premodern *and* modern realms, where they represented the worst of both worlds.

PAHO urged public health authorities to regulate the circulation of information about cholera, pressing them to make public announcements, create special informational programs, and "conduct special workshops and briefings to keep the media well-informed and advised, to prevent dissemination of misinformation, erroneous concepts, or inappropriate reaction [sic] to cholera."[74] The organization reported that it obtained $2.1 million from the Netherlands to create a "social communications program."[75] Such statements suggested that the voice of science could provide the knowledge and means for charting modern, rational reactions to cholera, while those of politicians, social movements, and the public simply provided obstacles.[76]

Characterizing health education as "probably the most important component of a cholera control program," PAHO pointed to the failure of educational efforts. It placed this assessment in the voice of regional governments themselves, noting that eighteen countries had reported to the organization that education regarding water and sanitation were "in general insufficient" and that eight "considered this to be a serious shortcoming."[77] In some cases this failure was seen as emerging from the way that politicians tied the hands of public health officials; in other cases it was blamed on citizens.[78] In Peru, for instance, "the disease was then spread via contaminated seafood, which, despite an intensive public health campaign, the patients had continued to eat raw, claiming that it was difficult to get fuel to cook their food and boil their water."[79] This statement revealed a disjunction between educational messages and the class standing and economic possibilities of the afflicted population. PAHO noted that it promoted radio spots in Spanish, Quechua, and Aymara that "assured people that '¡El remedio contra el cólera está en tus manos!'" (The cure for cholera is in your hands!),[80] thereby individualizing the problem and overlooking the structural issues that made it difficult for many to get their hands on the cure.

PAHO imagined the poor as being able to exercise free choice in regard to the basic conditions of their poverty. Qualifying this resistance as a "claim" implied that PAHO rejected the analysis that identified economic inequities as the limiting factor for the effectiveness of educational campaigns. These popular responses could have offered PAHO a lesson about misplaced agency.

PAHO failed to appreciate the potential of civil society for creating socially situated and effective prevention messages. Julia Paley richly documents the work of a small collective that operated in a poor periurban community in Santiago, Chile. When cholera cases were reported in that city, the group mounted its own anti-cholera campaign. The women demedicalized cholera, placing it within the broader political and economic situation faced by residents. While the health ministry's posters projected decontextualized images, the group's poster displayed images with which their neighbors could connect. Insofar as it depicted the epidemic as the failure of citizens to heed anti-cholera messages and downplayed the effects of broader political-economic factors, PAHO made it easier for Chilean elites to draw on an "ideology of racial superiority" that blamed cholera on the reluctance or inability of "the majority, nonwhite and nonmodern" to align itself with the "Chilean miracle" associated with Pinochet-era neoliberal reforms.[81]

Individual images of Latin American populations were connected in a number of ways. Tauxe and Blake argued in the *Journal of the American Medical Association* that "the urban fabric itself appears to be a major contributing factor" in the "extreme vulnerability" of the Peruvian population to cholera.[82] Contemporary epidemiologists favor models that focus on the interrelations of persons, places, and times.[83] In representations of the cholera epidemic, these linkages were built on powerful images of Latin Americans that circulated in a wide range of popular and scholarly contexts in the United States, Europe, and elsewhere, converting images into "social factors" in epidemiological models and raising them to the level of scientific descriptions.

In another article in the *Journal of the American Medical Association*, "Like Attacker Probing Defenses, Cholera Threatens U.S. Population from Elsewhere in This Hemisphere," Charles Marwick characterized cholera as a new "threat" to the U.S. population by depicting a broad contrast between the premodern south and the modern north and incorporating a lexicon of war and violence. Marwick suggested that Latin America not only had failed to undertake the sanitary revolution that enabled North America to "essentially" eliminate cholera in the early 1900s but was headed backward.[84]

Tauxe argued that even though water and sewage infrastructures in the United States would shield it from the "fury" of the epidemic, the likelihood was that more cases would be imported and could even spread and that cholera would "no longer be a remote and exotic disease for some Americans and their physicians."[85] Tauxe and Blake stated, "Our advanced sewerage and water treatment systems are not available to the entire U.S. population, and cholera could be transmitted in the United States among a homeless, destitute, or migrant farm labor population."[86] Tauxe included "the immigrants in 'colonias' along the U.S./Mexican border" as a potential locus for a cholera outbreak.[87]

The CDC warned professionals to be on the lookout for cholera cases crossing the border from the south. This message was underlined by reports of outbreaks in the United States caused by crabmeat brought into the country in the suitcases of immigrants who had visited their Latin American homelands.[88] The story of the Argentine airliner that created "a large outbreak" by feeding Los Angeles–bound passengers cold seafood salad is retold in epidemiological accounts and in the movie *Contagious*.[89] To be sure, real epidemiologists, unlike their Hollywood impersonators, were quick to assert that a secondary transmission of the sort imagined in the film had not been documented. Nevertheless, allusions to the importation of shellfish, contamination of oyster beds, and release of ballast water in U.S. ports by freighters from Latin America created images of infectious diseases swarming from poor brown and black bodies to those middle-class and white.

Government negligence, poverty, and cultural difference were not the only factors cited to explain the epidemic. Tauxe and Blake asserted that a lack of previous exposure to cholera and a history of infection with *H. pylori* might constitute "biologic factors [that] may also increase the susceptibility of the affected population."[90] They stated that persons with group O blood seemed to be more susceptible to cholera, to develop more severe symptoms, and to have less resistance following infection than persons of other blood groups. Three-quarters of Peruvians are purportedly of this blood group, which suggested a form of genetic predisposition to the disease. Although biologically based racial variation was cited much less frequently than were contrasts in culture or national policies, it seems clear that—just as in Delta Amacuro—cultural reasoning did not entirely displace physiological conceptions of difference.

It would be wrong to suggest that the images that circulated in PAHO's *Epidemiological Bulletin* and other professional journals were constructed *tout fait* in the United States and Europe. Some representations of social inequality that originated within Latin America acquired transnational sta-

tus in these publications; the story of Ecuadorian *indígenas* is one example. Many of the international epidemiologists whom I have quoted traveled to Latin America during the epidemic and heard accounts there of what was taking place and why. PAHO was constantly receiving information from its representatives in Latin American countries, and the agency sometimes placed its epidemiologists alongside employees of national ministries of health in labs and clinics. Latin American public health authorities also visited Washington. Some of the articles I have cited involved collaborations between international epidemiologists and their colleagues in national health ministries.[91] Images and explanations of the epidemic cycled from north to south as national epidemiologists received copies of the *Epidemiological Bulletin* and *WER* and the information they contained was reprinted or summarized in national epidemiological bulletins, manuals, and other publications. Briefings and reports by PAHO and WHO officials were relayed by international press services for publication in Latin American as well as in European and North American newspapers.

As constructions of social inequality circulated among international, national, and regional public health agencies, other government institutions, and the press, they were contextualized in accord with the institutional settings and the economies of race, gender, class, and nationality that predominated at each site. The medicalization of denigrating images and their global circulation deepened and extended social inequality, rendering it even more lethal. To be sure, leading practitioners embedded these images in scientific research that formed part of conscientious efforts to improve health conditions among the poor. This fact makes it all the more important to trace the circulation of these images and identify their lethal effects.

CONTESTED CLAIMS TO MODERNITY

Some of the most consequential constructions of our time—the notions of global and local, modern and premodern, First World and Third World—are imagined, made to seem real, and used in regulating access to power, capital, information, goods, and justice. The accounts produced by journalists, public health officials, physicians, and politicians constructed the epidemic as a problem that could be contained within simple modernist narratives. The distribution of cholera cases defined a dichotomy between modernity and its opposite, whether the latter was labeled premodern, traditional, *indígena*, uncivilized, Latin American, or Third World. Thus, the victims of cholera were people who lacked the knowledge, will, and resources to help themselves. They were "premoderns," incapable of taking advantage of modern

initiatives and, sometimes, actively resisting them when they were available. By failing to embrace modernity when the stakes were high, they proved that they could never become part of the modern world, at least not anytime soon. They had proved themselves, perhaps irredeemably, to be unsanitary subjects.

This relationship between modernity and cholera is invented—and dangerous. Daniel Rodríguez and María Vargas saw themselves as representatives of modernity, waging heroic struggles against politicians, merchants, and *indígenas* who, to varying degrees, represented a traditional, backward world. The tools that played a key role in their strategies, such as quarantines, cordons sanitaires, and chemoprophylaxis (treating entire communities with antibiotics), were depicted by officials at PAHO and WHO as the quintessence of premodern, irrational responses to a cholera epidemic. The relationship between modernity and cholera is also fragile. Magdalena Benavides, the foremost public health official in Delta Amacuro at the time of the epidemic, blamed the epidemic on the *indígenas'* belief in spirits and consultation with "shamans," yet she was believed to be a practitioner in the spirit possession "court" of María Lionza. The *60 Minutes* scandal suggested that any individual and any institution could be pegged as premodern, even WHO.

The stories that international epidemiologists told rested on the assumption that cholera is a medically simple disease, one for which we have the answers, and that its persistence was a problem of politicians and populations. A number of mysteries, however, lurk beneath the scientific surface.[92] Why didn't cholera turn up in Latin America in the 1970s, when the disease was so prevalent in Africa, or in the 1980s, when so many countries experienced economic collapse and cuts in social services? Gangarosa and Tauxe state that the reasons "defy explanation."[93] Why did cholera persist just off the coast of Louisiana and Texas without causing epidemics in the Gulf of Mexico? How did cholera reach Latin America?

Leading scientists could only present a range of possible explanations when cholera first appeared in Peru.[94] Similarly, when cholera was widely reported in Latin America, officials at PAHO and such leading epidemiologists as Tauxe and Blake were certain that it would appear in Caribbean countries and lead to similar epidemics there.[95] Why didn't this happen? Think of Trinidad, some seven miles from the delta: it has plenty of rural poverty and an active contraband trade through the delta, and its population has a taste for delta crabs, yet cholera did not appear there. A new variety of cholera, *Vibrio cholerae* 0139, emerged in Bangladesh and India in 1992 and 1993. Why? And why did cases of this new cholera begin to taper off after

the disease had emerged so rapidly?[96] Work published in recent anthologies has suggested that many questions persist, including important ones about the ecology and epidemiology of the disease.[97] Members of the "critical epidemiology" school in Latin America have argued that the work of "hegemonic epidemiology" is based on erroneous conceptions of social relations and political economy, which cloud understanding of the distribution of disease and the factors that shape it.[98] Timeworn stereotypes are hardly a good source for modern scientific research. Nevertheless, epidemiologists and public health officials have not seemed inclined to qualify the authority of their interpretations.

A number of the people we interviewed suggested, ironically, that cholera epidemics could be beneficial for public health. Dr. Feliciana García, head of WHO's Global Task Force on Cholera Control, stated, "I prefer to have an epidemic of cholera, in that we can at least succeed in mobilizing resources, we can succeed in changing the mentality of physicians, so that they are concerned and they do something. But the threat of cholera is not sufficient—we need a big epidemic!" At the other end of the institutional hierarchy, officials often applauded the epidemic for providing them with new visibility and clout in their efforts to bring modern sanitation and hygiene to the region and in discrediting *indígena* "witches."

I have reached a different conclusion. Responses to the epidemic in Delta Amacuro, regardless of the resources and energy they brought to the delta, were never intended to be more than short-term. No serious efforts were undertaken to change health and sanitary infrastructures or to provide systematic health education in the fluvial region, let alone to address issues of institutional racism, economic oppression, or a lack of respect for political and human rights. The long-term impact of institutional responses to the epidemic significantly *damaged* social, economic, and health conditions in the delta. Serious studies of nineteenth-century epidemics suggest that the success of efforts to improve water and sewage infrastructures depended more on debates regarding the role of the state in social life, explanations of social inequality, and broad schemes for regulating the lives of the poor than cholera-inspired exhortations by public health physicians.

Talking about sanitary reform may have helped some officials in Delta Amacuro, such as Vargas, save their jobs and even advance their careers, but the experience of Benavides, who was fired at the height of the epidemic, suggests that this rhetoric did not have consistent value even as a defensive strategy. Public health professionals didn't consciously invent this historical narrative to cover their tracks, but the story became so deeply ingrained in professional identities and forms of authority that officials failed to seek

alternative strategies for effecting change. If today public health officials or other parties genuinely wish to improve sanitary infrastructures and over-all health conditions, the rhetorical and political locus of such efforts can-not be based on the "positive effects" of the terror associated with cholera.

In the stories told by many people who survived cholera, the disease and modernity are connected in a very different way: cholera is the quintessential disease *of* modernity. If we equate modernity with the penetration of the nation-state into the delta and the lives of its residents, with transnational commerce, and with resource exploitation by national and transnational cor-porations, then cholera was precisely part of the experience of modernity. Just as alternative explanations for the epidemic were dismissed as fanciful conspiracy theories, this account of the cholera-modernity connection could be rejected out of hand because it reflects a lack of historical or global knowl-edge. The disease becomes a quintessential embodiment of the "violence of modernization."[99]

This shift in how we define cholera socially and politically brings the history of cholera pandemics into sharper focus. Writers dispute whether *Vibrio cholerae* 01 was present prior to the nineteenth century, but it is clear that the first half of the nineteenth century witnessed successive pandemics that caused tremendously high mortality in the Americas, Europe, Asia, and the Middle East. This was, of course, a period in which modernity reshaped the lives of peoples in all of these areas through colonialism, resource ex-traction, urbanization, industrialization, and the economic exploitation of workers. A central feature of the expansion of economic, social, and politi-cal modernity during the nineteenth century was the emergence of more extensive systems of transportation and travel. In other words, cholera pan-demics are not features of the premodern world but products of modernity itself. Moreover, modern sanitation promoted cholera epidemics through the development of systems for extracting feces from the sites where growing urban populations deposited them, transporting this waste through urban areas, and dumping it in rivers and oceans.[100]

It would be tempting to reverse the fundamental premise on which cholera stories rest by declaring that cholera is *caused* by modernity and sanitation, but this would only reposition the dichotomy that sustains con-structions of inequality in the modern world. The sanitary revolution nar-rative pretends to be egalitarian and inclusive; it suggests that all people can become part of a world in which diseases such as cholera will be part of the past. The eradication of naturally occurring smallpox, of course, stands as the great success story. But notions of sanitary citizenship produce exclu-sion and hierarchicalization. They assert the scientific, moral, political, and

social superiority of those individuals, communities, nations, and continents that have the resources to eradicate the conditions that harbor cholera and other infectious diseases. As representations of cholera and infected populations circulated, they helped legitimize medical profiling of racialized and poor communities in Latin America, countries in the region, and immigrant, homeless, and destitute segments of the U.S. population. Indeed, cholera narratives created new ideological connections between a broad range of practices of social subordination. By separating questions of sanitation and citizenship, and by ensuring that health and disease do not become grounds for social, racial, and political subordination, international public health institutions and their national counterparts could more effectively accomplish their own agendas. And they could end their complicity—however involuntary—in the stigmatization of poor and racialized communities.

13 Virulent Aftermath
The Consequences of the Epidemic

Institutions had a central role in shaping the course of the cholera epidemic in Delta Amacuro. Complex linkages among regional, national, and international organizations crucially affected what took place in Mariusa, Tucupita, Caracas, and Geneva, and powerful institutional structures molded how statistics, manuals, reports, epidemiological analyses, laboratory results, and press reports were produced and circulated. After all was said and done—in Geneva, Washington, Atlanta, Caracas, and Tucupita—it was the *indígenas* who overwhelmingly experienced the direct effects of the disease and its discursive shadow.

Cholera continued to influence life even after its power to cause death had dissipated. Wakanoko, a community previously consisting of some thirty-five adults near Guayo (see map 1, page 2), provides a striking example. A few clusters of houses set back into the forest, it is perched on both sides of a small tributary. If you didn't know it was there, you could pass right by it. In 1994 Tirso Gómez and I (Charles Briggs) visited Ramón Salas, a thin, tall man of about sixty with an unassuming manner. As his voice filled with sadness and apprehension, Salas described how nearly a third of the adults in Wakanoko died in a single night in 1992 from a previously unknown disease. The principal *wisidatu* died, followed by his son, who was also a healer. Another third of the community departed, too sad and scared to stay where no one seemed safe.

Salas's fear that cholera might return pervaded our conversation. Initially, the antibiotics and oral rehydration salts that had been handed out in the clinic in Guayo had provided a sense of security, but these medications had long since disappeared. The reaction of Pedro Salas, Ramón's older brother and the current leader of the community, was quite different; he was nonplussed: "The doctors [in Guayo] said, 'We'll let you know when cholera has returned, so that you will know, so that you will be informed. We'll hear about it soon here in the clinic, and we'll have medicine. We'll give you some.'"[1] Unfortunately, the two physicians who had made this promise back in 1992 had left the delta, and the current physician knew nothing about it.

A short way downriver we interviewed the *wisidatu*'s relatives—the two wives of the father who died and the only remaining son. They were the most abject people I have ever encountered. As Avilia Rodríguez, the younger wife, told a moving account of the sudden deaths, Carmen Flores, the older wife, could only weep. Rodríguez concluded, "I still weep. I can't leave, I can't go very far away. . . . I think about it all the time. My husband died only yesterday, maybe a month ago—it certainly hasn't been a year." "Yes," added Francisco Moreno, the surviving son, "about a month."[2] These deaths had taken place some two years before we spoke, but the women's *sanas* continued to reverberate through the forest. Time had been arrested by grief. Life, haunted by the ghosts of cholera, would never be the same.

Efforts to understand and control cholera could have exerted positive effects on health in the delta. Cooperation between vernacular and institutional practitioners, combined with greater incorporation of preventative techniques such as chlorinating or boiling water, could have reduced incidences of diarrheal disease. For example, between 1993 and 1996 Clara and I set up a pilot project in Mariusa. In addition to bringing a nurse to the community, Clara developed collegial relations with each of the vernacular practitioners who worked there. Instead of competition and distrust, healers, nurse, and physician exchanged patients and reinforced one another's ability to prevent and cure disease. Unfortunately, the effects of the cholera epidemic on health, social, and political conditions in the fluvial area overall were not so positive. Cholera continued to be an impetus for heated contestation regarding race, rights, and resources.

The epidemic increased friction between vernacular and institutional practitioners. Physicians, public health officials, missionaries, and politicians celebrated the perceived demise of "shamans" and the new ascendance of institutional medicine. Rafael Quintero, the director of ORAI in Tucupita after the epidemic, decided that the solution was to regulate healers by standardizing their practices, formalizing pedagogy, and laying down guidelines as to what sorts of therapeutic techniques would be permitted.[3] Healers were forced to assume a low public profile.

Another result of institutional responses to the epidemic was a tremendous rise in self-medication. Officials passed out substantial quantities of antibiotics to prevent delta residents from fleeing. Although envelopes of oral rehydration solution were also distributed, less emphasis was placed on this clinically crucial aspect of treating diarrhea and, accordingly, Bactron, a brand name for trimetoprim sulfametoxazol, became lodged in cultural memory as a magic bullet. When we traversed the delta in 1994 and 1995, some people told us that they were less worried about cholera because "if our stomach starts to hurt, we take one or two Bactron." One or two capsules of an antibiotic is far from an adequate course of treatment for diarrheal diseases, and it does nothing to rehydrate the patient. A false sense of security can lead to what physicians complain about the most in the delta: substantial delays in transporting patients to the clinic. Moreover, taking only one or two doses of an antibiotic is an excellent means of creating antibiotic-resistant strains of bacteria, including cholera.

Once the epidemic was officially declared to have ended, emergency allocations of medical resources disappeared. Having been stigmatized as an incorrigible premodern population and a serious political liability for the regional government, delta communities became an even lower priority. Many clinics had to turn away patients for want of even basic medicines. When supplies of Bactron ran out and MSAS refused to provide more, unscrupulous pharmacists sold large amounts of the drug, diverting funds that could have been used for food. Delta residents became disillusioned, and institutional medicine also lost a great deal of its legitimacy. In the years following the epidemic, Clara and I noted a pattern according to which delta residents would visit both the clinic and the local lay practitioner, sometimes with a visit to a *criollo curandero*, a spirit possession healer, or a Trinidadian healer in town thrown in. Rather than combining the potential benefits of these contrastive therapeutic techniques, patients often moved rapidly between practitioners in a desperate search for help, failing to follow a full course of treatment prescribed by any one. We watched in anguish as the one-year-old daughter of close friends died after being treated by a long series of practitioners, leaving the parents bitter and distrustful.

CHOLERA'S SILENT RETURN

This deterioration of the *indígenas'* way of life was certainly not confined to their health. Thousands fled to the mainland to be closer to clinics and farther from cholera, and many refused to return. Several hundred Mariusans settled along the *malecón* in Barrancas, much to the chagrin of local politicians (photograph 36). Officials in Tucupita and Barrancas were hardly welcoming, and few jobs were available. Many *indígenas* resorted to begging (photograph 37). Groups of *indígenas* began to travel to cities throughout Venezuela, including Caracas, Ciudad Guyana, Maracay, and Valencia.

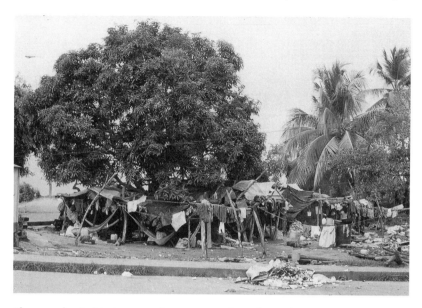

Photograph 36. Mariusan settlement across from the *malecón* in Barrancas.
Photograph by Charles L. Briggs.

It became common to see a hundred former residents of Winikina and Mariusa in Caracas, begging on downtown streets and spending the night on the
patio of the Goodyear tire store across from Paseo Vargas (photograph 38).

For Caracas residents, whose primary exposure to *indígenas* had been
through schoolbooks and television programs, throngs of people emerging
from the rainforest seemed exotic, and their presence became a media event.
As words and pictures of delta residents were plastered on the front pages of
newspapers and beamed nationwide on the evening news, a scandal erupted.
Opposition politicians joined reporters in decoding these images of impoverishment as a clear sign that government policies had failed. Local and national politicians called officials in Delta Amacuro and angrily ordered them,
"Take care of your Indian problem!"

As the scandal grew, people were rounded up at night—when no reporters
were watching—and taken by military transport to Delta Amacuro. A decision was made by the states of Delta Amacuro and Monagas to forcibly
prevent individuals whose bodies, clothing, and beaded jewelry led to their
categorization as *indígenas* from traveling to Caracas and other cities unless they carried a letter of permission from ORAI. The Guardia Nacional
was instructed to check all vehicles. The racialization of the *indígena* body
was, once again, the locus of surveillance and control. This practice blatantly

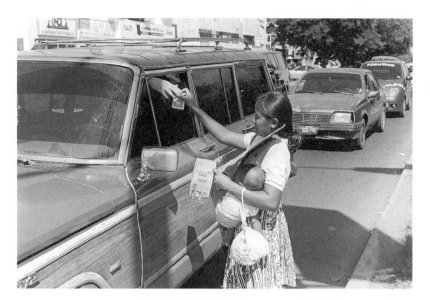

Photograph 37. Woman from Delta Amacuro asking for handouts in Puerto Ordaz, Bolívar state. Photograph by Charles L. Briggs.

violated the constitutional right to freedom of movement within Venezuela for these citizens. When Clara and I joined Vicente Medina and others who were protesting this policy, we were told that constitutional guarantees had been suspended. Officials warned us that our efforts to document and call attention to these restrictions were not subject to constitutional guarantees either, meaning that we could be arrested.

Officials cited a wide range of theories to justify these restrictions. Diego Escalante Castro, the mayor of Barrancas, suggested that the motive for *indígena* trips to large urban centers was frivolous, reflecting a desire for "an adventure, an outing *[paseo]*." Quintero reported that during a meeting with *indígena* leaders he told them that the government was simply trying to save them from a situation "that discredited them as a people, because it was humiliating."[4] His statement echoed the way that politicians and reporters characterized *indígena* motives for undertaking the protests of September 1992. Politicians often repeated an account that was originally offered, I was told, by an anthropologist, Gabriela Velásquez, who had long worked in the delta: because the Warao are traditionally gatherers, contact with modernity had induced them to change their traditional gathering practices from extracting food from the forest to gathering handouts from urban motorists.

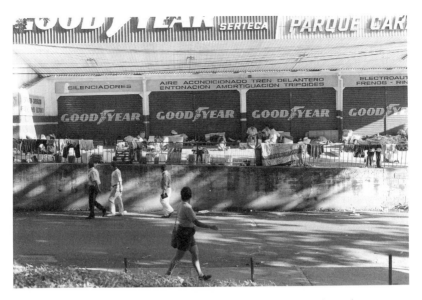

Photograph 38. People from Winikina and Mariusa camped in the early-morning hours in front of a Goodyear tire store in downtown Caracas, catching the eye of passersby. Photograph by Charles L. Briggs.

Nomadism was often cited as an explanation, and geography and climate were mentioned as well. These cultural and environmental discourses merged when the mayor of San Félix rationalized her decision to remove people camped on the edge of the bus terminal in the middle of the night—which *Notidiario* characterized as "rape"[5]—by arguing that "the ideal solution was to transport the Warao back to their natural habitat," given that they were "completely dislocated from their natural environment" when living on the mainland.[6] Here the discourses that had been finely tuned in efforts to blame *indígenas* for the cholera epidemic were recontextualized for use in a new institutional and political crisis.

The familiar discourse of the *mano peluda* (hairy hand)—the idea that *criollos* were secretly directing *indígena* actions—emerged over and over in statements by politicians, the police, and the military. Representative Bernardi repeated these questions on the floor of the Caracas municipal legislature: "How do they get here? How does such a large number of people travel if they don't even have the resources to stay in their area? Who could be financing the expenses associated with their travel?" Another official asserted with respect to this issue that "the *indígenas* don't respond, that they refuse to do so or elude the questions."[7] Assuming that this perceived silence of the subaltern provided a pretext for the state to speak, officials proposed a number of answers. Many argued that the exodus constituted a "traffic in *indígenas*" undertaken by someone who was charging for the service. It was, once again, easier to imagine the bodies of *indígenas* as objects of *criollo* intrigues than the *indígenas* as political agents.

Politicians soon fixed on the most powerful rhetoric of criminalization that circulates in Latin America. Lorenzo Díaz, the second highest official in Delta Amacuro, articulated the government's position. I interviewed him in November of 1994: "I have proof that . . . the most irresponsible, important authors of this grave situation were in the drug trade; these people were being used as mules in the transportation of drugs from other regions to here and back, understand? They had a connection with the Mafia, a kind of Mafia that was connected to the people in Colombia, well, a chain [from] Colombia–Caracas, Caracas–Delta Amacuro, with Delta Amacuro being the exit point for the drugs."[8] If they had not put a stop to this operation, he asserted, it would have led to the "complete extinction" of the Warao.

The purported Colombian connection helped to construct the presence of some hundred *indígenas* as a "massive exodus" that constituted a threat to public order and state security, according to Asdúbal Aguiar, governor of Caracas.[9] In a high-level meeting, Aguiar suggested that the exodus was one of the most critical problems of the day.[10] The assertion that some children coming from the delta were infected with measles and leprosy—another disease that evokes fear and powerful associations of poverty and ignorance—helped construct the refugees as a security threat.[11] The ranks of the homeless in Caracas and other cities were legion—indeed, the majority of Venezuelans live in poverty—yet the addition of a hundred ragged bodies that were racialized as *indígenas* suddenly became a threat to public order and national security.[12]

How did delta residents get to Caracas? José Félix Alvarez, the Mariusan healer who worked alongside Ricardo Campins in Tortuga, reported that his family sold hammocks and baskets to raise the cash. A key figure in the exodus was Sol María Moya, a short, white-haired woman of some sixty years of age who lived in Yakariyene. She was often seen around Tucupita, gathering aluminum cans for sale, asking for handouts, and addressing everyone she met in a no-nonsense tone of voice. Her command of Spanish and her outspoken character made her an instant media star, and she was featured prominently in television and newspaper reports. She noted that she had told military officials who questioned her, "I am able to speak forcefully. I can talk well. I'm not afraid—I'm going to speak without fear. I came here because I was dying from hunger, and my grandchildren had nothing to eat. There is no work."[13] She told me that a member of the Guardia Nacional threatened her with a beating and four months of prison if she spoke to the press again.

The press quoted Jaime López, whom they dubbed the "*cacique* of the Warao," constantly. Well-dressed, mustached,, and thoroughly bilingual, López is articulate and politically sophisticated. He had met with Bernardi and other officials and had addressed the National Congress. He was in his mid-thirties when we interviewed him in 1994. He blamed "politicians" for the deaths of so many *indígenas*: "Politicians ask for funds in our name and then steal the money. It's their fault. When the disease first came, they hid it—they knew it had arrived. . . . The governor does not provide jobs, clinics, or hospitals. Millions and millions of *Bolívares* were sent from afar in our name, for the Warao of the Delta Amacuro of the lower Orinoco. But where is that money?"[14] He stressed that the trips to Caracas were geared from the start to obtain cash *and* to protest inhumane conditions.

Delta residents were unable to get their cholera narratives into the media, where biomedical and institutional voices were privileged. Begging on urban streets, however, was just as visible, and they learned that their bodies, wracked by hunger and pain, could be powerful sites for the representation of poverty and inequality. This action was not initiated by leading activists. López, Moya, and other refugees from Barrancas and Tucupita—people who lacked education and social position—used the racialization process to create a context in which it was impossible for the nation-state to ignore the consequences of the cholera epidemic. Some used the situation to voice related concerns. Vicente Medina denounced forced assimilation and the expropriation of 90 to 95 percent of the funds earmarked for *indígenas*. Clara brought statistics on infant and child mortality in delta communities to the attention of the national press.[15] Anthropologist and activist Nelly Arvelo-Jímenez criticized land expropriation, aggressive missionization, and economic exploitation with regard to *indígenas* in Venezuela as a whole.[16] Unfortunately, although these voices challenged the dominant narratives in the media, images of *indígenas* as passive dupes or criminal surrogates continued to legitimate repressive policies.

Although the substantial infusion of medical resources into the fluvial region in 1992 and 1993 effectively contained the disease, it was not aimed at producing any long-term impact on health conditions. The control of information suppressed international awareness of the epidemic and helped to deflect the blame onto the people who suffered the most from not only cholera but also other infectious diseases and the malnutrition that is so prevalent in the region. Clara was repeatedly chastised by Venezuelan politi-

Table 2. Cholera in Venezuela and the Americas, 1994–1997

Year	Americas		Venezuela	
	Cases	Deaths	Cases	Deaths
1994	113,684	1,107	0	0
1995	85,809	845	0	0
1996	24,643	351	269 (6i)	9
1997	17,760	225	2,551	59

i = imported

SOURCES: Data drawn from World Health Organization, "Cholera in 1994/Le choléra en 1994," *Weekly Epidemiological Record/Relevé épidémiologique hebdomadaire* 70, nos. 28–29 (1995): 201–211; "Cholera in 1995/Le choléra en 1995," *Weekly Epidemiological Record/Relevé épidémiologique hebdomadaire* 71, no. 21 (1996): 157–163; "Cholera in 1996," *Weekly Epidemiological Record/Relevé épidémiologique hebdomadaire* 72, no. 31 (1997): 229–235; "Cholera in 1997," *Weekly Epidemiological Record/Relevé épidémiologique hebdomadaire* 73, no. 27 (1998): 201–208.

cians and public health authorities for suggesting that infrastructural changes and a serious health education campaign would be necessary to prevent subsequent epidemics. Rather than considering plans for long-range prevention following the 1992–1993 outbreak, officials in Delta Amacuro state concentrated on suppressing further references to cholera.

Given their failure to make significant infrastructural changes and cholera's penchant for estuarial environments, the return of cholera was inevitable. As table 2 shows, Venezuela did not report any cholera cases in 1994 and 1995, even as new epidemics were reported in the Americas as a whole. By February 1996, WHO's *WER* reported that cholera was present in fourteen Venezuelan states as well as in Caracas.[17] Venezuela was specifically mentioned in WHO's annual report on cholera: "Venezuela had several outbreaks in 1997. Whereas in 1996 cholera was reported for the first time in two years with a total of 254 cases, in 1997 a total of 2551 cases were registered with 59 deaths (CFR 2.3%)."[18] The attention of readers around the world was drawn to a case fatality rate (2.3 percent) that was more than double the acceptable levels and was almost double the figure for the Americas (1.3 percent). Welcome back to cholera country! Cases were reported in Delta Amacuro in 1996 and 1997, and history began to repeat itself. A third epidemic began in October 1998. In June 1999 the office of the regional epidemiologist received laboratory confirmation of cases in the Pedernales area at the same time that the new director of the Regional Health Service was telling the press that there was no cholera in Delta Amacuro.

Once again Mariusans were blamed for starting an epidemic, even though cases were concentrated in the Pedernales area.[19] Several members of their community died, and Mariusans again fled to Barrancas. Local authorities responded as they had before, complaining to Delta Amacuro officials that "their Warao" were jeopardizing the health of Barrancas residents. Reporting that two Mariusans had died from cholera in Barrancas in January 1997, Dr. Julio Mondragón, then the director of the Regional Health Service in Tucupita, told the press that these deaths "obligate us to immediately impose a sanitary barrier [*cerco sanitario*] in the remote population of Mariusa, . . . with strict instructions to impede the exodus of *indígenas* from Mariusa toward Barrancas del Orinoco."[20] Again the Mariusans were rounded up, forcibly returned to the delta, and, this time, distributed among various rural clinics.

The new epidemics differed from the first in one crucial way. The discourses that equated cholera with *indígenas* and the delta had been deployed so successfully in the first epidemic and its aftermath that the disease had become just another of the diarrheas that "kills the Indians this time of the year," to use the phrase that was often heard in regional institutions. Facing no threat to their legitimacy, public health and other institutions deemed it unnecessary to rush physicians, medicines, boats, or gasoline into the delta. Delta residents were clearly aware that the cholera patients required prompt medical attention, but many communities had even fewer resources to transport their members to clinics than they had in 1992 and 1993. The delta had become more economically and politically isolated.

CULTURAL LOGIC, GLOBAL INITIATIVES

When cholera re-emerged in Delta Amacuro, institutional officials and delta communities commanded a broad range of malleable narrative forms that could accommodate the reoccurrence of suffering and death. Responses to the cholera epidemic were part of a broader project of constructing social inequality in which the intersections between forms of subordination based on race, class, and gender were crucial.[21] Although the specifics of this story relate to cholera and Delta Amacuro, the lives of billions of people throughout the world are being reshaped today by the effects of globalization on institutions and social inequality. I want to explore these broader issues in the context of the cholera epidemic because the death and indignity that delta residents experienced can teach us to challenge the policies that endanger lives and augment suffering in other places and situations. The cholera epidemics in Delta Amacuro state offer a frighteningly perfect place to scrutinize how globalization can change relationships between nation-states, global forces, and poor citizens. The neoliberal policies imposed by the World Bank, the International Monetary Fund, the governments of wealthy countries, and transnational corporations to structure trade and labor have greatly increased the gap between the rich and the poor, both among and within nation-states. From 1960 to 1991 the portion of the world's wealth enjoyed by the poorest 20 percent of its population dropped from 2.3 to 1.1 percent. Although only one-fifth of the world's population lived in countries with the highest incomes, these people accounted for 86 percent of expenditures for private consumption worldwide; the poorest 20 percent accounted for only 1.3 percent.[22] Such social inequality has serious implications for health.[23] Most of the countries that reported substantial numbers of cholera cases in 1991 were struggling with economic crises marked by high unemployment, inflation, and the weakening or elimination of "social safety nets" that helped protect the poor.

Venezuela, rich in oil and a host of other natural resources, provides one of the most striking examples. Even when the economies of other Latin American nations were characterized as chaotic and collapsing, Venezuela enjoyed relative prosperity, and income was distributed more equitably. Many Latin American governments were authoritarian, but Venezuela had been governed by a constitutional democracy since 1958. Venezuela had claimed a place on the threshold of the First World, but then the *Bolívar*'s value against the dollar began to slip steadily, dropping from 4.5 to 1 in 1983 to nearly 700 to 1 in 2000. Fluctuations in oil prices and production quotas and the weakening currency complicated service payments on Venezuela's $30 billion foreign debt. Inflation rose. Bankers took their earnings—and huge sums of their clients' savings—to Miami in 1994. Efforts to balance the budget included substantial cuts in public services, which clearly affected the availability of health services. Public expenditures on health, which had previously reached a high of 5.2 percent of the gross domestic product, lay at 2.56 percent in 1991.[24] The percentage of the population living in poverty increased from 24 percent in 1981 to 59.2 percent in 1990.[25] The Venezuelan government suggested that the figure actually stood at about 80 percent in 2000.

Nowhere else in Latin America, with the possible exception of Chile, had structural adjustment signaled such a radical increase in poverty.[26] Although the national economy improved in the opening years of the 1990s, the benefit to poorer Venezuelans was less clear. Many Venezuelans believed that the country was still in crisis. Hugo Chávez Frías, leader of the attempted coups in 1992, was lionized by large segments of the working class. Although popular sectors did not take to the streets in the massive insurrection that Chávez had anticipated, his words and actions did speak to widespread distrust of the government and its institutions.

Cholera mapped this social inequality in Venezuela in crucial ways. As was the case in the nineteenth century, cholera outbreaks today tend to be concentrated among the poor. This situation can transform epidemics into debates over the causes and ethical implications of social inequality and the nature of modernity itself. As economic restructuring simultaneously cast more people into poverty *and* disseminated the idea that everyone had access to a global "flow" of information, technology, capital, goods, and culture, the bodies of people who were dying from a classic premodern disease became a site for debating the politics of inequality.

Saskia Sassen has argued that globalization is less usefully characterized as a "flow" of capital, goods, culture, information, and people across borders or as the eclipse of the nation-state than as a process that transforms institutions within countries in ways that render them useful to transnational capital.[27] In Latin America in the 1990s, as elsewhere, even governmental agencies that had no direct relationship to global markets, such as legal, penal, medical, and public assistance agencies, were often forced to make radical and abrupt changes in their guiding ideologies and practices. Powerful and entrenched bureaucracies could no longer take their access to power and resources—or even their ability to pay their civil servants—for granted. Latin American governments came under particular pressure when the U.S. foreign policy's emphasis on "fostering democracy" in electoral politics came to focus on "reforming" institutions. Globalization also enhanced the role of nongovernmental organizations and increased the circulation of discourses of human rights, thereby enhancing efforts by persons with less access to power and material resources to transform notions of citizenship and participation and to challenge institutions of the nation-state.[28]

The tremendous increases in social inequality that have been fostered by globalization have augmented the role of institutions that police the lives of the poor. During the epidemic, institutions were called upon to provide narratives that explained this growth of human misery not as a function of the consolidation of power and capital but as the result of individual choices, thus making it possible to shift the blame onto those who suffered the most. These are precisely the circumstances in which public health agencies became vital parts of the nation-state during nineteenth-century cholera epidemics. There is, of course, a big difference today. If cholera supposedly comes from having too little modernity, how can we explain the resurgence of the disease after modernity, including the establishment of public health institutions, had been firmly entrenched for more than a century?

The re-emergence of cholera presents us with this central theoretical challenge: we must develop a deeper understanding of the impact of globalization if we are to understand the shifting place of the poor. One view holds that globalization is producing new modes of inclusion that actually disrupt centralized control over the international flow of capital, people, goods, culture, and information. This view is one of a global egalitarianism in which powers such as the United States are no longer dominant and the poor can participate actively in shaping widely distributed imaginings of the social landscape. Although localization becomes more difficult, people can recover agency through a process of "indigenization" that was deployed in resisting colonialism.[29]

On the other hand, globalization can be seen as exclusionary: it exacerbates social differences based on access to capital, commodities, information, and culture. Groups that have purportedly failed to be incorporated into the social, cultural, and economic patterns that are considered progressive and "modern" are fixed in space and denied unrestricted access to the capital and culture that others enjoy.[30] According to this account, some people become localized while others become globalized.[31] Such localization produces a loss of agency and freedom, creating passive local viewers of global actors.[32] Cultural reasoning fits this process perfectly by virtue of the way that it places subaltern populations in ecological niches.[33] In this way globalization produces social fragmentation, differentiation, and inequality.

The full power of globalization was released in the delta when the Venezuelan government, prompted by international lending organizations, reopened its territory to transnational petroleum corporations. British Petroleum gained the right to exploit several existing oil wells in Pedernales in 1992. In 1996 Amoco entered into an agreement with PDVSA (the Venezuelan oil conglomerate) that accorded it exploration and exploitation rights for an area that included Mariusa, and the Delta Centro Operating Company (formed by two U.S. companies, Louisiana Land and Exploration and Benton Oil and Gas, and one Canadian firm, Norcen Energy Resources) obtained rights to 526,000 acres of the delta. "Exploration" entailed clearcutting forested areas, detonating powerful blasts in the course of seismic surveys, and drilling test wells, which involved the use of toxic chemicals.

Petroleum extraction endangered the economic base of delta communities. Because of the estuarial ecology of the delta, contaminants can spread over an extensive area and remain in the water for long periods, killing fish and other wildlife and threatening the only source of drinking water. An oil spill would be disastrous. Delta residents were not informed, let alone consulted, before leases were offered, bids accepted, or, in most cases, huge numbers of workers and amounts of technology arrived. Discovering this request for bids from oil companies via the Internet, we alerted delta residents, activists, and regional, national, and international environmental and indigenous rights organizations.

Residents in the region where British Petroleum was operating envisioned cholera as a poison that was placed in the water by the oil workers and dispersed by the explosions that these workers caused.[34] In 1999, as workers, helicopters, and equipment moved in and out of this area and as people began dying from cholera, narrators all over the delta suggested that foreign oil companies were driving fish from the waters and game from the land and planting cholera in the rivers to kill all *indígenas*.[35] These stories reflected the growing transfer of economic and political might from the nation-state to multinational corporations that goes by the names of "privatization" and "foreign investment." These new "conspiracy theories" mapped power and inequality on a global basis in ways that were closely tied to historical reality. Delta residents were not the only ones to link cholera to globalization. Roberto Guzmán, the assistant regional epidemiologist, was convinced that the outbreak in 1996 was started by an oil worker, probably from Zulia state (where cholera cases were being reported at the time).[36] Guzmán's efforts to draw attention to the health risks associated with petroleum exploration and exploitation apparently did not meet with much interest elsewhere in the Dirección Regional de Salud, which was receiving funding from oil companies. Globalization introduced barriers that restricted the circulation of cholera narratives and silenced cries of protest.

Cholera may well have been closely related to the "oil boom" in Delta Amacuro from the beginning. The massive rallies in 1992 against land expropriation, environmental degradation, and denial of political, legal, and human rights were part of a hemispheric social movement that was linking Native American groups and rights organizations. This activism might well have jeopardized quiet plans to invite foreign capital and technology into the region. As delta residents became increasingly stigmatized as filthy, ignorant, superstitious, and passive, the cultural logic that made these depictions seem cohesive, inescapable, and scientific became more ingrained in institutional practices. Further withdrawals of capital and services left activists with fewer resources for organization and mobilization. The ability of the government to disseminate its narratives in the media, to send them abroad, and to suppress tales of genocide created a powerful sense of the coercive power of the state and the seeming impossibility of opposing it.

INSTITUTIONALIZING INEQUALITY

Globalization—that is, neoliberal economic and social policies, the compression of geographical distance through electronic communication and rapid modes of transporting people and goods, and the growing hegemony of corporations and financial sectors—is transforming nation-states, their functions, and the types of power that they wield. Industrialized countries, corporations, and such international organizations as the World Bank, the International Monetary Fund, and the World Trade Organization exert especially forceful pressures on so-called peripheral states. Globalization also fosters the emergence of new social movements and the worldwide circulation of discourses on human rights, thereby providing subaltern subjects with access to ideologies and organizations that can help them effectively challenge state agencies. Nevertheless, bureaucracies worldwide have assumed the job of generating ideologies and practices that construct inequality in ways that transfer responsibility for human misery from international organizations, states, and corporations onto the shoulders of poor citizens.[37]

So many deaths from a preventable and curable infectious disease could have led public health officials and their colleagues in other agencies to make changes in ideologies, strategies, and daily practices that would have transformed some of the worst health conditions in the world. I have argued that the key reason that authorities opted instead for stopgap measures, information control, and rhetorics of blame was rooted in the way that spatializing, temporalizing, and racializing practices came together in institutional contexts. The result was to make a race ("the *indígenas*"), a space (the delta), and a bacteria *(Vibrio cholerae)* seem synonymous. A central mechanism for connecting these logics and for joining a host of scientific and popular discourses was cultural reasoning.

It is important to understand why cultural reasoning was such a useful tool for defending institutions and schemes of social inequality. An analogy might help. In the nineteenth century compiling statistics became crucially important to many state agencies when their legitimacy was threatened; their use of statistics was, in other words, a defense mechanism.[38] In the latter part of the twentieth century, officials found another agent that could dilute their responsibility in a similar way: to paraphrase Shakespeare, so let it be with culture. As globalization simultaneously threatened the legitimacy of institutions and presented them with new possibilities for controlling poor, politically marginalized populations, cultural reasoning provided an excellent means for playing both ends against the middle. Having been forged in academic battles against racism, the concept of culture retained its liberal and scientific patina—even when it was used illiberally in institutional contexts. State agencies could publicly declare the cultural sensitivity of their everyday practices, claiming to be responsive to the characteristics, needs, and rights of the populations they served. In Venezuela, officials could adopt an anti-racist, anti-imperialist, and anti-institutional stance that would seem to align them with the subaltern and against U.S. domination.

Global economic restructuring, the adoption of neoliberal policies by nation-states, and such things as cholera epidemics can upset the already unstable equilibriums, including those of race, that characterize economies of inequality.[39] Culture is widely used to create and control these fragmentations of social relations. Cultural arguments are commonly invoked in public health institutions worldwide in the face of epidemics of AIDS, tuberculosis, and other infectious diseases.[40] Programs promoting "cultural sensitivity" can cloak assertions of the superiority of biomedical interpretations and denigrations of alternative and resistant views as backward and pathological in the guise of a celebration of ethnic identity.[41] Rebecca Martínez argues in a study of cervical cancer in Venezuela that physicians often cited culture as a risk factor for the disease; here notions of cultural difference and a lack of culture, used in this sense as a stand-in for education and class standing, were involved in blaming patients for their condition.[42] Cultural reasoning helps make medical profiling invisible.

Cultural images of the residents of inner cities in the United States assist in squashing protests, imposing new regimes of segregation, and making high rates of incarceration for minority populations seem legitimate.[43] The U.S. Immigration and Naturalization Service uses cultural arguments to construct a double standard: human rights discourses may be used to condemn gender-based discrimination and female genital mutilation as barbaric, yet denials of refugee protection to individuals seeking to escape them are justified as a need to respect the cultural norms of the home country.[44] A number of studies suggest that cultural arguments are extensively used in criminal and civil proceedings that involve people of color in the United States.[45]

Cultural reasoning provides fertile ground for reimagining, extending, and naturalizing schemes of social inequality. It produces concrete images that seem to correspond directly to specific and often dramatic events, such as a cholera epidemic or an earthquake, even as it recycles age-old stereotypes. When the concept of culture is used to characterize racialized populations, its capacity to essentialize, exoticize, totalize, and dehistoricize is powerfully unleashed, reducing complex social phenomena to timeless sets of premodern traits that purport to provide a self-evident and exhaustive interpretation applicable to all "bearers."[46] Because cultural and overtly racial discourses are both capable of achieving these effects, even invocations of culture that are anti-racist can racialize populations effectively, and they wield their power without enabling target populations to make the sorts of appeals to liberal sentiment that would be prompted by overt public attributions of biological or intellectual inferiority.[47]

In anthropological investigations of culture, "diverse experiences and facts are selected, gathered, detached from their original temporal occasions, and given enduring value in a new arrangement."[48] The formulations these studies produce are perfect tools for turning partial, situated, and contested representations of complex social communities into totalizing constructions that can be adapted to fit particular institutional ideologies, practices, and projects in a range of contexts. Such rhetorics provide institutions with excellent means of capitalizing on the opportunities and uncertainties presented by globalization—the use of the cholera stigma in order to pave the way for petroleum exploration in the delta is only one example. Cultural reasoning characterizes racialized populations as being, in anthropologist Arjun Appadurai's rich phrase, incarcerated by culture—unable to escape the constraining effects of a rigid and narrow worldview—and institutions are taking advantage of this strategy for containing bodies and the politics of race.[49]

MSAS was not the only institution that used cultural reasoning to deflect political fallout and to attempt to maintain control over a racial landscape that had been upset by the protests of 1992 and the massive influx of cholera refugees into Tucupita and Barrancas. In September 1992, the second month of the cholera epidemic, Higinia Gómez, a sixteen-year-old woman working as a domestic in Tucupita, felt abdominal pains and was taken to the Luís Razetti Hospital in the middle of the night. Without examining her, the physician on duty gave her a powerful sedative and sent her home. Awakened near dawn by intense cramping, she went to the bathroom, seated herself on the toilet, and gave birth to a girl, which fell into the toilet bowl. On seeing the infant the young woman fainted, and the newborn apparently drowned. Later that morning the woman's employer reportedly discovered blood in the bathroom, found the dead infant in the trash, and took the mother and infant to the hospital. Based on a purported confession (produced through verbal and physical abuse), medical testimony, and other affidavits submitted by the prosecution, the mother was convicted of homicide.[50]

In finding the defendant guilty of culpable homicide (*homicidio culposo*), the judge explained the homicidal act in the following terms: "In her condition as a woman of the Warao *étnia,* giving birth for the first time, completely inexperienced in these affairs, she believed, according to her version, that the newborn was dead, for which reason she opted to put paper in its mouth, place it in a bag and throw it in the garbage."[51] Lawyers, anthropologists, and psychiatrists who argued in the woman's defense also focused on the question of *"indígena* culture." A lawyer hired by the National Office of Indigenous Affairs suggested that since Venezuelan laws are promulgated for people who form part of a "(more or less) homogeneous social-cultural milieu," they cannot be used in meting out punishment to people who act in accordance with "totally distinct cultural references." He stated that "taking into consideration her status as an *indígena Warao,* . . . it is necessary to establish up to what point this factor (WARAO CULTURE) contributes to explaining the failure to realize the importance of these acts."[52]

An ORAI anthropologist testified that the Warao "ethnolegal system" and cultural norms regarding motherhood would have rendered Gómez incapable of committing such an act; at the same time, since she was raised in a different culture, she could not possibly understand the norms regarding pregnancy, childbirth, and infanticide of the dominant culture. Moreover, this cultural clash "produced in [the defendant] a process of depersonalization, self-depreciation, and maladjustment." Arguing that living in town deprived *indígenas* of a "perpetual vital harmony between NATURE-MAN-CULTURE," he echoed the apartheid-like reasoning offered by public health officials.[53] These cultural arguments did not succeed in reversing the homicide conviction. In prison she was raped, impregnated, and nearly killed by a guard who attempted an abortion. She was released to keep a scandal from erupting during an election year. The cultural defense served as a basis for arguing that *indígenas* could only operate effectively within their own "ethnolegal system," not the political life of the nation-state. Many *criollos* read the case as clear proof that "the Warao" were not ready for political integration into the national society.

By fashioning Gómez into the quintessence of the bad *indígena* mother, the criminal proceedings and popular debate surrounding the case played squarely into institutional efforts to use cultural reasoning to blame cholera on *indígenas.* When the court covered up the hospital physician's malpractice, it helped public health institutions conceal the institutional racism embodied in official indifference to everyday health conditions in the delta. At the same time, affidavits by physicians and pathologists in the trial helped legal institutions counter charges that access to justice in Delta Amacuro was based on race.

This case resonates with María Vargas's inspections of *indígena* food preparation and Magdalena Benavides's claim that *indígena* mothers have no "affection for life" and fail to protect the health of their children or to lament their deaths. These examples point to the way that cultural reasoning and racialization practices often depend upon a patriarchal logic that pins the blame on women. Visions of poor, incompetent mothers juxtapose gender and class to generate the sense that the objects of these representations exhibit unnatural emotions and behaviors. The supposedly universal dimensions of motherhood reflect the political-economic position of white, middle-class women; poor mothers thus seem to be defective or unnatural deviations from these norms.[54] The mother who is callous toward the death of her own children is a widely dispersed image. When it is deployed in areas where infant and child mortality are high, as it frequently seems to be, it becomes a political tool for covering up the structural factors that lead to high infant mortality. Since a woman's duties as a citizen seem to include procreation for the benefit of the state, women who do not succeed in keeping their children alive can be seen as failing their citizenship duties.[55]

These constructions echo a Euro-American pattern that depicts the sexuality of women of color quite differently from that of white women.[56] Benavides's claim that *indígena* women do not mourn the death of their children revolves, in part, around her implicit claim that they are excessively fertile, having one baby after another. I have often heard public health officials suggest that the high infant mortality rate in the delta does not pose a serious problem because *indígenas* are so fertile. The bad-mother image draws on a common stereotype of *indígena* women as lacking respect for and control over their own sexuality, wantonly (and perhaps promiscuously) having babies one after another. Women who appear to fail so miserably at such a "natural" task as loving their children, nurturing them, and mourning their loss seem less than fully human. The fall from complete humanity can easily be extended to the "group" or "race" as a whole, making *indígenas* in general seem incapable of ever becoming sanitary citizens.

Cholera narratives provide insight into how cultural reasoning found institutional homes in Delta Amacuro. ORAI anthropologists and sociologists were sometimes assigned to public health agencies; public health professionals read published works by anthropologists; interinstitutional task forces such as the anti-cholera committee generated hybrid institutional languages. Informal discussions between professionals were of crucial importance. For example, Venezuela's census of indigenous people brought Caracas anthropologist Leonora Vásquez into the home of physician Manuel Mato on numerous evenings, thereby providing him with a mini-course on

"Warao culture." Finally, as anthropologists and public health authorities made statements to the press, their specialized perspectives became part of the public cholera discourse, which fostered the production of hybrid rhetorics. Accordingly, any professional could claim the right to speak for culture (although anthropologists are sometimes granted greater authority in this domain). As cultural reasoning was incorporated into diverse specialized discourses, cultural assertions became increasingly decontextualized and, accordingly, objectified both as common knowledge and as institutional ideology.[57] I note wryly that practitioners who think they can become amateur anthropologists would be very unlikely to accept anthropologists as amateur physicians in clinics!

At the same time that it circulates freely within, between, and beyond institutions, cultural reasoning adapts to the specific contours of the sites in which it is used. Cultural discourses create rough parallels between exotic beliefs and practices on the one hand and specific areas of expertise controlled by agencies on the other. Public health officials pointed to religious, ritual, healing, kinship, culinary, and hygienic practices in *indígena* communities as corresponding, in negative or inverted terms, to those recommended by medical practitioners. Their characterizations of consuming crabs, finding and storing water, and eliminating body wastes were objectified as activities that related directly to epidemiological hypotheses regarding routes of transmission. The anthropologist who submitted an affidavit on behalf of Gómez could draw (without citation) on my own work on dispute mediation in the delta to formulate an "ethnolegal system" that could be directly compared to—and certainly contrasted with—the Venezuelan legal system.[58] This forced me to reflect on how my research played a role in producing and circulating the forms of cultural reasoning that I am tracing in this book.

A second source of the malleability, scope, and specificity of cultural reasoning lies, as Etienne Balibar has suggested, in the status that notions of culture have "as the semantic 'horizon' of all the discourses that try to signify identity in a world of nations."[59] Discourses of identity embody "four major categorical polarities" in that they appear simultaneously (1) as "objective structures" and "a principle or a process of subjectivization," (2) as an expression of the singularity of "groups" and part of "the question of universality or universalization," (3) as defined by scientific, technical, and literary "experts" and as framed in popular culture, and (4) as being both permanent and evolving.[60] To these I would add a fifth polarity: identities are construed not only as self-constructions of the individuals and groups who bear them but also as labels imposed by dominant institutions.

The illusion that cultural identities are bounded, homogeneous, and singular—such as the hegemonic construction of the *indígena* category—is produced through the management of profound contradictions and the juxtaposition of heterogeneous discourses. The double-voiced nature of culture and cultural identities[61] enables institutions to use scientific language to impose supposedly universal categories and schemes while respecting the particular experiences of members of a specific population. The liberal patina helps to disguise timeworn stereotypes and institutional agendas. Cultural reasoning operates like historical narratives that permit practitioners to imagine social life and then imbue their constructions with the feel of the real.[62] Once naturalized and scientized through the use of cultural reasoning, these official constructions of identities can become the basis for racial profiling, medical and otherwise. Images backed by cultural reasoning often shape cultural memory of crucial events, drowning out other ways in which pasts, presents, and futures can be imagined. They accordingly help the state assert control over the production of history.[63] The fact that institutions in Delta Amacuro largely escaped criticism for failing to take any substantive action against the spread of cholera—despite the second and third epidemics—brings this message home.

IMAGINING MODERNITY

We thus come again to the crucial role of institutions in the lives of the poor. Our goal is not to pin blame on either the public health policies and practices that were in place in Venezuela in 1992 and 1993 (which are now being revised) or particular individuals, institutions, or countries for causing or misrepresenting the epidemic. This position does not spring from an "I'm okay, you're okay" stance—some of the words spoken and written and the actions taken in the epidemic were *not* okay. Our goal is, rather, to show that disease and social inequality are linked in public health rhetorics and practices and that these rhetorics and practices are partially responsible for the worsening status of poor people worldwide, particularly poor people of color, given their basis in and their effects on political and economic relations. Even good people with good intentions who do their jobs well participate in this process.

We think that it would be very difficult to come away from this study with the impression that public health officials, physicians, or politicians in Venezuela were generally incompetent or indifferent or to conclude that such failings explain why a cholera epidemic occurred there. It is not our intention to simply reverse the process of pointing fingers. The international epidemiologists and public health officials that we cite were selected precisely because their work is exemplary. They are leaders in their fields and have made important contributions to reducing the incidence of cholera.

Since the nineteenth century, public health discourses on infectious diseases have provided the perfect medium for cultivating imaginings of modernity. The opposition between civilization and barbarism is deeply written into the project of European modernism and its Latin American manifestations.[64] By suggesting that some cultures center on science, hygiene, democratic values, technological progress, and economic advancement while others rest on superstition, ritual, and unsanitary bodily practices, official rhetorics have been able to place populations on opposing sides of a great divide formed by the opposition of modernity—in particular, the advent of the sanitary revolution—and tradition.[65] Modernity's false claims to inclusiveness, rationality, and universality and its role in the creation of social inequality have perhaps been hardest to reveal and challenge when they were couched in terms of hygiene and public health.

Cholera was identified as the quintessential premodern disease. The descriptions of cholera that were offered by public health officials and disseminated by the media sustained the premodern ghosts that modernity needs to seem real, desirable, and necessary. Stigma, writes Erving Goffman, centrally involves external marks—"defective" physical, linguistic, or behavioral features—that seem to provide visual signs of a pervasive internal failing.[66] The horrible symptoms of cholera marked bodies indelibly as bearers of all that is antithetical to the modern world: dirt, ignorance, poverty, and backwardness. Because they contracted cholera, Mariusans were branded as threats to modern social and sanitary order, a stigma that antibiotics, quarantine, and even residence on the mainland could not erase. But this stigma was even harder to contain than *Vibrio cholerae*. The people who labeled their neighbors as cholera-ridden unsanitary subjects and officials who branded members of the public in this fashion often caught cholera's stigma themselves. Since denigrating images travel so well, medical profiling tends to return to haunt those who use it.

We have detailed the way that cholera continued to carry out the function in the late twentieth century that it served during much of the nineteenth—defining sanitary citizenship and identifying unsanitary subjects. This is a logic of opposition that works at three levels. First, nations are imagined as consisting of distinct populations, some of which are comprised of sanitary citizens—those who contribute to the body politic by internalizing scientific understandings of health, disciplining their bodies, and sanitizing their environments. Opposite these populations are other populations that threaten the health of sanitary citizens. Second, formal arrangements between nation-states and international public health organizations turn access to health care and sanitary infrastructures into a question of sanitary citizenship, granting the state the power to define health rights, shape access to health care, and hold a virtual monopoly over legitimate representations of people in relationship to disease. Even the individuals who enjoy the status of sanitary citizens get locked within the ideological and institutional parameters established by their governments—and, increasingly, by corporate providers of health care. Third, some nation-states get blamed for failing to turn their populations into sanitary citizens; they get branded as unsanitary states. Some of the accounts produced by international epidemiologists in the United States and Europe suggest that sanitary citizens are few and far between in Latin America.

Narratives told in the delta challenge the stigmatization of residents as unsanitary subjects. They counter the image of a benevolent state that provides *indígenas* with a wealth of opportunities and patiently waits for them to become sufficiently civilized to take advantage of them. They imagine the state in a complex range of ways: as distributing services along racial lines, as stealing funds earmarked for delta communities, as actively seeking to kill *indígenas* in order to take their lands, and, also, as sending physicians and medicines to save their lives. Toward the end of the 1990s, *indígena* activists throughout the country started placing health issues at the top of their agendas. Community leaders, regional representatives, and members of the Comisión Permanente para los Pueblos Indígenas (Permanent Commission for Indigenous Peoples) of the National Assembly—which includes the *indígena* representatives elected under the 1999 Bolivarian Constitution—are now making demands on the minister of health and social development for more adequate health care, and they are demanding a voice in the selection of public health officials and the drafting of laws and regulations that shape institutional practices.

Insofar as their efforts give them access to power, they might do well to counter the normalizing tendencies that often emerge when excluded groups finally gain a seat at the table. In particular, they should consider important issues raised by the cholera narratives: why some people have the power to assign sanitary citizenship, and how rights and stigmas in general are distributed.[67] As "narratives of self and community that do not look to the state/citizen as the ultimate construction of sociality,"[68] and as evidence of the racializing practices of the state and the effects of transnational capital and international relations, cholera stories show us that little is gained when struggles for health justice are primarily couched within the parameters of the sanitary citizenship paradigm.

As we begin the twenty-first century, discourses of cholera, sanitation, hygiene, and public health continue to exclude a huge segment of the world's population from access to its benefits. This situation raises issues of "biopower"—that is, who gets to shape how people think about bodies and health, not only their own but others'.[69] At the same time, these discourses help to sustain the egalitarian promise of modernity. If modernity and modern hygiene are essentially connected with ways of thinking about the body and the world and ways of scooping out water, washing hands, and cooking food, it would seem that anybody can be modern. The corollary is, of course, that if an individual doesn't become modern, it's her fault. Mariusans were dismissed, albeit often through a romantic idiom, as living passively within nature. In modern eyes they were doomed to extinction.

Using cholera to claim that you represent modernity presents several problems. First, the strategy is fallible—someone else is bound to come along and label your practices premodern and irrational. Second, the process of affirming one's own modernity by denying it to others reproduces social inequality, thereby helping to create the conditions in which cholera, tuberculosis, malaria, AIDS, and other diseases flourish. Finally, the rhetoric of modernity is becoming increasingly obsolete; as globalization forces more and more people into poverty, the idea that modernity and progress are just around the corner is becoming a hard sell.[70]

Rethinking the question of modernity has led to new insights into how it is produced and legislated. Some scholars argue that its emergence cannot be characterized simply as a unidirectional flow from European and North American cores toward peripheries. The process of modernization is, rather, a dynamic and decentered one that generates multiple modernities that sometimes compete and conflict with one another. One might say, then, that Venezuela and other "developing countries" are carving out paths to an alternate modernity—a distinct way of defining a break with the past and a vision of a more enlightened future—rather than aspiring to a Euro-American modernity.[71] It may be that the creation of multiple, interrelated modernities in Latin America goes hand in hand with the ongoing production of alternative traditionalities—distinct ways of maintaining continuities with the past—that not only inform but also shape their modern counterparts.[72] Venezuelan cholera narratives dramatize this process at the same time that they point out important limitations. Alternative forms of modernity and tradition would seem to be quintessentially embodied in biomedicine and vernacular healing, which have usually defined themselves by describing their opposition. In Venezuela, however, the need to project images of scienticity and objectivity—to echo the voices of MSAS, PAHO, and WHO—in order to gain authority and respond to criticism limited the generation of alternative modernities in the realm of medicine and public health. This formulation, which was supposedly universalistic and impartial, was indexically (that is, contextually) connected to nationalism, class, and race, linking the dominant narratives to a host of discourses with long historical trajectories. Some of these discourses circulated in the direction of the so-called center, supplying international epidemiologists with new images of *indígenas,* barrios, fiestas, and poverty. The passage of statistics to this center also helped shape how modernity and its absence could be spatialized, quantified, and explained.

It is also crucial to point out, however, that supposedly universal modernities generated along Euro-American models are no less fractured, contextually produced, or contradictory than those produced by either public health practitioners or *indígenas* in Venezuela. Similarly, I am not sure that the cholera narratives generated by officials in the CDC, PAHO, or WHO were any less haunted by multiple and contradictory discourses and "prescientific" notions or any less shaped by "local" institutional and political realities than were those generated by their Venezuelan counterparts.

Critics failed to examine the political economy that shapes how representations circulate. Profound critiques of the cholera-equals-premodernity thesis emerged in narratives told in delta communities, but these stories seldom made it out of the region. Here racialization, the power of the nation-state, and the centrality of official public health discourses converged to squash *indígena* stories and their challenge to the ways that cholera, modernity, and social inequality were imagined and regulated. These same discursive and political practices contained the nation-state's exposure to surveillance and criticisms over health conditions among *indígenas* and ensured that little would be done to change them. Thus, to speak of multiple or insurgent modernities without looking at who actually enjoyed access to the discursive and political arenas that shaped them can strengthen the role of elites (including scholars) and hide the effects of globalization on the poor, particularly poor people of color.

When people in the delta died without reaching a medical facility, their deaths became invisible. Other cases were converted into ordinary cases of "diarrhea and vomiting" through the lack of an authoritative signature. Most of the remaining cases were removed from public scrutiny through the rhetorical magic of requiring laboratory confirmation. The press was provided with the numbers that made it through this institutional gauntlet. Public health officials provided descriptions of *indígenas* that were sure to be repulsive to readers and viewers and imbued them with the scientific and liberal aura of culture. Newspapers produced visual images of suffering and quotes that emanated, it seemed, from the dying bodies themselves, construing patients and their kin as helpless victims.

As these images circulated, they followed a number of routes of de- and re-contextualization. Statistical techniques, epidemiological modes of explanation, commercialization of media representations, and political discourses on *indígenas* objectified these images, severing them from the complex institutional, social, political, and historical circumstances in which they were generated, turning them into immutable mobiles.[73] The farther this ironic combination of subjectivities and objective facts traveled and the longer it circulated, the more useful it was for producing and legitimating schemes of social inequality. This process also extended the images' ability to stand for (and thus imagine) entire races, classes, genders, sexualities, and nations. These kinds of appropriations have shaped the way that journalists and public health officials project social suffering worldwide.[74] There are, if you will, many deltas around the world, including some in rich countries.

Venezuelan scholars sometimes complain that discussions of *indígenas* have little relevance to contemporary Venezuela, in that they represent only some 2 percent of the population. It is important to reposition this question. If our central concern is how the 60 to 80 percent of Venezuelans living in poverty (according to different estimates) are affected by globalization and the nation-state, then constructions of *indígenas* provide a crucial site for addressing the theoretical and political issues at hand. By setting the limits for what counts as acceptable modes of describing and treating the most expendable populations, the racial economy determines what can be done to citizens whose "marginality" is defined primarily vis-à-vis conceptions of poverty and criminality rather than race. By failing to challenge projections of the social and spatial "marginality" of *indígenas* as a natural indicator of their political, legal, economic, social, and moral subordination and as a marker of the failure to become part of the modern project, critics accept a key element of the discourses and practices that legitimate structural violence against other Venezuelans, whether they are defined as "peasants," "residents of marginal barrios," or "street children."

Since "the Warao" of Delta Amacuro and "the Yanomami" of Amazonas state occupy center stage in Venezuelan imaginings of *indígenas*, they provide an essential means of defining the borders of modernity and "the national society" and setting the parameters for treating communities that do not qualify for substantive citizenship. Yanomami have long been seen as defenseless against the gold miners who usurp their lands, contaminate their water with mercury, spread malaria, and even massacre communities that stand in their way. Their depiction as helpless victims was furthered by the scandal caused by the publication of Patrick Tierney's *Darkness in El Dorado*, which charged that *indígenas* had been exploited by unethical anthropologists and other scientists.[75] The conditions that lead to the deaths of about half of the children did not become an important part of the debate.[76] As discussions about the *indígenas'* situation were reduced to widely publicized battles over reputations and book sales, efforts by Yanomami activists to press for access to rights of citizenship, including adequate health care, were neatly erased.

ACHIEVING SOCIAL JUSTICE

Do the effects of globalization on the poor provide real access to the production and consumption of goods and culture, or do they lead to a double exclusion from the postmodern world?[77] Neither picture is entirely adequate. Delta residents have not been excluded from modernity or globalization. Indeed, they seem to have a greater capacity for connecting the dilemmas they face in their own lives and localities with global forces than do the politicians, public health officials, physicians, anthropologists, and missionaries who have projected a gap between *indígenas* and modernity. Although mediated images such as those of the Persian Gulf War and Bill Clinton make it into the delta, delta residents have little control over whether their constructions of cholera, poverty, neoliberal economics, racism, oil wells, human rights abuses, and land expropriation make it out of Delta Amacuro—and they seldom do.

Like other discourses on social inequality, those used in the cholera campaign constructed categories of citizenship and enabled institutions to use them in defending themselves and regulating people's lives. These discourses constructed bodies—that is, it imbued bodies with social and political meanings. The power of public health discourse to categorize these bodies and then, at times, to misuse the invented categories to subordinate their bearers was painfully evident in Clara's account of how nurses at Pedernales "gave" Christian names to traumatized patients in the middle of the night and then taunted them in the morning for failing to remember them. Perhaps forgetting was a challenge to the nation-state's power to construct them in this way rather than evidence of their ignorance and intractability. Cultural reasoning was supposed to save the world from racism, but public discourses of culture absorbed racist categories that emerged in private conversations, where explicitly biological accounts of difference are permissible. Clara exposed some of these leaks from the private to the public sphere in her account of conversations over coffee in the Regional Health Service headquarters. Even when difference is imagined in liberal, cultural terms, the echo of biological reasoning and bald racism is often audible.[78]

Discourse is not a free-floating chain of signifiers: the signifiers produced by people who lack access to power and material resources seldom float beyond their own locality. This is not because they think or act locally—we have tried to show that the opposite is the case—but because institutional and political-economic barriers prevent these signs from becoming global. Notwithstanding the significance of Bob Marley's revolutionary black consciousness in reggae, Rubén Blades's ballads of rural violence, or rap lyrics that depict police violence against African-American youth, we should not take the circulation of selected subaltern forms to indicate a general absence of informational barriers.[79] Contrary to what many globalization theorists seem to believe, the "deterritorialization" of capital, culture, and communication has not broken down these barriers. Media networks and new technologies disseminate images, information, and discourses of culture around the globe in seconds, but globalization has made opportunities to successfully communicate one's side of the story profoundly unequal.

It is true that international discourses on human rights, the efforts of transnational nongovernmental organizations, and new communication technologies have created new openings for discussion and reform. Yet globalization also presents new possibilities for the surveillance and regulation of increasingly poor populations. Although many people in the delta suggested that the government's failure to prevent a cholera epidemic constituted genocide, their opinions carried little weight: international specialists and organizations determine which cases can be investigated, publicized, and prosecuted as possible acts of genocide. These individuals were unlikely to conclude that the institutional racism that exacerbated the epidemic constituted an act "committed with intent to destroy, in whole or in part, a national, ethnical, racial or religious group," to quote the definition that the U.N. General Assembly approved in 1948.[80]

If we are to disrupt transnational systems that exacerbate suffering, we need to know how, when, and where to intervene. Discerning these transnational circuits and the institutional frameworks that structure them is thus a crucial part of an activist agenda. How do we begin? WHO and other international epidemiologists have recently taken several steps that could help disrupt the processes we have described. Feliciana García of WHO noted that officials realize that "with regard to cholera, we don't have a valid reflection of what is going on in the world" and that the threat of economic sanctions leads countries to hide outbreaks of cholera in order to avoid "a vicious cycle of cholera, poverty, and cholera."[81] Officials assisted in the creation of an electronic list called ProMED, which circulates epidemiological information informally. Many of the postings refer readers to publications by WHO, PAHO, and other agencies or to articles appearing in newspapers around the world.[82] The list provides a potential means of circumventing the official channels that create a closed circuit between national public health authorities and WHO, increasing the possibility that information that governments do not want to acknowledge will still be disseminated. Each message carries this statement: "If you do not give your full name and affiliation, it may not be posted." We hope that this does not signal the exclusion of members of communities who lack access to professional positions and institutional affiliations and who already face such obstacles as limited access to computers and Internet links and literacy in English.

WHO is also attempting to change long-standing reporting requirements contained in International Health Regulations.[83] The idea is to provide access to resources and expertise that could be used to control epidemics and minimize the likelihood of negative effects on tourism and exports. National epidemiologists thus would be more likely to provide accurate reports if reporting cholera cases were no longer obligatory and stigmatized labels were no longer used. Efforts to address the problem of underreporting more explicitly and creatively and particularly to interrupt the circulation of cholera stigmas is to be applauded. We hope that the position of communities such as those in Delta Amacuro would be borne in mind when considering such changes. If cholera had not been such a volatile subject and international reporting of cholera cases had not been obligatory, MSAS might not have worked so hard in 1992 and 1993 to stop the epidemic. The threat of international scrutiny can be a tremendous resource for people who have been thrust into the realm of unsanitary subjects by calling attention to the conditions that they face and to their lack of access to medical care. As we saw with the second and third epidemics in the delta, when cholera simply becomes another disease that kills *indígenas* at a particular time of the year, extensive efforts to save lives become far less likely. WHO, and other institutions making laudable efforts, must consider explicitly how to challenge the differentials of power, sources, and specialized training that exclude the communities that face the worst health conditions from shaping the circulation of epidemiological information.

The anthropological tactic of attempting to expose social suffering by bringing local worlds to the attention of global audiences runs the risk of legitimating social inequality if it fails to challenge the global pretensions of elite accounts, to bring out the global critiques often found in the narratives of poor and racialized populations, and to confront the gatekeeping mechanisms that provide broad audiences for some narratives and restrict others to home.[84]

The solution does not lie in producing more authoritative or sophisticated or scientific definitions of culture or modes of cultural analysis. These formulations are likely to be appropriated as more powerful institutional representations of social inequality. Many students of globalization do not seem to appreciate sufficiently that both localization and globalization are less social processes than powerful illusions.[85] Just as the "local world" of cholera patients in the delta was shaped by the way that they theorized and critiqued the Gulf War and the actions of transnational oil companies, cholera narratives and the practices of WHO officials were constrained by the local institutional and political worlds they inhabit.

We must challenge the objectification of images of social inequality in epidemiology, demography, and social science. We must insist on keeping images of inequality closely linked to the social, political, and historical circumstances in which they were produced.[86] We must continue to expose and challenge master oppositions—for example, between modernity and premodernity, science and superstition—particularly when they are used to create authority and power for one group over another. Insight into the way that this process works to the detriment of all parties can help persons on the privileged side of a social divide be more responsible to those on the other side who are struggling to overcome structural violence and achieve social justice.

Supporting the struggle of the poor to secure access to health, legal protection, education, and economic well-being entails challenging institutional responses that sustain perhaps the most deadly fiction of all: that social justice can be achieved without uprooting the distribution of wealth and human dignity according to hierarchies of race, class, gender, sexuality, and nation. Dipesh Chakrabarty writes, "Nowhere is this irony—the undemocratic foundations of 'democracy'—more visible than in the history of modern medicine, public health, and personal hygiene, the discourses of which have been central in locating the body of the modern at the intersection of the public and the private (as defined by, and subject to, negotiations with the state)."[87] Fortunately, the work of critical epidemiologists in Latin America, critical race theorists in the United States, those engaged in subaltern studies, other social theorists on the subcontinent, and other communities of scholars and activists have provided us with the tools for challenging the naturalization of social inequality in practices of the nation-state. Unfortunately, few governmental and international institutions have followed their lead, and more and more of the resources they once controlled are being turned over to corporations and investors.

All parties must collaborate in identifying and expunging efforts to pass blame and stigma downward along lines of power and institutional authority in favor of creating a global partnership in which everyone's capacities and responsibilities are recognized and respected. Particular attention must be paid to how cultural reasoning is used in epidemiology, health education, the training of medical personnel, policy formulation, and press statements. The resocialization process that taught María Vargas, a dedicated, exacting, and well-trained physician, to accept racial inequality and its fatal effects can and must be reversed. "Cultural competence" is now stressed in many medical schools, but it can easily become a crash course in stereotypes that can further the destructive uses of cultural reasoning that we have documented here. In-depth training focused on identifying and expunging forms of racism and other practices of intolerance and dialogues between medical and public health practitioners and the communities they serve about issues of power, class, gender, sexuality, race, *and* culture are much more likely to improve patient care and health outcomes. Easy generalizations about culture will not do the trick—they can easily be converted into bases for medical profiling. An extensive review of studies on race and health care in the United States reports that even when their health insurance and incomes are similar, members of racialized minorities receive medical care inferior to the care that whites receive.[88] Medical profiling leads clinicians to make assumptions about patients based upon their race, thereby rendering it less likely that members of racialized minorities will receive life-saving procedures. It is vitally crucial to trace—as we have for Delta Amacuro—how clinicians and public health officials learn to engage in medical profiling, and its elimination must become a central priority of public health institutions worldwide.

With regard to health education, changing content is not enough. The failure of programs is often ensured as much by the power relations that shape their planning and implementation as by the stigmatizing images they disseminate. Since 1985, WHO has stressed that "world health will improve only if the people themselves become involved in planning, implementing, and having a say about their own health and health care," and a number of practitioners have argued for the need to place "community organization" at the core of health education efforts.[89] Rather than simply recruiting community leaders—such as the *"caciques"* chosen in the delta by state officials—to attend meetings in which the same power-laden, biomedically driven policies are announced, medical personnel and public health authorities must be willing to abandon practices that monopolize authority and impose hierarchies of knowledge. These professionals must develop programs of education, prevention, and treatment that do not miss or denigrate their target populations and that build relations of cooperation, participation, and empowerment. To ask doctors and public health professionals to share power is not to be anti-science or to deny that modern medicine can save lives; power sharing can give them better means for meeting their own goals.

It is only fair, of course, that we turn the question on ourselves. By listening to stories in the delta and writing this book—and everything that happened in between—we became thoroughly embedded in the processes described here. We have found no vaccine to protect ourselves from the contradictions that beset all other participants in the process. We claim no superior, objective, or distanced epistemological, moral, or political position. Indeed, Venezuelans would immediately recognize such an assertion—particularly coming from a white, middle-class, U.S.-born anthropologist—as a colonialist, imperialist pretension. We do not claim the right to decide which worlds are local and which are global because that would mean placing ourselves as the players who choose positions for other participants in the game.

Rather than creating local stories for global consumption, we have shown how people in the delta put their bodies on the line in Caracas and elsewhere to bring their stories—and thus their lives, histories, and political agency—to the attention of national and international audiences. Nor does this mean that we see ourselves as neutral observers, whatever that might be. We are outraged by what took place during the epidemic and its aftermath. Our goal has been to detail how death in racialized and poor communities is hidden from public view and to describe the political and human stakes involved in the circulation of narratives without oversimplifying the position of any of the participants. To do so we have drawn new relationships between competing narratives and extended the transmission of stories that have been largely suppressed.

Our role is largely finished. Since completing this book we have turned our attention to documenting how petroleum exploration and exploitation in the delta is affecting people's lives. We are working to ensure that the new Bolivarian Constitution and the overhaul of the Venezuelan penal code result in greater legal protection and fewer abuses of human rights for people classified as *indígenas*. The transformation of the new Ministerio de Salud y Desarrollo Social (Ministry of Health and Social Development) in keeping with the Plan de Salud Integral (Integrated Health Plan) holds great potential for using biomedicine as a tool for challenging social inequality. We are inaugurating a program to eradicate tuberculosis in the delta, which has one of the worst rates of infection in the world, through a program of treatment and health education. The authors' royalties from this book will be used to further these and other projects aimed at enabling delta residents to make headway in their struggle for health and justice.

If the *indígenas'* stories are not retold, they will have little social or political force. Whether you, as the reader of these stories, choose to keep them in circulation and how you choose to do so will have real effects on poor populations around the world that are struggling to achieve medical justice. We have tried to show how stories about a catastrophe in one region can open up a broad exploration of how social inequality is produced and particularly how it gets rooted in institutions. We have discussed how images of sanitary citizens get developed and described how being relegated to the status of unsanitary subjects affects people's health and the way they are treated by the state. We have attempted to demonstrate that medical profiling is a prescription for institutional failure and human suffering.

People in the delta continue to tell stories about their lives and press for justice, and the same is true all over the world. As the human effects of social inequality grow more extensive and, often, more fatal, all of us are directly implicated in shaping what sort of reception such stories will receive and what type of action will be taken. The global complicity we have described is neither rhetorical figure nor moral dictum—it is a fundamental facet of health, disease, and death. As anthrax delivered in the mail kills U.S. citizens, the fear of death from technologies developed by powerful nation-states comes very close to home for people who thought they were on the winning side of the sanitary revolution. It is widely believed that even the great symbol of the power of public health—the eradication of smallpox—could be reversed. The cholera stories teach us that us-versus-them perspectives that use images of scary microbes in pitting good sanitary citizens against threatening racialized subjects only make matters worse for everyone.

The story ends, just as it began, in some uncertainty and a bit of terror. Our role in circulating these stories has largely ended. But yours has just begun. We ask that you look around and see who suffers the most from preventable and treatable diseases, who gets what sort of health care, and what sorts of stories are told about patients and "at risk" populations. As you retell these stories, we ask you to think about how they can be used to uproot denigrating stereotypes and challenge governmental and corporate practices that limit access to health care and blame people for the effects of structural violence. If we have been able to retell them adequately, the lasting impact of cholera narratives from Delta Amacuro will lie not in the dramatic character of the particular events they describe but in their ability to expose everyday ideologies and common practices that are, in the end, much more terrifying and fatal.

Notes

1. When referring to the political jurisdiction that includes Tucupita, the capital, I use the expression *Delta Amacuro* or *Delta Amacuro state*. I use the term *delta* to refer to the fluvial area, which includes parts of neighboring Monagas and Bolívar states. Tucupita lies on an island connected to the mainland; my use of the term *delta* does not include Tucupita or Barrancas.

2. See G. H. Rabbani and William B. Greenough III, "Pathophysiology and Clinical Aspects of Cholera," in *Cholera*, ed. Dhiman Barua and William B. Greenough III (New York: Plenum Medical, 1992), 209–228; and C. O. Tacket, G. Losonksy, J. P. Nataro, S. S. Wasserman, S. J. Cryz, R. Edelman, and M. M. Levine, "Extension of the Volunteer Challenge Model to Study South American Cholera in a Population of Volunteers Predominantly with Blood Group Antigen O," *Trans. Royal Soc. Trop. Med. Hygiene* 89 (1995): 75–77. Many persons infected with *Vibrio cholerae* are asymptomatic, and many cases are mild.

3. This figure is for Delta Amacuro state; see Oficina Central de Estadística e Informática, *Censo*, 1: 13. It thus includes the high ground south of the Orinoco River and excludes parts of the fluvial area that lie in Monagas state.

4. For studies of this epidemic, see P. D. Rodríguez Rivero, *Epidemias y sanidad en Venezuela* (Caracas: Tip. Mercantil, 1924); and Germán Yépez Colmenares, "La epidemia de cólera morbus o asiático de 1854 a 1857 y sus efectos sobre la sociedad venezolana," *Anuario del Instituto de Estudios Hispanoamericanos de la Facultad de Humanidades y Educación* 1, no. 1 (1989): 151–180.

5. Each excerpt from an interview is identified by the place and date on which it was recorded. When providing additional material from the same interview in the same chapter, however, we do not repeat this identifying information unless the two portions of the transcript are widely separated.

6. The racializing process that divided the population in Delta Amacuro state into *indígena* (indigenous person) and *criollo* (Creole, or nonindigenous person) played a key role in shaping the cholera epidemic. By retaining the Spanish terms *indígena* and *criollo*, we draw the reader's attention to the status of these terms as powerful constructions. *Warao* refers to the *indígena* population of the Orinoco delta. It is a term of pride for many delta residents. Nevertheless, it is also used in enforcing a strict separation of *criollos* and *indígenas* and in discriminating against *indígenas*. We place the term in quotation marks occasionally as a means of reminding readers of its problematic status. Population data are from Oficina Central de Estadística e Informática, *Censo Indígena de Venezuela, 1992,* 1 (Caracas: Oficina Central de Estadística e Informática, 1993).

7. Anna Tsing suggests that "flow" and "circulate" make problematic developments (such as globalization) seem like natural processes; "The Global Situation," *Cultural Anthropology* 15, no. 3 (2000): 327–360. We use *circulation* to describe how narratives, statistics, etc. travel. This process is certainly not as benevolent as, for example, the circulation of blood. We have, however, been unable to find a term that would not create other metaphorical problems. We ask readers to remember that this "circulation" follows institutional structures that channel and constrain what moves, prevent other narratives from traveling, and configure the rights of parties to control this process.

8. Charles E. Rosenberg, *Explaining Epidemics and Other Studies in the History of Medicine* (Cambridge: Cambridge University Press, 1992), 279. On epidemics as social mirrors, see Shirley Lindenbaum, "Images of Catastrophe: The Making of an Epidemic," in *The Political Economy of AIDS,* ed. Merrill Singer (Amityville, N.Y.: Baywood, 1998), 33–58, and "Kuru, Prions, and Human Affairs: Thinking about Epidemics," *Annual Review of Anthropology* 30 (2001): 363–385. On illness narratives, see Arthur Kleinman, *The Illness Narratives: Suffering, Healing, and the Human Condition* (New York: Basic Books, 1988).

9. See Kai Erikson, *Everything in Its Path: The Destruction of Community in the Buffalo Creek Flood* (New York: Simon and Schuster, 1977); and Anthony Oliver-Smith, *The Martyred City: Death and Rebirth in the Andes* (Albuquerque: University of New Mexico Press, 1986).

10. On the process of racialization, see Michael Omi and Howard Winant, *Racial Formation in the United States: From the 1960s to the 1990s* (New York: Routledge, 1994). Our thinking about race and racism has also been shaped by critical race theory and by the largely European Critical Discourse Analysis (CDA), which brings a range of linguistic approaches to bear on the study of racism. For overviews of CDA, see Norman Fairclough, *Discourse and Social Change* (Cambridge: Polity, 1992); Teun van Dijk, *Elite Discourse and Racism* (Newbury Park, Calif.: Sage, 1993); R. Wodak and M. Reisgl, "Discourse and Racism: European Perspectives," *Annual Review of Anthropology* 28 (1999): 175–199; and Jan Blommaert and Chris Bulcaen, "Critical Discourse Analysis," *Annual Review of Anthropology* 29 (2000): 447–466.

11. See Stuart Hall and David Held, "Citizens and Citizenship," in *New Times: The Changing Face of Politics in the 1990s*, ed. Stuart Hall and Martin Jacques (London: Verso, 1990), 175.

12. This is T. H. Marshall's classic division, as presented in his essay "Citizenship and Social Class," in *Class, Citizenship, and Social Development*, ed. Seymour Martin Lipset (Westport, Conn.: Greenwood Press, 1964), 65–122. For Marshall, the civil element refers to "liberty of the person, freedom of speech, thought, and faith, the right to own property and to conclude valid contracts, and the right to justice" (71). The social element ranges from questions of "economic welfare and security to the right to share to the full in the social heritage and to live the life of a civilized being according to the standards prevailing in the society," and he suggests that this element is tied most closely to educational and social service institutions (72).

13. See William V. Flores and Rina Benmayor, eds., *Latino Cultural Citizenship: Claiming Identity, Space, and Rights* (Boston: Beacon, 1997), especially the introduction; and Renato Rosaldo, "Cultural Citizenship, Inequality, and Multiculturalism," in Flores and Benmayor, eds., *Latino Cultural Citizenship*, 27–38.

14. We comment on this debate in chapter 13.

15. Some individuals were interviewed more than once.

CHAPTER 1. PREPARING FOR A BACTERIAL INVASION

1. Michael Taussig, *The Nervous System* (New York: Routledge, 1992).

2. Ministerio de Sanidad y Asistencia Pública, *Manual de normas y procedimientos para la prevención y manejo de enfermedades diarréicas y cólera* (Caracas: Division de Enfermedades Transmisibles, Dirección de Epidemiología y Programas, Dirección General Sectorial de Salud, Ministerio de Sanidad y Asistencia Social, 1991), 1. MSAS also published a set of *Environmental Sanitation Measures to Avoid Cholera* in May, and it continued to create booklets and pamphlets and distribute them nationally during the coming months.

3. Ludmila Vinogradoff, "El cólera nació en la India," *El Nacional*, 17 April 1991, C-4. When no author is listed, we cite articles under the newspaper's title. In a few cases, we use clippings taken from MSAS archives or the personal archives of officials that do not indicate the page on which an article appeared; in such cases, no page numbers appear in the bibliography.

4. See, for example, Alberto Arébalos, "El cólera se propaga por América Latina," *El Nacional*, 12 April 1991, A-11.

5. "El cólera abre otro frente: el estado Bolívar," *El Nacional*, 20 November 1991, C-4.

6. "Cólera y dengue en Venezuela admite Sanidad," *El Mundo*, 14 November 1991, 1.

7. Teresita Hernández, "El asesino a la puerta," *El Nacional*, 28 April 1991, C-4.

8. See "Alerta nacional contra cólera y dengue."

9. See Peter L. Berger and Thomas Luckmann, *The Social Construction of Reality: A Treatise in the Sociology of Knowledge* (Garden City, N.Y.: Doubleday, 1966).

10. Amilcar Bracamonte, "303 casos de cólera detactados en el país," *El Mundo,* 10 August 1991, 7.

11. Marielba Nuñez, "Sociedad de Salud Pública pide más vigilancia del SAS ante el cólera," *El Nacional,* 18 February 1991, D-15.

12. "Cordón fronterizo contra el cólera," *El Nacional,* 15 February 1991, A-1.

13. See, for example, Hernán Mena Cifuentes, "Extreman medidas de control anticólera en Puerto La Guaira y en Maiquetía," *El Nacional,* 7 July 1991, D-6.

14. "Inminente el cólera en Venezuela," *El Nacional,* 9 August 1991, D-4.

15. "Cerrar la frontera piden los caraqueños," *El Nacional,* 29 April 1991, C-1.

16. In Argentina, cholera stories became central vehicles for anti-immigrant discourses. See Morita Carrasco, "Cólera, cultura y poder: La trama discursiva del cólera," in *Cultura, salud y enfermedad: Temas en antropología médica,* ed. Marcelo Alvarez and Victoria Barreda (Buenos Aires: Instituto Nacional de Antropología y Pensamiento Latinoamericano, 1995), 145–154.

17. Ministerio de Sanidad y Asistencia Pública, *Legislación sanitaria nacional: Acuerdos, leyes, decretos, reglamentos y resoluciones sobre sanidad nacional* (Caracas: Editorial Jurídical Venezolana, 1967), 454.

18. Hereafter, we simplify Dr. Echezuría's title to "national epidemiologist."

19. Articles often reported acts of communication between officials, above and beyond the content of a particular exchange (which was sometimes not even provided), as news. See, for example, Marlene Rizk, "Alerta en el país por dengue e inevitable entrada del cólera," *El Nacional,* 10 August 1991, C-4, in which Rizk describes Páez Camargo's "close communication with Colombia, and just a few minutes before receiving the press he got a telephone call from his Colombian counterpart, who keeps him up to date on information." Note the anthropomorphization of Colombia as a communicative partner.

20. Ministerio de Sanidad y Asistencia Pública, "Cólera," *Boletín Epidemiológico Semanal* 46 (1991): 66–75.

21. Verónica Díaz Hung, "El cólera no debería llegar de incógnito," *El Nacional,* 22 May 1991, C-4, reported, "The doctor [the director of the INH] defines as detective work the job performed by the bacteriological team. It is as if cholera acted like a delinquent who wants to come into the country, knowing that because of the crimes he has committed his entry has been denied."

22. Díaz Hung, "El cólera."

23. See Michel Foucault, *Power/Knowledge: Selected Interviews and Other Writings, 1972–1977,* trans. Colin Gordon et al. (New York: Pantheon, 1980), for his notion of a regime of truth.

24. See Bruno Latour, *The Pasteurization of France,* trans. Alan Sheridan and John Law (Cambridge, Mass.: Harvard University Press, 1988).

25. Aliana González, "Con el cólera en las puertas," *El Nacional,* 15 February 1991, C-2.

26. Asdrubal Barrios, "93 naciones atacadas por el cólera," *El Nacional*, 14 March 1991, C-2.

27. "Ningún país latinoamericano está ajeno a epidemia del cólera," *El Nacional*, 12 March 1991; Arébalos, "El cólera."

28. See Ian Hacking, *The Taming of Chance* (Cambridge: Cambridge University Press, 1990); Theodore Porter, *Trust in Numbers: The Pursuit of Objectivity in Science and Public Life* (Princeton, N.J.: Princeton University Press, 1995); Alain Desrosières, *The Politics of Large Numbers: A History of Statistical Reasoning*, trans. Camille Naish (Cambridge, Mass.: Harvard University Press, 1998).

29. "El cólera alcanzará a Panamá," *El Nacional*, 4 June 1991, A-10. *El Mundo* reported the figures for July; *El Nacional* reported the figures for December.

30. Marlene Rizk, "El 83% de los venezolanos es vulnerable al cólera," *El Nacional*, 29 April 1991, C-1.

31. Quoted in Bracamonte, "303 casos."

32. "El cólera nació en la India," *El Nacional*, 17 April 1991, C-4.

33. See Edward Said, *Orientalism* (New York: Pantheon, 1978).

34. See Dhiman Barua, "History of Cholera," in *Cholera*, ed. Dhiman Barua and William B. Greenough III (New York: Plenum Medical, 1992), 1–36.

35. I am using "the poor" and the concept of "poverty" itself to refer not to stable, transparent aspects of the social world but to the social constructs that emerged in cholera narratives. As with my use of *indígena* and "Warao," I have refrained from placing "the poor" and "poverty" in quotes each time, in keeping with editorial conventions. I ask the reader to keep the constructing, shifting, and problematic status of these terms in mind.

36. "La epidemia de cólera dejará 40,000 muertos," *El Nacional*, 20 April 1991, A-9.

37. As noted by Marcos Cueto, *El regreso de las epidémias: Salud y sociedad en el Perú del siglo XX* (Lima: Instituto de Estudios Peruanos, 1997).

38. Ludmila Vinogradoff, "72 barrios de Caracas serían presas del cólera," *El Nacional*, 13 April 1991, C-1.

39. "El 83% de los venezolanos," *El Nacional*, 29 April 1991.

40. Hacking, *Taming Chance*, and Porter, *Trust in Numbers*, trace the way that statistics became a crucial part of the daily practices of institutions of the nation-state in the nineteenth century. Desrosières, *The Politics of Large Numbers*, argues that the emergence of systematic efforts to use statistics as a tool for keeping large populations under surveillance and for planning public policies helped shape the nature of modern states and for some (such as Germany) played a role in their creation. Geoffrey C. Bowker and Susan Leigh Star, *Sorting Things Out: Classification and Its Consequences* (Cambridge, Mass.: MIT Press, 1999), extend this argument to include state-to-state relations, international organizations, and transnational corporations as well.

41. Paul Farmer, *AIDS and Accusation: Haiti and the Geography of Blame* (Berkeley: University of California Press, 1992).

42. "Suramerica en tiempos del cólera," *El Nacional*, 5 May 1991, A-2.

43. Ibid.

44. Reported in "El cólera es una infección típica de las personas de bajos recursos," El Mundo, 27 November 1991, 13.

45. Thanks to Francisco Armada, M.D., for his discussion of this point (personal communication, 1999).

46. See Arturo Escobar, Encountering Development: The Making and Unmaking of the Third World (Princeton, N.J.: Princeton University Press, 1995).

47. See Fernando Coronil and Julie Skurski, "Dismembering and Remembering the Nation: The Semantics of Political Violence in Venezuela," Comparative Studies in Society and History 33, no. 2 (1991): 288–337.

48. Asdrubal Barrios, "Alertan sobre posible estallido de cólera en Caracas," El Nacional, 23 February 1991, C-3.

49. Vinogradoff, "72 barrios."

50. Asdrubal Barrios, "El cólera está cerca," El Nacional, 22 October 1991, C-2.

51. Quoted in Verónica Díaz Hung, "La prevención del cólera disminuyó las diarreas," El Nacional, 19 September 1991, C-4.

52. I ask the reader to keep in mind that I am using the terms Waayú and Guajíro to refer to the dominant racial construct of a bounded, homogeneous, and culturally isolated étnia.

53. Raúl Gómez V., "En peligro étnia waayu por aparición del cólera en el Estado Zulia," El Mundo, 5 December 1991, 32.

54. Alonso Zambrano, "Aumentaron a 67 casos de cólera en la frontera," El Nacional, 18 November 1991, D-6.

55. Charles Rosenberg argues that this monopoly was largely established in the United States in the course of nineteenth-century cholera epidemics. See The Cholera Years: The United States in 1832, 1849, and 1866 (Chicago: University of Chicago Press, 1962).

56. See Stuart Hall, Chas Critcher, Tony Jefferson, John Clarke, and Brian Roberts, Policing the Crisis: Mugging, the State, and Law and Order (London: Macmillan, 1978), 58, on the role of institutions as "primary definers" of news topics. I rely on their excellent book at several points in this section.

57. "Medidas para evitar el cólera," El Nacional, 10 August 1991, C-4.

58. Cindy Patton, Fatal Advice: How Safe-Sex Education Went Wrong (Durham, N.C.: Duke University Press, 1996).

59. This is what Néstor García Canclini refers to as an elemento autoritario (authoritarian element). See his Culturas híbridas: Estrategias para entrar y salir de la modernidad (Mexico City: Grijalbo, 1989).

60. See Aliana González, "Descartarán cólera en placton costero," El Nacional, 26 July 1991, C-4.

61. Gustavo Azocar, "Táchira se prepara para enfrentar el cólera," El Nacional, 20 November 1991, C-4.

62. Aliana González, "Juramentado el voluntariado para la lucha anticólera," El Nacional, 4 May 1991, C-2.

63. Modesto Rivero G., "Acerca del cólera," El Mundo, 1 June 1991, 4. The

original reads: "Cada ciudadano debe convertirse en fiscal de su propio hogar, centro de estudio o de trabajo, y de su comunidad, para exigir el cumplimiento de las normas emanados, y cuando produzcamos que el vecino se proteja adecuadamente, nos estamos protegiendo nosotros mismos." The Cámara de Diputados was, under the 1961 constitution, the lower house of Congress.

64. González, "Juramentado."

65. Díaz Hung, "La prevención."

66. See, for example, Howard Leventhal and Linda Cameron, "Persuasion and Health Attitudes," in *Persuasion: Psychological Insights and Perspectives*, ed. Sharon Shavitt and Timothy C. Brock (Boston: Allyn and Bacon, 1994), 219–249.

67. Marilyn Nations and Cristina Monte make this point in their study of cholera education efforts in Brazil. See "'I'm Not Dog, No!': Cries of Resistance against Cholera Control Campaigns," *Social Science and Medicine* 43, no. 6 (1996): 1007–1024.

68. See Fernando Coronil, *The Magical State: Nature, Money, and Modernity in Venezuela* (Chicago: University of Chicago Press, 1997).

69. Venezuelan authorities were hardly alone in this regard. Peruvian public health officials also adopted this sort of strategy in programs aimed at countering the cholera epidemic there; see Cueto, *El regreso de las epidémias*, 211.

70. "El cólera: Medio año después," *El Mundo*, 27 August 1991, 5.

71. Barrios, "El cólera."

72. Ibid.

73. Marlene Riz[k] and Graciela García, "El cólera viaja en comidas ambulantes," *El Nacional*, 18 April 1991, C-4.

74. See Marlene Rizk, "Controlarán ventas ambulantes," *El Nacional*, 23 April 1991, C-1.

75. Datanalisis, an economic consulting firm, estimated that 39 percent of the population worked in the informal sector in 1992; by January 2001, that figure had risen to 56 percent. See Eduardo Camel Anderson, "Indice de informalidad económica se elevo a 56% de la población activa," *El Nacional* (web version), 9 March 2001.

76. See Néstor García Canclini, *Culturas híbridas*.

77. Marlene Rizk, "Pese al caso de cólera no estamos en emergencia," *El Nacional*, 5 December 1991, C-4. Epidemiologists commonly distinguish "imported" from "autochthonous" cases. Nation-states fully enter the geography of cholera only once they report "autochthonous" cases, thereby admitting that the disease is spreading within their borders.

78. "Un indígena sería la primera víctima mortal del cólera," *El Nacional*, 14 December 1991, C-14.

79. Marlene Rizk, "Confirman primera muerte de cólera en Maracaibo," *El Nacional*, 17 December 1991, C-4.

80. Ibid.

81. María Victoria Cristancho, "Emergencia sanitaria por cólera," *El Mundo*, 17 December 1991, 2.

82. Alonso Zambrano, "Donde murió niña guajira crean cordón sanitario," *El Nacional,* 18 December 1991, C-4.

83. "Cuatro casos de cólera diarios en Venezuela," *El Mundo,* 9 March 1992, 23.

84. Luís R. García, "Es necesario incrementar la campaña educativa contra el cólera," *El Nacional,* 27 February 1992, C-4.

85. "Los casos de cólera que se han presentado están sanos y salvos," *Notidiario,* 18 February 1992, 22.

86. Elsy García, "25 nuevos casos de cólera en el Zulia," *El Mundo,* 16 March 1992, 29.

87. Yelitza Linares, "No hay suero ni decreto que detenga el cólera," *El Nacional,* 24 December 1991, C-4.

88. Acianela Montes de Oca, "Aún es un enigma origen de casos de cólera en Caracas," *El Nacional,* 22 January 1992, C-4.

89. Acianela Montes de Oca, "Nuevo caso en el Zulia," *El Nacional,* 21 January 1992, C-4.

90. Acianela Montes de Oca, "El cólera nos acompañará hasta el próximo siglo," *El Nacional,* 26 March 1992, C-1.

91. Montes de Oca, "Nuevo caso."

92. See Coronil, *The Magical State.*

93. María Eugenia Villalón reported to me that Pérez's statement was broadcast in a radio news program before the first cases were reported in Venezuela (personal communication, 1995).

94. For example, Páez Camargo declared that "[t]he information that appeared in some Caracas dailies yesterday, which pointed to the appearance of the first case of cholera in the country, is incorrect." "Sanidad niega caso de cólera," *El Nacional,* 17 May 1991, A-1.

95. "Plan de la OPS contra el cólera," *El Nacional,* 11 July 1991, C-5.

96. See Marlene Rizk, "El cólera llegó al país per el MSAS lo oculta," *El Nacional,* 12 July 1991, C-4.

97. "Los venezolanos creen que el SAS no tomará las medidas necesarias," *El Nacional,* 15 February 1991, C-3. It is tempting to think that women were more skeptical because the cholera education campaign placed the potential blame primarily on their shoulders.

98. "Alerta máxima contra el cólera en el Zulia," *El Nacional,* 28 April 1991, A-1.

99. Douglas González, "Gobierno dice haber controlado el cólera," *El Nuevo País,* 18 August 1992, 2.

100. See Vicente Navarro, "Neoliberalism, 'Globalization,' Unemployment, Inequalities, and the Welfare State," *International Journal of Health Services* 28, no. 4 (1998): 607–682; and Richard G. Wilkinson, *Unhealthy Societies: The Afflictions of Inequality* (London: Routledge, 1996). Other scholars have challenged the figures they use and their interpretations of them; see K. Judge, "Income Distribution and Life Expectancy: A Critical Appraisal," *British Medical Journal* 311, no. 7015 (1995): 1282–1285.

101. Colin McCord and Harold Freeman, "Excess Mortality in Harlem," *New England Journal of Medicine* 322, no. 3 (1990): 173–177.

102. As Amartya Sen has powerfully argued; see *Commodities and Capabilities* (Amsterdam: North-Holland, 1985), *Poverty and Child Health* (Oxford: Radcliff Medical Press, 1996), and *On Economic Inequality,* expanded ed. (Oxford: Clarendon Press, 1997).

103. "Prioridad: Atacar el cólera," *2001,* 17 August 1992, 5.

CHAPTER 2. EPIDEMIC AT THE DOOR

1. See Oficina Central de Estadística e Informática, *El Censo 90 en Delta Amacuro* (Caracas: Oficina Central de Estadística e Informática, 1995), 5; and "Para evitar el cólera prohiben consumo de alimentos crudos y hielo," *Notidiario,* 22 February 1992, 23.

2. "Instruye a médicos rurales sobre prevención del cólera," *Notidiario,* 16 May 1991, 5.

3. According to the 1992 indigenous census; see Oficina Central de Estadística e Informática, *Censo.*

4. Asdrubal Barrios, "Las bocas del Orinoco (I): Un delta empobrecido pide ayuda al Parlamento," *El Nacional,* 20 August 1991, C-1.

5. Quoted in Asdrubal Barrios, "Las bocas del Orinoco (II): Coexistencia moral con la civilización," *El Nacional,* 21 August 1991, C-1. For this balance, see also H. Dieter Heinen and Kenneth Ruddle, "Ecology, Ritual, and Economic Organization in the Distribution of Palm Starch among the Warao of the Orinoco Delta," *Journal of Anthropological Research* 30, no. 2 (1974): 116–138.

6. This trickster-like ability to identify resources available for re-appropriation and to be the first to devise a strategy capable of securing them is admired by many. The only problem with cholera was that the stakes were too low, that it only held the key to unlocking a fairly modest set of resources.

CHAPTER 3. STORIES OF AN EPIDEMIC FORETOLD

1. A school was constructed in 1998 by the community using funds provided by the Amoco Corporation, which was exploring for oil in the vicinity; the Ministry of Education sent two teachers to the community in that year.

2. See Mary Louise Pratt, *Imperial Eyes: Travel Writing and Transculturation* (London: Routledge, 1992), for her discussion of contact zones.

3. Again, this statement must be amended to reflect the establishment of a public school constructed with Amoco funds in 1998.

4. Interviewed in Mariusa Akoho on 12 October 1994.

5. Michele Goldwasser details the history of this interaction between delta residents and Trinidadians. See "The Rainbow Madonna of Trinidad: A Study in the Dynamics of Belief in Trinidadian Religious Life," Ph.D. diss., University of California, Los Angeles, 1996.

6. All equivalents are to American dollars.

7. Johannes Wilbert has written extensively about Warao curing; see "Tobacco and Shamanistic Ecstasy among the Warao of Venezuela," in *Flesh of the Gods: The Ritual Use of Hallucinogens*, ed. Peter Furst (New York: Praeger, 1972), 55–83, and *Mystic Endowment: Religious Ethnography of the Warao Indians* (Cambridge, Mass.: Harvard University Center for the Study of World Religions, 1993). Also see Dale A. Olsen, *Music of the Warao of Venezuela: Song People of the Rain Forest* (Gainesville: University Presses of Florida, 1996).

8. Interviewed in Mariusa Akoho in 2000.

9. "Bajó en un noventa por ciento demanda de pescado en Tucupita," *Notidiario*, 17 August 1992, 17.

10. Interviewed in Mariusa Akoho on 8 October 1994.

11. Ibid.

12. Interviewed at Yakariyene in Tucupita on 12 November 1992.

13. This figure is for Mariusa, Boca de Macareo, and Boca de Cocuina, and comes from a census undertaken by SOCSAL; see their "Registro sociodemográfico Warao de Punta Pescador," photocopy [1998].

14. See Werner Wilbert, *Fitoterápia Warao: Una teoría pnéumica de la salud, la enfermedad y la terápia* (Caracas: Instituto Caribe de Antropología y Sociología, Fundación La Salle de Ciencias Naturales, Instituto Caribe de Antropología y Sociología, 1996), for an extensive study of the use of plants in vernacular healing in the Winikina area.

15. See Charles L. Briggs, "'Since I Am a Woman, I Will Chastise My Relatives': Gender, Reported Speech, and the (Re)production of Social Relations in Warao Ritual Wailing," *American Ethnologist* 19 (1992): 337–361, and "Personal Sentiments and Polyphonic Voices in Warao Women's Ritual Wailing: Music and Poetics in a Critical and Collective Discourse," *American Anthropologist* 95 (1993): 929–957.

16. Charles Briggs has developed this argument in a number of publications. Relevant here, in addition to the essays on wailing ("'Since I Am a Woman,'" and "Personal Sentiments"), are his discussions of dispute mediation ("Conflict, Language Ideologies, and Privileged Arenas of Discursive Authority in Warao Dispute Mediation," in *Disorderly Discourse: Narrative, Conflict, and Social Inequality*, ed. Charles L. Briggs [Oxford: Oxford University Press, 1996], 204–242), gossip ("'You're a Liar—You're Just Like a Woman!' Constructing Dominant Ideologies of Language in Warao Men's Gossip," in *Language Ideologies: Practice and Theory*, ed. Bambi Schieffelin, Kathryn A. Woolard, and Paul V. Kroskrity [New York: Oxford University Press, 1998], 229–255), and the performance of "ancestral narratives" ("Generic versus Metapragmatic Dimensions of Warao Narratives: Who Regiments Performance?" in *Reflexive Language: Reported Speech and Metapragmatics*, ed. John A. Lucy [Cambridge: Cambridge University Press, 1993], 179–212).

17. The word *wisidatu* is not marked for the singular-versus-plural distinction; we add an *-s* to plural uses in order to assist the reader.

18. Interviewed in Nabaribuhu on 29 July 1990.

19. Briggs, "'You're a Liar,'" analyzes a gossip session in which Rivera and Torres jointly sought to discredit sorcery accusations that had been made about them.

20. See Johannes Wilbert, *Textos folklóricos de los indios Warao* (Los Angeles: Latin American Center, University of California, Los Angeles, 1969), and *Folk Literature of the Warao Indians* (Los Angeles: Latin American Center, University of California, 1970); and Claude Lévi-Strauss, *The Raw and the Cooked: Introduction to a Science of Mythology*, trans. John and Doreen Weightman (New York: Harper and Row, 1969). Missionaries Basilio Barral and Julio Lavandero have also published extensive collections; see Rev. P. Fr. Basilio Barral, *Guarao guarata: Lo que cuentan los indios guaraos* (Caracas: Editorial Salesiana [1961]); and Julio Lavandero Pérez, ed., *Ajotejana I: Mitos* (Caracas: n.p., 1991), *Ajotejana II: Relatos* (Caracas: n.p., 1992), and *Uaharaho: Ethos narrativo* (Caracas: Hermanos Capuchinos, 1994). H. Dieter Heinen and I have presented *dehe hido* or *dehe kwaimotane abane*, "stories of recent times," that speak with equal poignancy about the way that the power of the nation-state is felt, courted, and resisted; see H. Dieter Heinen, *Oko Warao: Marshland People of the Orinoco Delta* (Muenster: Lit Verlag, 1988); and Briggs, "Conflict, Language Ideologies, and Privileged Arenas," and "'You're a Liar.'"

21. See Briggs, "Generic versus Metapragmatic Dimensions" and "'You're a Liar.'"

22. See Charles L. Briggs, "Emergence of the Non-Indigenous Peoples," in *Translating Native Latin American Verbal Art: Ethnopoetics and Ethnography of Speaking*, ed. Kay Sammons and Joel Sherzer (Washington, D.C.: Smithsonian Institution Press, 2000), 174–196.

23. See Michael Taussig, *Shamanism, Colonialism, and the Wild Man: A Study in Terror and Healing* (Chicago: University of Chicago Press, 1987).

24. William Labov and Joshua Waletsky, "Narrative Analysis," in *Essays on the Verbal and Visual Arts*, ed. June Helm (Seattle: University of Washington Press, 1967), 12–44.

25. Jonathan Culler, *The Pursuit of Signs* (London: Routledge & Kegan Paul, 1981).

26. Jerome S. Bruner, *Acts of Meaning* (Cambridge, Mass.: Harvard University Press, 1990), 43.

27. Paul Ricoeur, *Hermeneutics and the Human Sciences*, trans. John B. Thompson (Cambridge: Cambridge University Press, 1981), 284; see also Paul Ricoeur, *Time and Narrative*, trans. K. McLaughlin and D. Pellauer, vol. 1 (Chicago: University of Chicago Press, 1984).

28. See Richard Bauman, *Story, Performance, and Event: Contextual Studies of Oral Narrative* (Cambridge: Cambridge University Press, 1986); for the contrasting argument, see Labov and Waletsky, "Narrative Analysis."

29. Marita Sturken, *Tangled Memories: The Vietnam War, the AIDS Epidemic, and the Politics of Remembering* (Berkeley: University of California Press, 1997). Elinor Ochs and Lisa Capps, *Living Narrative: Creating Lives in*

Everyday Storytelling (Cambridge, Mass.: Harvard University Press, 2001), lucidly explore the role of everyday storytelling in creating memory.

30. See Hayden White, *Tropics of Discourse: Essays in Cultural Criticism* (Baltimore: Johns Hopkins University Press, 1978), on the role of narrative structures in shaping cultural memory.

31. See Avery F. Gordon, *Ghostly Matters: Haunting and the Sociological Imagination* (Minneapolis: University of Minnesota Press, 1997).

32. Sigmund Freud, "Screen Memories," in *The Standard Edition of the Complete Psychological Works of Sigmund Freud,* trans. James Strachey (London: Hogarth Press, 1962), 3: 301–322.

33. See Briggs, "Personal Sentiments and Polyphonic Voices."

CHAPTER 4. FIGHTING DEATH IN A REGIONAL CLINIC

1. The quotations included in this chapter were not tape-recorded; they are thus approximations drawn from the memory of the author (Clara Mantini-Briggs). This conversation took place in Tucupita on 2 August 1992.

2. She is referring here to the three leading political parties at the time.

3. Cruz José Marín, *Estampas deltanas* (Tucupita, Venezuela: privately published, 1977), 79.

CHAPTER 5. TURNING CHAOS INTO CONTROL

1. Interviewed in Tucupita on 14 January 1994.

2. Interviewed in Tucupita on 17 May 1995.

3. Interviewed in Tucupita on 1 November 1994.

4. Conversation with Charles Briggs in Caracas on approximately 10 November 1992. This quote is taken from memory, as the exchange was not recorded.

5. Interviewed, along with Elizabethe Pérez de Silva, in Tucupita on 18 April 1995.

6. Jacques Derrida calls this the metaphysics of presence; see *Of Grammatology,* trans. Gayatri Chakravorty Spivak (Baltimore: Johns Hopkins University Press, 1974).

7. "ORAI emprende campaña contra el cólera en zonas indígenas," *Notidiario,* 8 August 1992, 23.

8. "Se extiende el cólera en el Delta por migración de los indígenas," *Notidiario,* 12 August 1992, 2.

9. Nolasco Guarisma Alvarez, "Sub-Comisión congresal visita sectores afectados por el cólera en el Delta," *Notidiario,* 21 August 1992, 2.

10. "Se extiende."

11. "Alerta roja por cólera en el estado Delta Amacuro," *Notidiario,* 8 August 1992, 1.

12. "Instalan en Tucupita laboratorio de microbiología," *Notidiario,* 19 August 1992, 3.

13. These cases, which are listed in the regional epidemiologist's summary of laboratory-confirmed cases in 1992 and 1993 (see Ministerio de Sanidad y Asistencia Pública, Departamento de Epidemiología, Estado Delta Amacuro, "Casos de cólera, positivos," typescript, 1993), were described to Charles Briggs by Rodríguez.

14. "Criollos temen contagiarse del cólera," *Notidiario*, 21 August 1992, 23.

15. "La sombra del cólera," *Notidiario*, 6 August 1992, 1; and "Pánico en el delta," *Notidiario*, 6 August 1992, 24.

16. "Delta Amacuro llamando al SAS S.O.S.," *Notidiario*, 7 August 1992, 1.

17. "17 casos de tuberculosis en el hospital Razetti," *Notidiario*, 8 August 1992, 23.

18. "A la Isla Tortuga llevaron a 251 Waraos," *Notidiario*, 18 August 1992, 1.

19. Patton, *Fatal Advice*. She is commenting here on HIV/AIDS education in the United States during the 1980s.

20. As argued with reference to portrayals of AIDS patients by Sturken, *Tangled Memories*, 160–163; and Paula Treichler, "AIDS, Homophobia, and Biomedical Discourse: An Epidemic of Signification," in *AIDS: Cultural Analysis/ Cultural Activism*, ed. Douglas Crimp (Cambridge, Mass.: MIT Press, 1988), 31–70, and "AIDS, Gender, and Biomedical Discourse: Current Contests for Meaning," in *AIDS: Burdens of History*, ed. Elizabeth Fee and Daniel M. Fox (Berkeley: University of California Press, 1988), 190–266. Steven Epstein argues that AIDS activists accordingly rejected victimhood in favor of political engagement and power sharing; see *Impure Science: AIDS, Activism, and the Politics of Knowledge* (Berkeley: University of California Press, 1996).

21. See Gordon, *Ghostly Matters*, 4.

22. On these concepts, see Charles L. Briggs and Richard Bauman, "Genre, Intertextuality, and Social Power," *Journal of Linguistic Anthropology* 2, no. 2 (1992): 131–172.

23. González, "Gobierno dice haber controlado el cólera."

24. "49 casos de cólera registra el SAS de Delta Amacuro," *Notidiario*, 19 August 1992, 3.

25. "Hambre, vomito [*sic*] y diarrea extingue [*sic*] la raza warauna," *Notidiario*, 6 August 1992, 19.

26. "Declarado en emergencia sanitaria Delta Amacuro por brote de cólera," *Notidiario*, 12 August 1992, 3.

27. "121 nuevos casos."

28. "Grupo de socorristas de la Cruz Roja llega a Delta Amacur," *Notidiario*, 17 August 1992, 23.

29. See Elizabeth Cohen, "Programa de ayuda a Waraos ofreció Comunidad Económica," *El Nacional*, 15 September 1992; "Holanda financiará en Venezuela un proyecto masivo de la Comunidad Lucha contra el Cólera," *Notidiario*, 15 October 1992, 20.

30. See Lawrence W. Green and Marshall W. Kreuter, *Health Promotion Planning: An Educational and Ecological Approach* (Mountain View, Calif.: Mayfield, 1999); N. Pearce, "Traditional Epidemiology, Modern Epidemiology,

and Public Health," *American Journal of Public Health* 86 (1996): 678–683; and M. Terris, "Epidemiology and the Public Health Movement," *Journal of Public Health Policy* 7 (1987): 315–329.

31. See, for example, Leventhal and Cameron, "Persuasion and Health Attitudes."

32. This brochure bears the logos and names of both MSAS and regional and local governments in Delta Amacuro.

33. See Charles Taylor, *Multiculturalism: Examining the Politics of Recognition,* ed. and intro. Amy Gutmann (Princeton, N.J.: Princeton University Press, 1994).

34. "Autoridades del SAS salieron a buscar recursos contra el cólera," *Notidiario,* 7 September 1992, 17.

35. Although the slogan was used frequently in health education programs undertaken during the epidemic, this billboard was installed after it ended.

36. Sturken, *Tangled Memories,* suggests that events of trauma in particular expose the structures and fractures of culture in a way that renders them powerful sites for the construction of cultural memory.

37. I have changed the name of this community.

38. "ORAI emprende campaña."

39. "Establecen puente aéreo entre Tucupita y Caracas," *Notidiario,* 19 August 1992, 3.

40. Interviewed in Tucupita on 17 May 1995.

41. José Gómez Zuloaga, "Controlado el cólera en Barrancas," *El Diario de Monagas,* 2 September 1992. Interviewed in Tucupita on 14 January 1994.

42. Interviewed in Tucupita on 14 January 1994.

43. "Por nada del mundo regresaremos a los sitios que dejamos en el Delta," *Notidiario,* 17 August 1992, 12.

44. "A 837 ascienden los casos de cólera en Delta Amacuro," *Notidiario,* 2 September 1992, 1.

45. González, "Gobierno dice haber controlado el cólera"; "Controlado brote de cólera en el Delta," *El Diario de Monagas,* 18 August 1992, 3; and "Continua avanzando el cólera en el estado Delta Amacuro," *Notidiario,* 18 August 1992, 24.

46. José María García Gómez was the *caudillo,* or political boss, of Delta Amacuro in the 1980s and 1990s. He resigned as governor in 1992 in order to be able to run in the first official elections for the office in December of that year. Although he officially won the contest, Movimiento al Socialismo candidate Bernardo Alonzo challenged the election in court and was declared governor in 1993.

47. "Llaman a comisión indigenista en zona afectada por cólera," *Notidiario,* 4 September 1992.

48. "El cólera en el Delta Amacuro está asociado a la baja calidad de la vida," *Notidiario,* 17 August 1992, 15. Candidate Abraham Gómez similarly asserted that a visit to the lower delta revealed that the people had been waiting for years for a response, presumably from the government, to their sadness and poverty; he relayed residents' complaints regarding the lack of facilities for sewage and

potable water and medicine; see "Abraham Gómez recorrió el bajo Delta," *Notidiario*, 19 August 1992, 5.

49. See M. M. Bakhtin, *The Dialogic Imagination: Four Essays,* trans. Caryl Emerson and Michael Holquist, ed. Michael Holquist (Austin: University of Texas Press, 1981).

50. See Yolanda Salas, "La dramatización social y política del imaginario popular: el fenómeno del bolivarismo en Venezuela," in *Estudios latinoamericanos sobre cultura y transformaciones sociales en tiempos de globalización,* ed. Daniel Mato (Buenos Aires: Consejo Latinoamericano de Ciencias Sociales, 2001), 201–221. Yolanda Salas de Lecuna demonstrated that Bolívar continues to provide a central symbolic resource for structuring relations of social and political domination and resistance in Venezuela; see *Bolívar y la historia en la conciencia popular* (Caracas: Instituto de Altos Estudios de América Latina, Universidad Simón Bolívar, 1987).

51. Interviewed in Nabasanuka on 8 July 1995.

52. We want to note clearly the limitations of our sources here. The authors interviewed Gómez and nurses who work in Nabasanuka, and the priest who served the Nabasanuka mission provided an eyewitness account. Nevertheless, we were not able to interview the visiting physician, and the doctor who was in residence in Nabasanuka was not in the community at the time the incident took place. As a result, our assessment of the physician's position is based on accounts provided by others.

53. Interviewed in Nabasanuka on 8 July 1995.

54. See Omi and Winant, *Racial Formation in the United States.* They define a racial project as a concrete set of activities that are *"simultaneously an interpretation, representation, or explanation of racial dynamics, and an effort to reorganize and redistribute resources along particular racial lines"* (56; original emphasis).

CHAPTER 6. CONTAINING AN INDIGENOUS INVASION

1. This figure is from the 1990 census. See Oficina Central de Estadística e Informática, *El censo 90 en Monagas* (Caracas: Oficina Central de Estadística e Informática, 1995).

2. See Yépez Colmenares, "La epidemia de cólera," 165.

3. *Notidiario* provided this figure; see "Por nada del mundo regresaremos a los sitios que dejamos en el Delta," 17 August 1992, 12–13. Note that the figure given below in María Vargas's story is slightly higher.

4. "Por nada del mundo regresaremos," 12–13.

5. As Russian linguist and literary critic V. N. Volosinov has suggested; see *Marxism and the Philosophy of Language,* trans. Wladislav Metejka and I. R. Titunik (New York: Seminar Press, 1973).

6. "Por nada del mundo regresaremos," 13.

7. As Mary Douglas argues; see *Purity and Danger: An Analysis of the Concepts of Pollution and Taboo* (London: Routledge & Kegan Paul, 1966).

8. See Otto Santa Ana, *Brown Tide Rising: Metaphors of Latinos in Contemporary American Public Discourse* (Austin: University of Texas Press, 2002). With respect to the notion of an "invasion" by *indígenas,* Sontag argues that military metaphors, also common in this context, are dangerous in that they authorize the nation-state (the sole authorized war-making body) to take counter-measures of whatever scale it deems necessary; see Susan Sontag, *Illness as Metaphor and AIDS and Its Metaphors* (New York: Doubleday, 1990).

9. Several of the officials who had been closely connected with cholera control efforts expressed this eagerness to tell their story.

10. This figure differs significantly from that in the records at the Regional Health Service in Tucupita.

11. As suggested by the Italian political theorist Antonio Gramsci. Gramsci has argued that the power of the nation-state and elites is primarily effected through what he referred to as *hegemony;* see *Selections from the Prison Notebooks of Antonio Gramsci,* trans. Quintin Hoare and Geoffrey Nowell Smith (New York: International, 1971).

12. Susan Chase found that women who become superintendents of public school systems in the United States tell narratives in which they cast themselves as struggling individually to overcome obstacles; see *Ambiguous Empowerment: The World of Narratives of Women School Superintendents* (Amherst: University of Massachusetts Press, 1995).

13. The manual, following Michael Taussig, takes the form of a montage, a juxtaposition of heterogeneous elements; see Taussig, *Shamanism.*

14. *Manual de normas y procedimientos,* 11. These guidelines were taken directly from the "Rules Regarding Obligatorily Reportable Diseases" enacted by presidential decree on 14 August 1939; see *Legislación sanitaria nacional,* 453.

15. World Heath Organization, *WHO Guidance on Formulation of National Policy on the Control of Cholera* (Geneva: World Health Organization, 1992), 4; original emphasis.

16. PAHO distributes the WHO manuals to ministries of health in the Americas; the PAHO imprimateur appears on some editions. PAHO also issues a Spanish translation of each new edition of the American Public Health Association's *Control of Communicable Diseases Manual* as part of its own Scientific Publication series; see Abram S. Benenson, *Control of Communicable Diseases Manual,* 14th ed. (Washington, D.C.: American Public Health Association, 1990). These manuals are authoritative sources for physicians and public health officials in Latin America. In 1970, the manual suggested "the adoption of temporary measures . . . for the isolation and adequate treatment of the sick and in order to discover suspect cases. It can be convenient to identify and isolate carriers, but generally is impractical" (52). When the epidemic began in 1991, the fourteenth edition (published in English in 1985 and in Spanish in 1987) was in use. By then, doubt regarding the "practicality" of isolating possible carriers had been replaced by a clear statement: "Quarantine: None."

17. *Manual de normas y procedimientos,* 4.

18. "No se ha registrado casos de cólera."

19. Interviewed in Maturín, Monagas, on 31 March 1995.

20. Interviewed in Tucupita on 5 December 1994.

21. Interviewed in Tucupita on 18 April 1995.

22. Megan Vaughan illuminates how public health authorities in colonial Africa used it in naturalizing the epidemics of infectious diseases; see *Curing Their Ills: Colonial Power and African Illness* (Palo Alto, Calif.: Stanford University Press, 1991).

23. See Peter Stallybrass and Allon White, *The Politics and Poetics of Transgression* (Ithaca, N.Y.: Cornell University Press, 1986).

24. See Omi and Winant, *Racial Formation in the United States*.

25. See Pierre Bourdieu, *Outline of a Theory of Practice,* trans. Richard Nice (Cambridge: Cambridge University Press, 1977 [1972]).

26. *Yupari* and *Oyapari* are different spellings of the same name.

CHAPTER 7. EXILE AND INTERNMENT

1. "No se ha registrado casos de cólera."

2. Nolasco Guarisma Alvarez, "Indígenas de Mariusa y Winikina volvieron a sus lugares de origen," *Notidiario,* 4 September 1992, 9.

3. Ibid.

4. See Ricardo Hausmann, *Shocks externos y ajuste macroeconómico* (Caracas: Banco Central de Venezuela, 1990), 224; see also Ricardo Hausmann, *Dealing with Negative Oil Shocks: The Venezuelan Experience in the Eighties,* Working Paper Series, no. 307 (Washington, D.C.: Inter-American Development Bank, 1995). Anthropologist Fernando Coronil concurs with Hausmann's assessment; see *The Magical State.*

5. The similarity to the situation in the United States is striking. African-Americans and Latinos who obtain public assistance are particularly vulnerable to stereotyping, stigmatization, and the loss of fundamental rights, such as the right to have or raise children; see Dorothy Roberts, *Killing the Black Body: Race, Reproduction, and the Meaning of Liberty* (New York: Vintage, 1997).

6. Interviewed in Barrancas on 15 November 1994.

7. Interviewed in Caracas on 10 November 1994.

8. Guarisma Alvarez, "Indígenas de Mariusa y Winikina."

9. In the discourse of Monagas officials, *Tucupita* refers to the government of Delta Amacuro state. Common elsewhere as well, it seems to erase the presence of people who live in the fluvial area.

10. Guarisma Alvarez, "Indígenas de Mariusa y Winikina."

11. Interviewed in Tucupita on 14 September 1994.

12. From another section of the interview in Caracas on 10 November 1994.

CHAPTER 8. MEDICINE, MAGIC, AND MILITARY MIGHT

1. See Maurice Belrose, *La época del modernismo en Venezuela* (Caracas: Monte Avila, 1999), for a study of modernism in Venezuelan literature.

2. See Johannes Wilbert, *Tobacco and Shamanism in South America* (New Haven, Conn.: Yale University Press, 1987), *Mystic Endowment,* and "Tobacco and Shamanistic Ecstasy."

3. Interviewed in Nabaribahu on 16 February 1995.

4. Castañeda, Aranguren, Romero, Salazar, García, and other Tortuga residents interviewed on 12 February 1995.

5. Dipesh Chakrabarty has argued that this notion of the simultaneous existence of worlds that belong to distinct temporal realms, modern and premodern, plays a key role in constituting modern schemes of social inequality. See *Provincializing Europe: Postcolonial Thought and Historical Difference* (Princeton, N.J.: Princeton University Press, 2000).

6. See Bakhtin, *Dialogic Imagination.*

7. Johannes Fabian refers to this mode of creating distance as the "denial of coevalness" and suggests that it is the classic process whereby anthropologists have claimed distance from and superiority over the objects of their research, thereby contributing to colonial relations of power and domination. See *Time and the Other: How Anthropology Makes Its Object* (New York: Columbia University Press, 1983).

8. See Edward W. Soja, *Postmodern Geographies: The Reassertion of Space in Critical Social Theory* (London: Verso, 1989), 120.

9. A number of writers have argued that the production of space is both grounded in and in turn structures political-economic processes. See Henri Lefebvre, *The Production of Space,* trans. Donald Nicholson-Smith (Oxford: Blackwell, 1991); David Harvey, *The Condition of Postmodernity* (Cambridge: Blackwell, 1989); and Manuel Castells, *The Information Age: Economy, Society and Culture,* vol. 1: *The Rise of the Network Society* (Oxford: Blackwell, 1996).

10. Rather than cluttering the text with quotation marks around "civilized," "uncivilized," "savage," "natural man," "nature," and the like, I ask the reader to bear in mind that I am using these concepts as powerful social constructions, not invoking them as modes of social classification.

11. Jean-Jacques Rousseau, *Discourse on the Origin of Inequality,* trans. Franklin Philip (Oxford: Oxford University Press, 1994).

12. This picture is riddled with intriguing logical contradictions. While one of the defining features of the Mariusans is their nomadic character, the very way that they are defined and labeled—as Mariusans—rigidly spatializes them as inhabiting one part of the delta. Similarly, adapting oneself to a *changing* natural environment would seem to depict a cultural dynamism that undermines the image of people who live just as their ancestors lived "a hundred years ago."

13. See Etienne Balibar, "Is There a 'Neo-Racism'?" in *Race, Nation, Class: Ambiguous Identities,* Etienne Balibar and Immanuel Wallerstein (London: Verso, 1991), 17–28.

14. Taussig, *Shamanism.*

15. Recall the statement by the mayor of Barrancas regarding the cordon sanitaire in Tortuga that was intended to curtail "movement of *indígenas* who

are carriers of the cholera vibrio toward the southern part of Monagas"; see "No se ha registrado casos de cólera."

16. Interviewed in central Venezuela on 13 November 1994.

17. See Bruno Latour, *We Have Never Been Modern,* trans. Catherine Porter (Cambridge, Mass.: Harvard University Press, 1993).

18. Interviewed on 13 November 1994. This supports Etienne Balibar's characterization of cultural reasoning and its projection of cultural differences as insurmountable; see Balibar, "Is There a 'Neo-Racism'?"

19. Julio C. Salas, *Civilización y barbarie: Estudios sociológicos americanos* (Caracas: Fundación Julio C. Salas, 1998 [1919]), 174.

20. Ramón Rivera (with Diego González), Mariusa Akoho, 12 October 1994; the narrative appears in chapter 6.

21. José Rivera, Nabaribuhu, 16 February 1995; the narrative appears in chapter 7.

22. See Latour, *We Have Never Been Modern.*

23. As David Arnold has observed with respect to British colonial medicine in India; see *Colonizing the Body: State Medicine and Epidemic Disease in Nineteenth-Century India* (Berkeley: University of California Press, 1993).

CHAPTER 9. CULTURE EQUALS CHOLERA

1. My motives for separating the narratives into these two categories is largely expositional. I wish neither to imply any sort of temporal or epistemological priority nor to judge the political underpinnings and effects of either in advance. As Martha Kaplan and John D. Kelly suggest, setting up rigid analytic borders between hegemonic or complicit versus resistant discourses says more about the classificatory compulsions of academics than the complex workings of power in everyday life; see "Rethinking Resistance: Dialogics of 'Disaffection' in Colonial Fiji," *American Ethnologist* 21 (1994): 122–151. My goal is to trace these dynamics as they emerged in different sites and agendas and to assess the way that these explanations of a medical emergency came to shape a vast range of features of daily life—what Michel Foucault calls "positive productivity"; see *Discipline and Punish: The Birth of the Prison,* trans. Alan Sheridan (New York: Vintage, 1977).

2. "En el Delta Amacuro: Seis muertos por cólera al consumir cangrejos," *El Nacional,* 5 August 1992, D-19.

3. "Pánico en el delta"; added emphasis.

4. "Huyendo del cólera." The complete name of the institution is the Dirección General Sectorial de Saneamiento Socio Ambiental, Zona XXIII Malariología.

5. Rafael Luna Noguera, "Entre el hambre, la insalubridad y el cangrejo peludo transcurre la vida en el Delta Amacuro," *Ultimas Noticias,* 17 August 1992, 24.

6. "El miedo de los Waraos por los cangrejos azules rompe una tradición milenaria," *Notidiario,* 17 August 1992, 11.

7. "Instalan en Tucupita laboratorio de microbiología," *Notidiario,* 19 August 1992, 3. The term is written as both *nowara* and *noara.*

8. See I. Kaye Wachsmuth, Gracia M. Evins, Patricia I. Fields, Ørjan Olsvik, Tanja Popovic, Cheryl A. Bopp, Joy G. Wells, Carlos Carrillo, and Paul A. Blake, "The Molecular Epidemiology of Cholera in Latin America," *Journal of Infectious Diseases* 167, no. 3 (1993): 621–626.

9. As Aaron Cicourel suggests; see "The Interpenetration of Communicative Contexts: Examples from Medical Encounters," in *Rethinking Context: Language as an Interactive Phenomenon,* ed. Alessandro Duranti and Charles Goodwin (Cambridge: Cambridge University Press, 1992), 291–310.

10. See Julio Lavandero Pérez, *Noara y otros rituales* (Caracas: Universidad Católica Andrés Bello, 2000).

11. "El miedo de los Waraos."

12. White, *Tropics of Discourse,* suggests that dominant narratives imagine social reality, then use narrative strategies to legitimate these contradictions.

13. "Continua avanzando el cólera."

14. See Volosinov, *Marxism and the Philosophy of Language.*

15. For heteroglossia, see Bakhtin, *Dialogic Imagination.*

16. Interviewed in Tucupita on 29 March 1995.

17. "El cólera está matando a los Waraos del Delta," *Notidiario,* 14 August 1992, 12.

18. "Controlado brote de cólera."

19. Quoted in Mariela Nuñez, "Delta Amacuro, Sucre, D.F. y Monagas: Focos mas activos del cólera," *El Globo,* 18 August 1992, 45.

20. Interviewed in Maturín, Monagas, on 31 March 1999.

21. Quoted in a documentary on the Vietnam War directed by Peter Davis, *Hearts and Minds* (1974). I would like to thank Jorge Mariscal for pointing out this source for the quotation and Joseph Sherman-Villafañe for transcribing it.

22. Luna Noguera, "Entre el hambre."

23. Quoted in "Se extiende el cólera en el Delta."

24. See Rev. P. Fr. Basilio Barral, *Los indios guaraunos y su cancionero: Historia, religión, y alma lírica,* Biblioteca "Missionalia Hispanica," vol. 15 (Madrid: Consejo Superior de Investigaciones Científicas, Departamento de Misionología Española, 1964); Olsen, *Music of the Warao;* Wilbert, "Tobacco and Shamanistic Ecstasy," *Tobacco and Shamanism,* and *Mystic Endowment.*

25. See Briggs, "'Since I Am a Woman,'" and "Personal Sentiments."

26. "Se desplaza hacia Monagas brote epidémico de cólera," *Notidiario,* 20 August 1992, 2.

27. "Se extiende el cólera en el Delta."

28. Ibid.

29. "A más de mil ascienden casos de cólera en el Delta," *El Diario de Monagas,* 6 October 1992, 1.

30. Interviewed in Maturín on 31 March 1995.

31. Nineteenth-century cholera epidemics provided crucial sites for exerting the control of elites, the medical profession, and the nation-state over the lives

of the working class and communities of color. See Rosenberg, *The Cholera Years*, for the United States. For Europe, see Louis Chevalier, *Le choléra: La première épidémie du XIXe siècle* (Roche-sur-Yon: Imprimerie Centrale de l'Ouest, 1958); François Delaporte, *Disease and Civilization: The Cholera in Paris, 1832*, trans. Arthur Goldhammer (Cambridge, Mass.: MIT Press, 1986); Catherine J. Kudlick, *Cholera in Post-Revolutionary Paris: A Cultural History* (Berkeley: University of California Press, 1996); Michael Durey, *The Return of the Plague: British Society and the Cholera, 1831–32* (Dublin: Gill and Macmillan, 1979); Richard J. Evans, *Death in Hamburg: Society and Politics in the Cholera Years 1830–1910* (Oxford: Clarendon Press, 1987); and R. J. Morris, *Cholera 1832: The Social Response to an Epidemic* (New York: Holmes & Meier, 1976). For India, see Arnold, *Colonizing the Body*; and V. Prashad, "Native Dirt/Imperial Ordure: The Cholera of 1832 and the Morbid Resolutions of Modernity," *Journal of Historical Sociology* 7 (1994): 243–260; and for the Philippines, see R. C. Ileto, "Outlines of a Non-Linear Emplotment of Philippine History," in *Reflections on Development in Southeast Asia*, ed. L. T. Ghee (Singapore: ASEAN Economic Research Unit, Institute of Southeast Asian Studies, 1988), 130–159, and "Cholera and the Origins of the American Sanitary Order in the Philippines," in *Discrepant Histories: Translocal Essays on Filipino Cultures*, ed. Vincent L. Rafael (Philadelphia: Temple University Press, 1995), 51–81.

32. Interviewed in Tucupita on 17 May 1995.

33. See Francisco José Ferrándiz, "The Body in Its Senses: The Spirit Possession Cult of María Lionza in Contemporary Venezuela," Ph.D. diss., University of California, Berkeley, 1996; Angelina Pollak-Eltz, *María Lionza: Mito y culto venezolano* (Caracas: Instituto de Investigaciones Históricas, Universidad Católica Andrés Bello, 1972); and Salas de Lecuna, *Bolívar y la historia*.

34. See Arjun Appadurai, *Modernity at Large: Cultural Dimensions of Globalization* (Minneapolis: University of Minnesota Press, 1996); and Harvey, *The Condition of Postmodernity*.

35. See Niklas Luhmann, *The Differentiation of Society*, trans. Stephen Holmes and Charles Larmore (New York: Columbia University Press, 1982). Politicians who are always undergoing media scrutiny may be an exception.

36. I draw here on Emily Martin, *Flexible Bodies: Tracking Immunity in American Culture from the Days of Polio to the Age of AIDS* (Boston: Beacon Press, 1994), and "Mind-Body Problems," *American Ethnologist* 27, no. 3 (2000): 569–590.

37. See Michael Taussig, *The Magic of the State* (New York: Routledge, 1997).

38. Jaber F. Gubrium and James A. Holstein, *The New Language of Qualitative Method* (New York: Oxford University Press, 1997). In the United States, child protection and public service agencies, homeless shelters, police departments, courts, prison and parole officers, and others bring the lives of the poor, especially the racialized poor, under increasing scrutiny.

39. See Charles L. Briggs, "The Politics of Discursive Authority in Research on the 'Invention of Tradition,'" *Cultural Anthropology* 11, no. 4 (1996): 435–469. With regard to performances of cultural difference in Venezuela, see

David M. Guss, *The Festive State: Race, Ethnicity, and Nationalism as Cultural Performance* (Berkeley: University of California Press, 2000).

40. Interviewed in Tucupita on 6 December 1994.

41. "121 nuevos casos de cólera." The term *governmentality* is from Michel Foucault, *The Foucault Effect: Studies in Governmentality*, ed. Graham Burchell, Colin Gordon, and Peter Miller (Chicago: University of Chicago Press, 1991).

42. "Presencia de la Guardia Nacional contribuyó grandemente a combatir el mal," *El Diario de Monagas*, 19 August 1992, for example, asserts that "the geographic characteristics of Delta Amacuro . . . make sanitary or any other type of control in the region difficult."

43. Francis Bacon is often credited with inaugurating this instrumental approach to a distanced nature; see *Novum organum*, vol. 4 of *The Works of Francis Bacon*, ed. James Spedding, Robert Leslie Ellis, and Douglas Denon Heath (New York: Garrett Press, 1968).

44. Interviewed in Tucupita on 8 December 1994.

45. See Fabian, *Time and the Other*.

46. See Bakhtin, *Dialogic Imagination*.

47. "Instalado y juramentado Comité Regional de Lucha Contra el Cólera," *Notidiario*, 14 January 1997.

48. Interviewed in Koboina on 16 October 1994.

49. Interviewed in Caracas on 13 December 1994.

50. See George W. Stocking, Jr., *Race, Culture, and Evolution: Essays in the History of Anthropology* (New York: Free Press, 1968).

51. Franz Boas, *Race, Language, and Culture* (New York: Free Press, 1940). As Stocking, in *Race, Culture, and Evolution*, argues, Boas did not consistently use the term *culture* in its modern sense; nevertheless, he played a crucial role in thrusting cultural reasoning into prominence in social science.

52. Balibar, "Is There a 'Neo-Racism'?"

53. Interviewed in Tucupita on 14 January 1994.

54. Interviewed in Maturín on 31 March 1995.

55. "El cólera está matando."

56. "Entró el cólera a Delta Amacuro provocando muerte de los indígenas," *Notidiario*, 9 September 1992, 15.

57. See Roger I. Glass and Robert E. Black, "The Epidemiology of Cholera," in *Cholera*, ed. Dhiman Barua and William B. Greenough III (New York: Plenum Medical, 1992), 149.

58. See Martin, *Flexible Bodies*, who argues that the immune system constitutes a site at which biological rhetorics are joined to cultural reasoning in rationalizing social inequality in the United States.

59. Randall M. Packard, *White Plague, Black Labor: Tuberculosis and the Political Economy of Health and Disease in South Africa* (Berkeley: University of California Press, 1989), argues that biomedical arguments regarding the transmission of tuberculosis were used to justify segregating blacks in South Africa

in homelands outside urban centers. Initial discussions in the early twentieth century largely followed cultural arguments, and it was only after apartheid laws had been enforced for some time that biological reasoning became the driving ideological force.

60. Jane H. Hill has referred to this sort of relationship as a "leaky boundary"; see "Junk Spanish, Covert Racism and the (Leaky) Boundary between Public and Private Spheres," *Pragmatics* 5, no. 2 (1995): 197–212. Hill argues that mocking uses of Spanish by non-Latinos in the southwestern United States, including in the media and political discourse, link the covert use of racist symbols in public contexts with their overt use in other settings, where there are fewer constraints on the expression of anti-Latino sentiments.

61. For a rich discussion of these shifting relations in Peru, see Marisol de la Cadena, *Indigenous Mestizos: The Politics of Race and Culture in Cuzco, Peru, 1919–1991* (Durham, N.C.: Duke University Press, 2000).

62. See Latour, *Pasteurization of France.*

63. See Charles L. Briggs and Clara Mantini-Briggs, "'Bad Mothers' and the Threat to Civil Society: Race, Cultural Reasoning, and the Institutionalization of Social Inequality in a Venezuelan Infanticide Trial," *Law and Social Inquiry* 25, no. 2 (2000): 299–354. This logic has also been used with African-American women in the United States; see Roberts, *Killing the Black Body.* The construction of kinship and family relations provides a crucial locus for launching broad ideological and material projects; see Jane Fishburne Collier and Sylvia Junko Yanagisako, eds., *Gender and Kinship: Essays toward a Unified Analysis* (Palo Alto, Calif.: Stanford University Press, 1987).

CHAPTER 10. CHALLENGING THE LOGIC OF CULTURE

1. Again, we regret that we are not able to cite these works here; to do so would reveal his identity.

2. Medina referred here to anthropologists with extensive experience in delta communities. "Wilbert" might refer either to Johannes Wilbert, former director of the Latin American Studies Center of the University of California, Los Angeles, or his son Werner, who now teaches in the anthropology department of the Instituto Venezolano de Investigaciones Científicas (IVIC) in Caracas. H. Dieter Heinen, now retired, taught for many years at IVIC. Bernarda Escalante works at the Instituto Caribe de Antropología y Sociología of the Fundación La Salle in Caracas.

3. Gaining proficiency in chanting, smoking enormous palm leaf cigars, and performing therapeutic massage came to be something of a problem for me in later years as I, too, was occasionally accused of sorcery. Even *criollos* in Tucupita sometimes warned people to stay away from me, saying, "He's a witch!" Torres once thought that one of my dreams saved his life.

4. See Guardia Nacional, *Diálogo intercultural, líderes indígenas–Guardia Nacional,* mimeograph (Caracas: Guardia Nacional, Comite LV Aniversario, Sub-

Comité Actividades Indígenas, 1992). On the role of performances of cultural difference in sustaining state and corporate projects in Venezuela, see David Guss, *The Festive State: Race, Ethnicity, and Nationalism as Cultural Performance* (Berkeley: University of California Press, 2000).

5. See Olsen, *Music of the Warao*.

6. See Lisseth Boon Bartolozzi, "Indígenas exigen derecho sobre propiedad de la tierra," *El Diario de Caracas*, 16 July 1992, and "Comunidades indígenas del país tomaron el Congreso," *El Diario de Caracas*, 17 July 1992.

7. Briggs, "Politics of Discursive Authority," discusses the dance troupe and the "Intercultural Dialogue" in greater detail. Our account of these events is based on interviews with the organizers and others, including participants, a videotape of the performance in Caracas, newspaper articles, and the Guardia Nacional's *Diálogo intercultural*. We would like to thank Mauricio Albrizzio for help in researching the Caracas performance.

8. See Coronil and Skurski, "Dismembering and Remembering the Nation"; and Julie Skurski and Fernando Coronil, "Savage Capitalism: Redefining Citizenship in Venezuela," paper presented at Discourses of Genocide, University of California, San Diego, 12–13 April 1996.

9. Guardia Nacional, *Diálogo intercultural*.

10. For conspiracy theories in general, see Richard Hofstadter, *The Paranoid Style in American Politics and Other Essays* (New York: Random House, 1967).

11. Guevara noted later in the interview that he based his explanation on MSAS statements printed in newspapers and broadcast on the radio.

12. See, for example, Hernán Mena Cifuentes, "Aviones y barcos procedentes de Perú, Colombia y Ecuador bajo control anticólera," *El Nacional*, 5 April 1991, last page of D section; "Extrema medidas para impedir entrada del cólera," *El Nacional*, 14 February 1991, C-3.

13. See Goldwasser, "The Rainbow Madonna of Trinidad."

14. See Charles L. Briggs, "Emergence of the Non-Indigenous Peoples." Romero appears to contradict himself by referring to the crab vendors as both *criollos* and Trinidadians. The term *criollo* is used, however, in what linguists refer to as unmarked and marked senses; it refers in its broader sense to all humans who are not classified as *indígenas* and more specifically to non-*indígena* Venezuelans. In suggesting that cholera is a "*criollo* disease," he is rejecting its racialization as an *indígena* disease.

15. The contamination of air and water by petroleum also appeared in popular accounts of the origin of cholera in Peru; see Cueto, *El regreso de las epidémias*, 208.

16. In our survey of delta communities in 1994–1995, Clara and I found two *wisidatus* who did claim to have dealt successfully with cholera, and I will describe how they accomplished this success later in this chapter.

17. See Briggs, "Generic versus Metapragmatic Dimensions," and "Patterning of Variation."

18. Paul Farmer has made the same observation with respect to the relationship between Haitian vernacular healing and biomedical treatment; see *In-*

fections and Inequalities: The Modern Plagues (Berkeley: University of California Press, 1999).

19. See Bruno Latour, *We Have Never Been Modern,* trans. Catherine Porter (Cambridge, Mass.: Harvard University Press, 1993 [1991]).

20. To cite just one example, the stereotype of "bad mothers," much like Benavides's characterization of "Warao" mothers, has been found in a great deal of colonial and postcolonial discourse—see Kalpana Ram and Margaret Jolly, eds., *Maternities and Modernities: Colonial and Postcolonial Experiences in Asia and the Pacific* (Cambridge: Cambridge University Press, 1998)—as well as contemporary accounts of African-American women in the United States; see Roberts, *Killing the Black Body.*

21. "Alerta roja por cólera."

22. See Rita R. Colwell and William M. Spira, "The Ecology of Vibrio Cholerae," in *Cholera,* ed. Dhiman Barua and William B. Greenough III, 107–127 (New York: Plenum Medical, 1992).

23. See Marshall Sahlins, *Culture and Practical Reason* (Chicago: University of Chicago Press, 1976); and Stocking, *Race, Culture, and Evolution.*

24. This is what Paul Farmer refers to as "immodest claims of causal efficacy"; see *Infections and Inequalities.*

25. See Derrida, *Of Grammatology.*

26. For Fanon's observations, see "The Fact of Blackness," in *Anatomy of Racism,* ed. David Theo Goldberg, 108–126 (Minneapolis: University of Minnesota Press, 1990).

27. See Said, *Orientalism,* for Orientalist constructions.

28. See Gordon, *Ghostly Matters,* for complex subjects.

29. Clifford Geertz celebrated "local knowledge" as the desideratum of anthropology; see *Local Knowledge* (New York: Basic Books, 1985). For critiques of this project see James Clifford, *The Predicament of Culture: Twentieth-Century Ethnography, Literature, and Art* (Cambridge, Mass.: Harvard University Press, 1988); James Clifford and George E. Marcus, eds., *Writing Culture: The Poetics and Politics of Ethnography* (Berkeley: University of California Press, 1986); and George E. Marcus and Michael M. J. Fischer, *Anthropology as Cultural Critique: An Experimental Moment in the Human Sciences* (Chicago: University of Chicago Press, 1986).

30. Recall that "the Warao" constituted one of the classic examples for Claude Lévi-Strauss of "cold societies," the peoples whose cultures revolve around an ignorance or even a denial of history; see *Conversations with Claude Lévi-Strauss,* ed. Georges Charbonnier, trans. John and Doreen Weightman (London: Cape, 1969).

31. See Derrida, *Of Grammatology.*

32. See, for example, George E. Marcus, ed., *Paranoia within Reason: A Casebook on Conspiracy as Explanation* (Chicago: University of Chicago Press, 1999).

33. Hoftstadter argues that they accordingly take their adherents into the realm of the paranoid; see *Paranoid Style.*

34. Fredric Jameson, *The Geopolitical Aesthetic* (Bloomington: Indiana University Press, 1992), 3.

35. As Mark Fenster, *Conspiracy Theories: Secrecy and Power in American Culture* (Minneapolis: University of Minnesota Press, 1999), 61, suggests.

CHAPTER 11. LOCAL NUMBERS AND GLOBAL POWER

1. Pan American Health Organization, *Basic Documents of the Pan American Health Organization,* 15th ed., Official Document no. 240 (Washington, D.C.: Pan American Health Organization, 1991), 9.

2. See Ricardo Archila, *Historia de la sanidad en Venezuela* (Caracas: Impr. Nacional, 1956), 395–405. These and many other international documents, such as the Pan-American Classification of Causes of Death, are reprinted in MSAS's compilation of *Legislación sanitaria nacional* (Caracas: MSAS, 1967). Note that the Bolivarian Constitution ratified in 1999 replaced MSAS with the Ministry of Health and Social Development.

3. World Health Organization, *The First Ten Years of the World Health Organization* (Geneva: World Health Organization, 1958), 459.

4. Ministerio de Sanidad y Asistencia Pública, "Cólera," 71.

5. Latour, *The Pasteurization of France.*

6. World Health Organization, *International Statistical Classification of Diseases and Related Health Problems,* 10th rev. ed. (Geneva: World Health Organization, 1992). See Geoffrey C. Bowker and Susan Leigh Star, *Sorting Things Out: Classification and Its Consequences* (Cambridge, Mass.: MIT Press, 1999).

7. These statements refer to the situation in 1992–1993. Subsequently, as discussed in chapter 13, other circuits for the dissemination of information on epidemics have begun to break nation-state monopolies over the production of these statistics.

8. Ministerio de Sanidad y Asistencia Pública, Departamento de Epidemiología, Estado Delta Amacuro, "Casos de cólera, positivos."

9. World Health Organization, "Cholera in 1992/Le choléra en 1992," *Weekly Epidemiological Record/Relevé épidémiologique hebdomadaire* 68, no. 21 (1993): 151.

10. Bowker and Star, *Sorting Things Out,* 282.

11. See Latour, *The Pasteurization of France,* on "obligatory passage points." Here experience in Delta Amacuro seems to have recapitulated the history of the Pasteurian revolution in nineteenth-century France, as told by Latour. More than a century ago, microbiologically based conceptions of disease strengthened the hands of public health professionals, who greeted them enthusiastically, while the physicians were more reticent about subordinating their clinical knowledge in favor of techniques over which they had less control.

12. "25 muertos por cólera y 1138 casos en tratamiento," *Notidiario,* 16 September 1992, 3.

13. "El cólera diezma a étnia Warauna," *Notidiario,* 12 November 1992, 23.

14. World Health Organization, *Guidelines for Cholera Control* (Geneva: World Health Organization, 1993).

15. Interviewed in Washington, D.C., on 8 November 1999.

16. World Health Organization, *WHO Guidance on Formulation of National Policy,* 1.

17. Ministerio de Sanidad y Asistencia Pública, "Cólera," 70.

18. Ibid., 72; World Health Organization, *WHO Guidance on Formulation of National Policy,* 2.

19. Interviewed in Washington, D.C., on 8 November 1998.

20. Hacking argues that "the benign and sterile-sounding word 'normal' has become one of the most powerful ideological tools of the twentieth century"; see *Taming of Chance,* 169. On numbers and institutions, see also Alain Desrosières, *The Politics of Large Numbers: A History of Statistical Reasoning,* trans. Camille Naish (Cambridge, Mass.: Harvard University Press, 1998).

21. Porter, *Trust in Numbers.*

22. Bruno Latour, *Science in Action* (Cambridge, Mass.: Harvard University Press, 1987).

23. Bowker and Star, *Sorting Things Out.*

24. Porter, *Trust in Numbers,* 91, 198, 202–209.

25. As Rosenberg, *Cholera Years,* suggests.

26. See, for example, Porter, *Trust in Numbers.*

27. Bowker and Star, *Sorting Things Out.*

CHAPTER 12. SANITATION AND GLOBAL CITIZENSHIP

1. For this history, see Barua, "History of Cholera"; Norman Howard-Jones, *The Scientific Background of the International Sanitary Conferences 1851–1938* (Geneva: World Health Organization, 1975), and *Pan American Health Organization: Origins and Evolution* (Geneva: World Health Organization, 1981); and Miguel E. Bustamante, *The Pan American Sanitary Bureau: Half a Century of Health Activities, 1902–1954* (Washington, D.C.: Pan American Sanitary Bureau, 1953).

2. W. X. Shandera, B. Hafkin, D. L. Martin, et al., "Persistence of Cholera in the United States," *American Journal of Tropical Medicine and Hygiene* 32 (1983): 812–817.

3. As in other chapters, the names we use for the national and international officials whom we have interviewed are fictitious. The disadvantage in using pseudonyms here is that we cannot tie these individuals' publications to their recorded remarks. When we make reference to their writings, no connection is made to the interview materials.

4. These details are taken both from our interviews with PAHO officials and from the description provided in Pan American Health Organization, *Pro Salute Novi Mundi: A History of the Pan American Health Organization* (Washington, D.C.: Pan American Health Organization, 1992), 7.

5. As Gill Walt notes; see "WHO under Stress: Implications for Health Policy," *Health Policy* 24 (1993): 125–144.

6. See ibid., 135; Andrew Chetley, *The Politics of Babyfoods: Successful Challenges to an International Marketing Strategy* (London: Francis Pinter, 1986); Najmi Kanji et al., eds., *Drugs Policy in Developing Countries* (London: Zed, 1992); and Kathryn Sikkink, "Codes of Conduct for Transnational Corporations: The Case of the WHO/UNICEF Code," *International Organization* 40, no. 4 (1986): 817–840.

7. See Halfdan Mahler, "The Meaning of 'Health for All by the Year 2000,'" *World Health Forum* 3, no. 1 (1981): 5–22. For a critique of the ideological underpinnings of the Alma Ata declaration, see Vicente Navarro, "A Critique of the Ideological and Political Position of the Brandt Report and the Alma Ata Declaration," *International Journal of Health Services* 15, no. 4 (1984): 525–544.

8. As I write, after the passing of the "Year 2000," the current situation could be more accurately characterized as "Health for the Few in the Year 2000." See Jim Yong Kim, Joyce V. Millen, Alec Irwin, and John Gershman, eds., *Dying for Growth: Global Inequality and the Health of the Poor* (Monroe, Me.: Common Courage Press, 2000).

9. John M. Starrels, *The World Health Organization: Resisting Third World Ideological Pressures* (Washington, D.C.: The Heritage Foundation, 1985). See also R. Caplan and Scott L. Malcomson, "Giving the U.N. the Business," *The Nation* 16, no. 23 (1986): 109–111.

10. As Paul Taylor, "The United Nations System under Stress: Financial Pressures and Their Consequences," *Review of International Studies* 17, no. 4 (1991): 365–382, and Walt, "WHO under Stress," argue.

11. Pan American Health Organization, *Pro Salute Novi Mundi*, 6.

12. CBS News, "Why?" transcript of text for segment of *60 Minutes*, 4 December 1994, vol. 27, no. 13 (Livingston, N.J.: Burrelle's Information Services, 1994), 2, © CBS News.

13. This was subsequently replaced in an institutional reorganization.

14. CBS News, "Why?" 4–5.

15. World Health Organization, "Responding to the Threat of a Cholera Outbreak" (Geneva: WHO Programme for the Control of Diarrhoeal Disease, n.d.); original emphasis. Other materials in the Cholera Information Kit are listed as having been updated in 1992. We obtained our copy of the packet in 1994.

16. Paul Thomas, personal communication, 1995.

17. World Health Organization, "Cholera," *Weekly Epidemiological Record/ Relevé épidémiologique hebdomadaire* 66, no. 6 (1991): 40.

18. World Health Organization, "Cholera," *Weekly Epidemiological Record/ Relevé épidémiologique hebdomadaire* 66, no. 7 (1991): 48.

19. World Health Organization, "Cholera," *Weekly Epidemiological Record/ Relevé épidémiologique hebdomadaire* 66, no. 9 (1991): 61.

20. Bakhtin, *Dialogic Imagination*, 84.

21. James A. Trostle, "Early Work in Anthropology and Epidemiology: From

Social Medicine to the Germ Theory, 1840–1920," in *Anthropology and Epidemiology,* ed. Craig R. Janes, Ron Stall, and Sandra M. Gifford (Dordrecht: Reidel, 1986), 43.

22. Judith S. Mausner and Shira Kramer, *Epidemiology: An Introductory Text,* 2d ed. (Philadelphia: W. B. Saunders, 1985).

23. As Ronald Frankenberg argues; see "Risk: Anthropological and Epidemiological Narratives of Prevention," in *Knowledge, Power, and Practice: The Anthropology of Medicine and Everyday Life,* ed. Shirley Lindenbaum and Margaret Lock, 219–242 (Berkeley: University of California Press, 1993).

24. World Health Organization, "Cholera in 1991/Le choléra en 1991," *Weekly Epidemiological Record/Relevé épidémiologique hebdomadaire* 67, no. 34 (1992): 253.

25. Ibid.; and World Health Organization, "Cholera in 1992/Le choléra en 1992," *Weekly Epidemiological Record/Relevé épidémiologique hebdomadaire* 68, no. 21 (1993): 149–155.

26. World Health Organization, "Cholera in 1992," 151–152.

27. Cholera has formed a stable element of Orientalist representations of the subcontinent since the nineteenth century; see Arnold, *Colonizing the Body.* Interestingly, a new strain of cholera that was first reported in the Bay of Bengal in 1992 was named "*Vibrio cholerae* 0139 synonym Bengal." See Howard-Jones, *Scientific Background,* on cholera's "origin" in India.

28. The way that India was stigmatized by cholera is paralleled by how Africa was marked as the site of origin for AIDS; like "Indian cholera" or "Asiatic cholera," we get "African AIDS." See Richard C. Chirimuuta and Rosalind J. Chirimuuta, *AIDS, Africa and Racism,* rev. ed. (London: Free Association Books, 1989); Panos Institute, *AIDS and the Third World* (Philadelphia: New Society, 1989); Cindy Patton, *Inventing AIDS* (New York: Routledge, 1990); and Paula Treichler, "AIDS, Africa, and Cultural Theory," *Transitions* 51 (1991): 86–103. Our thanks to Steven Epstein for a fruitful discussion of the parallels between AIDS and cholera with regard to the question of origins; see Farmer, *AIDS and Accusation.* These associations have long historical trajectories, as the link between India and cholera suggests. Small wonder that the American or European origin of syphilis was debated so ardently; see Alfred W. Crosby, Jr., *The Columbian Exchange: Biological and Cultural Consequences of 1492* (Westport, Conn.: Greenwood Press, 1972); and William H. McNeill, *Plagues and People* (New York: Anchor Books, 1976).

29. See Bakhtin, *Dialogic Imagination.*

30. Ibid.

31. World Health Organization, "Cholera," no. 9 (1991): 61.

32. Ibid.

33. Ibid.

34. See Martin, *Flexible Bodies,* on military metaphors in popular medical discourses. Arnold, *Colonizing the Body,* 168, suggests that we should not dismiss military metaphors as merely metaphorical.

35. Military metaphors can lead to popular resistance. Marilyn K. Nations

and Cristina M. G. Monte suggest that the "War against Cholera" in north-eastern Brazil was seen as a war on the *diseased;* some refused medication and hid symptoms in order to avoid being stigmatized by the "dog's disease"; see "'I'm Not Dog, No!': Cries of Resistance against Cholera Control Campaigns," *Social Science and Medicine* 43, no. 6 (1996): 1007–1024.

36. World Health Organization, "Cholera," no. 9 (1991): 61.

37. As James A. Trostle notes; see "Political, Economic and Behavioral Aspects of the Re-emergence of Cholera in Latin America," paper presented at the Annual Meeting of the American Anthropological Association, Washington, D.C., November 1995.

38. Robert V. Tauxe and Paul A. Blake characterize the drop in the case-fatality rate in Peru to "less than 1%" as "a laudable achievement"; see "Epidemic Cholera in Latin America," *Journal of the American Medical Association* 267, no. 10 (1992): 1389.

39. World Health Organization, "Cholera in 1992," 155.

40. For work that does not take nations as natural units, see M. M. Levine and O. S. Levine, "Changes in Human Ecology and Behavior in Relation to the Emergence of Diarrheal Diseases, Including Cholera," *Proceedings of the National Academy of Sciences* 91 (1994): 2390–2394.

41. Robert V. Tauxe, "Lessons of the Latin American Cholera Epidemic, 1992," *Atlanta Medicine* 66, no. 4 (1992): 42. Since I am citing the published writings of these epidemiologists, I have not used pseudonyms.

42. John Anderson, "Cholera in the Nineties," *CDC Briefs* 3, no. 4 (1992): 1. *CDC Briefs* is an official publication of the CDC in Atlanta, which forms part of the U.S. Public Health Service.

43. See Eugene J. Gangarosa and Robert V. Tauxe, "Epilogue: The Latin American Cholera Epidemic," in *Cholera,* ed. Dhiman Barua and William B. Greenough III (New York: Plenum Medical, 1992), 351–358. For Tauxe's biography, http://www.cdc.gov/ncidod/dbmd/biographies/rtauxe.htm.

44. Tauxe, "Lessons," 41–42.

45. Pan American Health Organization, "Cholera Situation in the Americas: An Update," *Epidemiological Bulletin* 12, no. 2 (1991): 6.

46. Pan American Health Organization, "Cholera Situation in the Americas," *Epidemiological Bulletin* 12, no. 1 (1991): 4.

47. *Nuevos conceptos y técnicas de investigación* (Quito: Centro de Estudios y Asesoría en Salud, 1994). See also E. Gotuzzo et al., "Cholera: Lessons from the Epidemic in Peru," *Infectious Disease Clinics of North America* 8 (1994): 183–205.

48. Norman Gall, *The Death Threat, Part of a Broader Study of Chronic Inflation as Systemic Failure: Latin America and the Polarization of the World Economy* (São Paulo: Fernand Braudel Institute of World Economics, 1993), 101.

49. Tauxe and Blake, "Epidemic Cholera," 1388.

50. Tauxe, "Lessons," 42.

51. Richard L. Guerrant, "Twelve Messages from Enteric Infections for Science and Society," *American Journal of Tropical Medicine and Hygiene* 51, no. 1 (1994): 27; see also Tauxe and Blake, "Epidemic Cholera," 1390.

52. Pan American Health Organization, "Cholera Situation in the Americas: An Update," *Epidemiological Bulletin* 12, no. 2 (1991): 10.

53. Pan American Health Organization, "Cholera Situation in the Americas: An Update," *Epidemiological Bulletin* 15, no. 1 (1994): 16.

54. Pan American Health Organization, "Cholera Situation in the Americas," *Epidemiological Bulletin* 12, no. 2 (1991), 10.

55. Ibid., 5.

56. See Guerrant, "Twelve Messages."

57. For Pacini, see Howard-Jones, *Scientific Background;* for Koch, see Evans, *Death in Hamburg.*

58. See Margaret Pelling, *Cholera, Fever, and English Medicine 1825–1865* (Oxford: Oxford University Press, 1978); Evans, *Death in Hamburg;* and Rosenberg, *Cholera Years.* In contrast, Barua, "History of Cholera," 24, and other experts argue that cholera led to sanitary reform.

59. See Tauxe, "Lessons," 43. For eighteenth-century reforms, see Suzanne Austin Alchon, "Disease, Population, and Public Health in Eighteenth-Century Quito," in *"Secret Judgments of God": Old World Disease in Colonial Spanish America*, ed. Noble David Cook and W. George Lovell, 159–182 (Norman: University of Oklahoma Press, 1992).

60. Pan American Health Organization, *Pro Salute Novi Mundi*, 7.

61. Pan American Health Organization, "Update: The Cholera Situation in the Americas," *Epidemiological Bulletin* 12, no. 3 (1991): 1.

62. Pan American Health Organization, "Cholera Situation in the Americas: An Update," *Epidemiological Bulletin* 12, no. 4 (1991): 13.

63. Pan American Health Organization, "Cholera Situation in the Americas," 15, no. 1 (1994), 14.

64. Pan American Health Organization, "Cholera Situation in the Americas," 12, no. 1 (1991), 4.

65. Pan American Health Organization, "Cholera Situation in the Americas," 15, no. 1 (1994), 14, 16.

66. See, for example, David L. Swerdlow, Eric D. Mintz, Marcela Rodríguez, et al., "Waterborne Transmission of Epidemic Cholera in Trujillo, Peru: Lessons for a Continent at Risk," *The Lancet* 340, no. 8810 (1992): 28–32.

67. Pan American Health Organization, "Cholera Situation in the Americas," 12, no. 1 (1991), 24.

68. Tauxe and Blake, "Epidemic Cholera," 1388.

69. Swerdlow et al., "Waterborne Transmission," 31.

70. Pan American Health Organization, "Cholera Situation in the Americas: An Update," 12, no. 2 (1991): 2–3.

71. Pan American Health Organization, "Cholera Situation in the Americas: An Update," 12, no. 4 (1991): 11.

72. Pan American Health Organization, "Cholera Situation in the Americas," 12, no. 1 (1991), 4.

73. Ibid., 23.

74. Pan American Health Organization, "Update: The Cholera Situation in the Americas," 12, no. 3 (1991), 14.

75. Pan American Health Organization, *Pro Salute Novi Mundi*, 14.

76. Pan American Health Organization, "Cholera Situation in the Americas," 12, no. 1 (1991), 12.

77. Ibid., 20.

78. Gangarosa and Tauxe, "Epilogue," suggest that implicating a municipal water source "can be politically explosive."

79. Pan American Health Organization, "Cholera Situation in the Americas," 12, no. 1 (1991), 9.

80. Pan American Health Organization, *Pro Salute Novi Mundi*, 10.

81. See Julia Paley, *Marketing Democracy: Power and Social Movements in Post-Dictatorship Chile* (Berkeley: University of California Press, 2001), on the women's collective; and Ricardo Trumper and Lynne Phillips, "Cholera in the Time of Neoliberalism: The Cases of Chile and Ecuador," *Alternatives—Social Transformation and Humane Governance* 20, no. 2 (1995): 165–193, on the responses of Chilean and Ecuadorian elites to the epidemic.

82. Tauxe and Blake, "Epidemic Cholera," 1388.

83. Frederick L. Dunn and Craig R. Janes, "Introduction: Medical Anthropology and Epidemiology," in *Anthropology and Epidemiology*, ed. Craig R. Janes, Ron Stall, and Sandra M. Gifford (Dordrecht: Reidel, 1986), 8.

84. "Like Attacker Probing Defenses, Cholera Threatens U.S. Population from Elsewhere in This Hemisphere," *Journal of the American Medical Association* 267, no. 10 (1992): 1314–1315.

85. Tauxe, "Lessons," 41.

86. Tauxe and Blake, "Epidemic Cholera," 1390.

87. Tauxe, "Lessons," 42.

88. See Lyn Finelli, David Swerdlow, Kristen Mertz, Halina Ragazzoni, and Kenneth Spitalny, "Outbreak of Cholera Associated with Crab Brought from an Area with Epidemic Disease," *Journal of Infectious Diseases* 166 (1992): 1433–1435.

89. See Gangarosa and Tauxe, "Epilogue," 356.

90. Tauxe and Blake, "Epidemic Cholera," 1388.

91. See, for example, Swerdlow et al., "Waterborne Transmission."

92. We would like to thank Veena Das for raising this question.

93. Gangarosa and Tauxe, "Epilogue."

94. See, for example, I. Kaye Wachsmuth, Paul A. Blake, and Ørjan Olsvik, *Vibrio cholerae and Cholera: Molecular to Global Perspectives* (Washington, D.C.: ASM Press, 1994).

95. See Pan American Health Organization, "Cholera Situation in the Americas: An Update," no. 2 (1991): 5, and 12, no. 4 (1991): 13; and Tauxe and Blake, "Epidemic Cholera," 1390.

96. See M. John Albert et al., "Large Epidemic of Cholera-Like Disease in Bangladesh Caused by *Vibrio cholerae* 0139 Synonym Bengal," *The Lancet* 342, no. 8868 (1993): 387–390, and "Large Outbreak of Clinical Cholera Due

to *Vibrio cholerae* non-o1 in Bangladesh," *The Lancet* 341, no. 8846 (1993): 704.

97. See B. S. Drasar and B. D. Forrest, eds., *Cholera and the Ecology of* Vibrio cholerae (London: Chapman and Hall, 1996); Gerald T. Keusch and Masanobu Kawakami, eds., *Cytokines, Cholera, and the Gut* (Amsterdam: IOS Press, 1996); and Wachsmuth, Blake, and Olsvik, *Vibrio cholerae.* Guerrant, "Twelve Messages," 28, states that the lessons that have been learned include "healthy measures of humility."

98. See Jaime Breilh, *Epidemiología: Economía, medicina y política* (Mexico: Editorial Fontamara, 1986), and *Nuevos conceptos y técnicas de investigación,* Serie Epidemiología Crítica, no. 3 (Quito: Centro de Estudios y Asesoría en Salud, 1994); and Asa Cristina Laurell, *La política social en la crisis: Una alternative para el sector salud* (Mexico City: Fundación Friedrich Ebert, 1990), and *Nuevas tendencias y alternativas en el sector salud* (Mexico City: Universidad Autónoma Metropolitana, 1994).

99. I draw here on Jean Franco, "Death Camp Confessions and Resistance to Violence in Latin America," *Socialism and Democracy* 2 (1986): 5–17.

100. See Abby A. Rockefeller, "Civilization and Sludge: Notes on the History of the Management of Human Excreta," *Capitalism, Nature, Socialism* 9, no. 3 (1998): 3–18.

CHAPTER 13. VIRULENT AFTERMATH

1. Interviewed in Waranoko on 20 October 1994.
2. Interviewed in Waranoko on 20 October 1994.
3. This material was provided in an interview conducted in Tucupita on 6 December 1994. The policy was never instituted.
4. Interviewed in Tucupita on 6 December 1994.
5. "Alcaldía de Caroní raptó a los Waraos," *Notidiario,* 20 August 1994, 24.
6. Ender Fuenmayor, "Los indígenas no fueron raptados," *Notidiario,* 23 August 1994, 23.
7. Quoted in Desiree Santos Amaral, "Tráfico de indígenas convertidos en mendigos investiga el Consejo," *Ultimas Noticias,* 24 August 1994, 19.
8. Interviewed in Tucupita on 14 November 1994.
9. Casto Ocando Hernández, "Continúan llegando contingentes de indígenas a Caracas," *El Universal,* 21 August 1994, 1–28; for Aguiar, see "Gobernador de Caracas responsabiliza al gobierno de Delta Amacuro por éxodo de indígenas Waraos," *Correo del Caroní,* 25 August 1994, D-1.
10. "Reunión de alto nivel discutió migración de indígenas a Caracas," *El Universal,* 12 September 1994.
11. Ocando Hernández, "Continúan llegando contingentes de indígenas"; Vaughan, *Curing Their Ills.*
12. On homelessness in Caracas, see Patricia C. Márquez, *The Street Is My Home: Youth and Violence in Caracas* (Palo Alto, Calif.: Stanford University Press, 1999).

13. Interviewed in Tucupita on 6 September 1994.

14. Interviewed in Barrancas on 10 September 1994.

15. Yira Yoyotte, "Huyendo de condiciones infrahumanas los indígenas acuden a las ciudades," *Ultimas Noticias,* 26 August 1994, 14.

16. *Notidiario,* 27 September 1994.

17. World Health Organization, "Infected Areas as at 22 February 1996/Zones infectés au 22 février 1996," *Weekly Epidemiological Record/Relevé épidémiologique hebdomadaire* 71, no. 8 (1996): 63.

18. World Health Organization, "Cholera in 1997," *Weekly Epidemiological Record/Relevé épidémiologique hebdomadaire* 73, no. 27 (1998): 204.

19. Our information is based primarily on interviews with Rudolfo Figueroa, who served as regional epidemiologist in December 1998; Sofía Méndez, who held the position in June 1999; and Roberto Guzmán, who had held the post of assistant regional epidemiologist for over five years. Guzmán was interviewed in 1997 and 1999.

20. "Muerto por cólera dos indígenas en el Delta," *Notidiario,* 20 January 1997, 16.

21. See Kimberle Crenshaw, "Mapping the Margins: Intersectionality, Identity Politics, and Violence against Women of Color," *Stanford Law Review* 43 (1991): 1241–1299.

22. United Nations Development Programme, *Human Development Report, 1998* (New York: Oxford University Press, 1998).

23. As suggested by Kim et al., *Dying for Growth;* Navarro, "Neoliberalism"; and Wilkinson, *Unhealthy Societies.*

24. See María Helena Jaén, *El sistema de salud venezolano: Desafíos* (Caracas: Ediciones IESA, 2001), 95.

25. This estimate is from Gustavo Márquez et al., "Fiscal Policy and Income Distribution in Venezuela," in *Government Spending and Income Distribution in Latin America,* ed. Ricardo Hausmann and Roberto Rigobón (Washington, D.C.: Inter-American Development Bank, 1993), 146, 155.

26. Samuel A. Morley and Carola Alvarez, *Poverty and Adjustment in Venezuela,* Working Paper Series, no. 124 (Washington, D.C.: Inter-American Development Bank, 1992), 38.

27. For Sassen's argument, see *Globalization and Its Discontents* (New York: New Press, 1998), and "Spatialities and Temporalities of the Global: Elements for a Theorization," *Public Culture* 12, no. 1 (2000): 215–232. Anna Tsing warns of the conceptual and political problems that follow from reliance on this hydraulic metaphor in talking about these complex phenomena; see "The Global Situation," *Cultural Anthropology* 15, no. 3 (2000): 327–360.

28. See Sonia E. Alvarez, Evalina Dagnino, and Arturo Escobar, eds., *Cultures of Politics/Politics of Cultures: Re-visioning Latin American Social Movements* (Boulder, Colo.: Westview Press, 1998).

29. Appadurai, *Modernity at Large,* 31; see also Arjun Appadurai, "Patriotism and Its Futures," *Public Culture* 2, no. 2 (1993): 411–430.

30. Michel-Rolph Trouillot argues that the shift to postmodern forms can

doubly displace people who were denied the status of modernity; see "Anthropology and the Savage Slot: The Poetics and Politics of Otherness," in *Recapturing Anthropology: Working in the Present*, ed. Richard G. Fox (Santa Fe: School of American Research, 1991), 17–44.

31. Zygmunt Bauman, *Globalization: The Human Consequences* (New York: Columbia University Press, 1998).

32. See Roland Robertson, *Globalization: Social Theory and Global Culture* (London: Sage, 1995).

33. Arjun Appadurai characterizes the way that anthropologists imagine subaltern populations as rooted in space in the following terms: "Natives are those who are somehow confined to places by the connection to what the place permits." He continues, "The intellectual operations of natives are somehow tied to their niches, to their situations." See "Putting Hierarchy in Its Place," *Cultural Anthropology* 3, no. 1 (1988): 37, 38.

34. Based on interviews conducted in Waranoko and Hohebura on 23 and 24 September 1994.

35. Based on interviews conducted in the Pedernales, Macareo, and Mariusa areas in 1999 and 2000.

36. Interviewed in Tucupita on 30 June 1999.

37. In the United States, for example, this process is apparent in the expansion of the prison-industrial complex and in the institutional schemas to "get people off welfare."

38. See Porter, *Trust in Numbers*.

39. On the notion of an unstable racial equilibrium, see Omi and Winant, *Racial Formation in the United States*.

40. See Paul Farmer, "Hidden Epidemics of Tuberculosis," and *Infections and Inequalities*; and Nina Glick-Schiller, "What's Wrong with This Picture? The Hegemonic Construction of Culture in AIDS Research in the United States," *Medical Anthropology Quarterly* 6, no. 3 (1992): 237–254.

41. See Vilma Santiago-Irizarry, "Culture as Cure," *Cultural Anthropology* 11, no. 1 (1996): 3–24.

42. "Medicine, Morality, and Hygiene: Social Configurations of a 'Woman's Disease' in Venezuela," Ph.D. diss., University of California, Irvine, 1998.

43. See Kristin Koptiuch, "Third-Worlding at Home," *Social Text* 9 (1991): 87–99.

44. See Jacqueline Bhabha, "Embodied Rights: Gender Persecution, State Sovereignty, and Refugees," *Public Culture* 9 (1996): 3–32.

45. See Jack Campisi, *The Mashpee Indians: Tribes on Trial* (Syracuse, N.Y.: Syracuse University Press, 1991); and Clifford, *The Predicament of Culture*, on Native American land claims. Roberts, *Killing the Black Body*, has documented the use of cultural reasoning and similar constructions in the criminalization of African-American women. Leti Volpp has focused squarely on the effects of the "cultural defense" in criminal trials of people of color; see "(Mis)identifying Culture: Asian Women and the 'Cultural Defense,'" *Harvard Women's Law Journal* 17 (1994): 57–101, "Talking 'Culture': Gender, Race, Nation, and the

Politics of Multiculturalism," *Columbia Law Review* 96 (1996): 1573–1617, and "Blaming Culture for Bad Behavior," *Yale Journal of Law and the Humanities* 12 (2000): 89–116.

46. See Appadurai, "Putting Hierarchy in Its Place."

47. See Lila Abu-Lughod, "Writing Against Culture," in *Recapturing Anthropology: Working in the Present*, ed. Richard G. Fox (Santa Fe, N.M.: School of American Research, 1991), 137–162; and Marisol de la Cadena, *Indigenous Mestizos: The Politics of Race and Culture in Cuzco, Peru, 1919–1991* (Durham, N.C.: Duke University Press, 2000).

48. Clifford, *The Predicament of Culture*.

49. Appadurai, "Putting Hierarchy in Its Place."

50. This case is documented in Charles L. Briggs, "Notes on a 'Confession': On the Construction of Gender, Sexuality and Violence in an Infanticide Case," *Pragmatics* 7, no. 4 (1997): 519–546; and Briggs and Mantini-Briggs, "'Bad Mothers.'"

51. Quoting from the *Expediente* filed in the Tribunal de Primera Instancia en lo Penal y de Salvaguarda del Patrimonio Público, Tucupita, 90, quoted in Briggs and Mantini-Briggs, "'Bad Mothers,'" 312.

52. Ibid., 168; original emphasis.

53. Ibid., 210.

54. For contrasting points of view on this issue in a Brazilian context, see Nancy Scheper-Hughes, *Death without Weeping: The Violence of Everyday Life in Brazil* (Berkeley: University of California Press, 1992); Marilyn K. Nations, "Illness of the Child: The Cultural Context of Child Diarrhea in Northeast Brazil," Ph.D. diss., University of California, Berkeley, 1982; and Marilyn K. Nations and Linda-Anne Rebhun, "Angels with Wet Wings Can't Fly: Maternal Sentiment in Brazil and the Image of Neglect," *Culture, Medicine, and Psychiatry* 12, no. 2 (1988): 141–200.

55. See Carole Pateman, *The Sexual Contract* (Palo Alto, Calif.: Stanford University Press, 1988), 11, on the "duty" of women to procreate for the state. Laura E. Gómez, *Misconceiving Mothers: Legislators, Prosecutors, and the Politics of Prenatal Drug Exposure* (Philadelphia: Temple University Press, 1997); and Roberts, *Killing the Black Body*, explores how U.S. courts criminalize African-American women for their purported failure to comply with legal obligations to their fetuses and newborns. Martha Fineman argues that rhetorical images of bad mothers constitute a "cross-over discourse." Owing to patriarchal assumptions about the nuclear family and the need for male power over wives and children, images of bad mothers move easily into new contexts and shape consequential understandings of women. See "Images of Mothers in Poverty Discourses," *Duke Law Journal* 1991, no. 1 (1991): 276.

56. See Kimberle Crenshaw, "Demarginalizing the Intersection of Race and Sex: A Black Feminist Critique of Antidiscrimination Doctrine, Feminist Theory and Antiracist Politics," *The University of Chicago Legal Forum* (1989): 139–168; and Gail Elizabeth Wyatt, "The Sexual Experience of Afro-American

Women," in *Women's Sexual Experience: Exploration of the Dark Continent,* ed. Martha Kirkpatrick (New York: Plenum, 1982).

57. Images embedded in cultural reasoning are much like statistics in that they come to be seen as objective facts and, approaching the status of immutable mobiles, are readily recontexualized.

58. See Briggs, "'You're a Liar,'" and "Conflict, Language Ideologies, and Privileged Arenas."

59. Etienne Balibar, "Culture and Identity (Working Notes)," in *The Identity in Question,* ed. John Rajchman (New York: Routledge, 1995), 179.

60. Ibid., 174–176.

61. See M. M. Bakhtin, "The Problem of Speech Genres," in *Speech Genres and Other Late Essays,* ed. Caryl Emerson and Michael Holquist (Austin: University of Texas Press, 1986), 60–102.

62. See White, *Tropics of Discourse.*

63. Prasenjit Duara, *Rescuing History from the Nation: Questioning Narratives of Modern China* (Chicago: University of Chicago Press, 1995).

64. See Fernand Braudel, *La historia y las ciencias sociales,* trans. Josefina Gómez Mendoza (Madrid: Alianza Editorial, 1968), and *A History of Civilizations,* trans. Richard Mayne (New York: A. Lane, 1994); and Rafael Humberto Moreno Durán, *De la barbarie a la imaginación: La experiencia leída* (Bogotá: Tercer Mundo Editores, 1988), who presents an extensive treatment of the way this opposition plays out in Latin American letters. Venezuelan modernities are discussed by Julio C. Salas, *Civilización y barbarie: Estudios sociológos americanos* (Caracas: Fundación Julio C. Salas, 1997 [1908]); and Maurice Belrose, *La época del modernismo en Venezuela* (Caracas: Monte Avila, 1999).

65. Balibar, "Is There a 'Neo-Racism'?" argues that this facet of "anthropological culturalism" has placed it in an intimate relationship with racism.

66. See Erving Goffman, *Stigma: Notes on the Management of Spoiled Identity* (New York: Simon and Schuster, 1963).

67. In his excellent study of HIV/AIDS activism in the United States, Steven Epstein argues that gay activist groups that gained a role in shaping research and treatment policies increasingly distanced themselves from more radical rhetorics and tactics; see *Impure Science.*

68. The quote is from Dipesh Chakrabarty, "Postcoloniality and the Artifice of History: Who Speaks for Indian Pasts?" *Representations* 37 (1992): 26.

69. *Biopower* is Michel Foucault's term; see *The History of Sexuality: An Introduction,* trans. Robert Hurley, vol. 1 (New York: Vintage, 1978).

70. See James Ferguson, *Expectations of Modernity: Myths and Meanings of Urban Life on the Zambian Copperbelt* (Berkeley: University of California Press, 1999).

71. See Coronil, *Magical State;* Enrique Dussel, "Eurocentrism and Modernity," *Boundary* 2 (1993): 65–76; Walter Mignolo, *The Darker Side of the Renaissance* (Ann Arbor: University of Michigan Press, 1995), and *Local Histories/Global Designs: Coloniality, Subaltern Knowledges, and Border Thinking*

(Princeton, N.J.: Princeton University Press, 2000); Aihwa Ong, *Flexible Citizenship: The Cultural Logics of Transnationality* (Durham, N.C.: Duke University Press, 1999); and Ella Shohat and Robert Stam, *Unthinking Eurocentrism* (New York: Routledge, 1994).

72. See García Canclini, *Culturas híbridas.* The Chiapas revolution in Mexico provides a striking example not only of how "tradition" can help redefine "modernity" but of the increasing arbitrariness of the borders that supposedly separate them.

73. See Latour, *The Pasteurization of France.*

74. As Arthur and Joan Kleinman have suggested; see "The Appeal of Experience, the Dismay of Images: Cultural Appropriations of Suffering in Our Times," *Daedalus* 125, no. 1 (1996): 1–23.

75. See Patrick Tierney, *Darkness in El Dorado: How Scientists and Journalists Devastated the Amazon* (New York: Norton, 2000).

76. While infant mortality officially stood at 19 per 1,000 in Venezuela as a whole in 1999, it was double that in Amazonas state; these figures are on file in the Ministerio de Sanidad y Asistencia Pública, Caracas. Infant and child mortality in the Yanomami population served by the Salesian missionaries' clinics was around 50 percent, much like the percentage in areas of Delta Amacuro; this figure is from an interview in Puerto Ayacucho with Father Rafael Narvaez, a Salesian missionary who has worked with Yanomami people for over twenty years. A former regional epidemiologist suggested that this figure was probably accurate.

77. Appadurai, *Modernity at Large,* argues the former; Trouillot, "Anthropology and the Savage Slot," the latter.

78. As Bakhtin, "The Problem of Speech Genres," has argued.

79. George Lipsitz warns us that the possibilities for appropriation and distortion are great in this global mix; see *Dangerous Crossroads: Popular Music, Postmodernism, and the Politics of Place* (London: Verso, 1994).

80. United Nations, *Convention on Genocide,* GAOR Resolution 260A (III), 9 December 1948, Article II (Geneva: United Nations, 1948). For a fuller discussion of accusations of genocide in the cholera narratives, see Charles L. Briggs and Clara Mantini-Briggs, "'The Indians Accept Death as a Normal, Natural Event': Institutional Authority, Cultural Reasoning, and Discourses of Genocide in a Venezuelan Cholera Epidemic," *Social Identities* 3, no. 3 (1997): 439–469.

81. Interviewed in Geneva on 27 July 1998.

82. For example, in 1997, David Coder, a microbiologist at the University of Washington, translated several articles on cholera in Venezuela from the pages of *El Nacional* and posted them on ProMED. See the http://www.promedmail.org posting of 22 September 1997 on "Cholera–Venezuela (15)."

83. For an update on the discussions inaugurated by the World Health Assembly in 1995, see World Heath Organization, "Revisions of the International Health Regulations: Progress Report, February 2001," *Weekly Epidemiological Record* 76, no. 8 (2001): 61–63.

84. For example, Kleinman and Kleinman issue such a call for incorporating "local worlds" into national and international discussions of social suffering; see "The Appeal of Experience," 18. Zygmunt Bauman argues, however, that getting characterized as local, fixed in space and culture, while others get globalized becomes "a sign of social deprivation and degradation"; see *Globalization*, 2. The notion of gatekeeping mechanisms comes from Frederick Erickson and Jeffrey Shultz, *The Counselor as Gatekeeper: Social Interaction in Interviews* (New York: Academic Press, 1982).

85. I would argue that this point applies to such leading works as Leslie Sklair, *Sociology of the Global System*, 2d ed. (Baltimore: Johns Hopkins University Press, 1995); Bauman, *Globalization;* Robertson, *Globalization;* and Castells, *The Information Age.*

86. As advocated by Michael Taussig, *The Nervous System* (New York: Routledge, 1992), 10.

87. Chakrabarty, "Postcoloniality," 21.

88. Brian D. Smedley, Adrienne Y. Stith, and Alan R. Nelson, eds., *Unequal Treatment: Confronting Racial and Ethnic Disparities in Health Care* (Washington, D.C.: National Academy Press, 2002).

89. World Health Organization, *Education for Health: A Manual on Health Education in Primary Health Care* (Geneva: World Health Organization, 1988); see also Meredith Minkler and Nina Wallerstein, "Improving Health through Community Organization and Community Building," in *Health Behavior and Health Education: Theory, Research, and Practice,* 2d ed., ed. Karen Glanz, Frances Marcus Lewis, and Barbara K. Rimer (San Francisco: Jossey-Bass, 1997), 241–268.

Bibliography

"Abraham Gómez recorrió el bajo Delta." *Notidiario,* 19 August 1992, 5.

Abu-Lughod, Lila. "Writing against Culture." In *Recapturing Anthropology: Working in the Present,* edited by Richard G. Fox, 137–162. Santa Fe: School of American Research, 1991.

Ackers, M. L., R. E. Quick, et al. "Are There National Risk Factors for Epidemic Cholera? The Correlation between Socioeconomic and Demographic Indices and Cholera Incidence in Latin America." *International Journal of Epidemiology* 27, no. 2 (1998): 330–334.

"A La Isla Tortuga llevaron a 251 Waraos." *Notidiario,* 18 August 1992, 1.

"Alarmante situación ante colera en región Goajira." *El Mundo,* 3 December 1991, 26.

Albert, M. John, et al. "Large Epidemic of Cholera-Like Disease in Bangladesh Caused by *Vibrio cholerae* 0139 Synonym Bengal." *The Lancet* 342, no. 8868 (1993): 387–390.

———. "Large Outbreak of Clinical Cholera due to *Vibrio cholerae* non-01 in Bangladesh." *The Lancet* 341, no. 8846 (1993): 704.

"Alcaldía de Caroní raptó a los Waraos." *Notidiario,* 20 August 1994, 24.

Alchon, Suzanne Austin. "Disease, Population, and Public Health in Eighteenth-Century Quito." In *"Secret Judgments of God": Old World Disease in Colonial Spanish America,* edited by Noble David Cook and W. George Lovell, 159–182. Norman: University of Oklahoma Press, 1992.

"Alerta máxima contra el cólera en el Zulia." *El Nacional,* 28 April 1991, A-1.

"Alerta nacional contra cólera y dengue." *El Nacional,* 14 August 1991, C-4.

"Alerta roja por cólera en el estado Delta Amacuro." *Notidiario,* 8 August 1992, 1.

Alvarez, Sonia E., Evalina Dagnino, and Arturo Escobar, eds. *Cultures of Politics/Politics of Cultures: Re-visioning Latin American Social Movements.* Boulder, Colo.: Westview Press, 1998.

"A más de mil ascienden casos de cólera en el Delta." *El Diario de Monagas*, 6 October 1992, 1.

"Amenaza el cólera en todo el país." *Notidiario*, 6 October 1992, 2.

Anderson, John. "Cholera in the Nineties." *CDC Briefs* 3, no. 4 (1992): 1–2.

Anonymous. "Prioridad: Atacar el cólera." *2001*, 17 August 1992, 5.

"A 837 ascienden los casos de cólera en Delta Amacuro." *Notidiario*, 2 September 1992, 1.

Appadurai, Arjun. *Modernity at Large: Cultural Dimensions of Globalization*. Minneapolis: University of Minnesota Press, 1996.

———. "Patriotism and Its Futures." *Public Culture* 2, no. 2 (1993): 411–430.

———. "Putting Hierarchy in Its Place." *Cultural Anthropology* 3, no. 1 (1988): 36–49.

Araujo, Elizabeth. "No estamos preparados para combatir al cólera." *El Nacional*, 30 April 1991, C-2.

Archila, Ricardo. *Historia de la sanidad en Venezuela*. Caracas: Impr. Nacional, 1956.

Arébalos, Alberto. "El cólera se propaga por América Latina." *El Nacional*, 12 April 1991.

Arnold, David. *Colonizing the Body: State Medicine and Epidemic Disease in Nineteenth-Century India*. Berkeley: University of California Press, 1993.

Aubrey, John. *Three Prose Works*. Edited by John Buchanan-Brown. Carbondale: Southern Illinois University Press, 1972.

"Aumentan a mil casos de cólera." *Notidiario*, 9 September 1992, 1.

"Autoridades del SAS salieron a buscar recursos contra el cólera." *Notidiario*, 7 September 1992, 17.

Azocar, Gustavo. "Táchira se prepara para enfrentar el cólera." *El Nacional*, 20 November 1991, C-4.

Bacon, Francis. *Novum organum*. Vol. 4 of *The Works of Francis Bacon*. Edited by James Spedding, Robert Leslie Ellis, and Douglas Denon Heath. New York: Garrett Press, 1968.

"Bajó en un noventa por ciento demanda de pescado en Tucupita." *Notidiario*, 17 August 1992, 17.

Bakhtin, M. M. *The Dialogic Imagination: Four Essays*. Translated by Caryl Emerson and Michael Holquist. Edited by Michael Holquist. Austin: University of Texas Press, 1981.

———. "The Problem of Speech Genres." In *Speech Genres and Other Late Essays*, edited by Caryl Emerson and Michael Holquist, 60–102. Austin: University of Texas Press, 1986.

Balibar, Etienne. "Culture and Identity (Working Notes)." In *The Identity in Question*, edited by John Rajchman, 173–196. New York: Routledge, 1995.

———. "Is There a 'Neo-Racism'?" In *Race, Nation, Class: Ambiguous Identities*, Etienne Balibar and Immanuel Wallerstein, 17–28. London: Verso, 1991.

Banerji, Debabar. "The Political Economy of Western Medicine in Third World

Countries." In *Issues in the Political Economy of Health Care,* edited by John B. McKinlay, 257–282. New York: Tavistock, 1984.

Barral, Rev. P. Fr. Basilio. *Diccionario Guarao-Español, Español-Guarao.* Caracas: Instituto Caribe de Antropología y Sociología, Fundación La Salle de Ciencias Naturales, 1957.

———. *Guarao guarata: Lo que cuentan los indios Guaraos.* Caracas: Editorial-Salesiana [1961].

———. *Los indios Guaraunos y su cancionero: Historia, religión, y alma lírica.* Biblioteca "Missionalia Hispanica," vol. 15. Madrid: Consejo Superior de Investigaciones Científicas, Departamento de Misionología Española, 1964.

———. *Mi batalla de Dios: Reflejos de la vida y afanes de un misionero.* Vigo, Spain: Artes Gráficas Galicia, 1972.

Barrett, Ronald, Christopher W. Kuzawa, Thomas McDade, and George J. Armelagos. "Emerging and Re-emerging Infectious Diseases: The Third Epidemiologic Transition." *Annual Review of Anthropology* 27 (1998): 247–271.

Barrios, Asdrubal. "Alertan sobre posible estallido de cólera en Caracas." *El Nacional,* 23 February 1991, C-3.

———. "Las bocas del Orinoco (I): Un delta empobrecido pide ayuda al Parlamento." *El Nacional,* 20 August 1991, C-1.

———. "Las bocas del Orinoco (II): Coexistencia moral con la civilización." *El Nacional,* 21 August 1991, C-1.

———. "El cólera está cerca." *El Nacional,* 22 October 1991, C-2.

———. "93 naciones atacadas por el cólera." *El Nacional,* 14 March 1991, C-2.

Barua, Dhiman. "History of Cholera." In *Cholera,* edited by Dhiman Barua and William B. Greenough III, 1–36. New York: Plenum Medical, 1992.

Barua, Dhiman, and William B. Greenough III, eds. *Cholera.* New York: Plenum Medical, 1992.

Basso, Ellen B. *A Musical View of the Universe: Kalapalo Myth and Ritual Performances.* Philadelphia: University of Pennsylvania Press, 1985.

Bauman, Richard. *Story, Performance, and Event: Contextual Studies of Oral Narrative.* Cambridge: Cambridge University Press, 1986.

Bauman, Richard, and Charles L. Briggs. *Modernizing Discourse: Language, Modernity, and the Politics of Inequality.* Cambridge: Cambridge University Press, 2002.

Bauman, Zygmunt. *Globalization: The Human Consequences.* New York: Columbia University Press, 1998.

———. *Legislators and Interpreters: On Modernity, Postmodernity and Intellectuals.* Ithaca, N.Y.: Cornell University Press, 1987.

———. *Modernity and Ambivalence.* Cambridge: Polity, 1991.

Becklund, Laurie. "Officials Expect Few New Cases of Cholera." *Los Angeles Times,* 23 February 1992, B-1, 5.

Benedict, Ruth. *Patterns of Culture.* Boston: Houghton Mifflin, 1934.

Benenson, Abram S. *Control of Communicable Diseases Manual.* Washington, D.C.: American Public Health Association, 1970.

————. *Control of Communicable Diseases Manual.* 14th ed. Washington, D.C.: American Public Health Association, 1990.

Berg, Marc. *Rationalizing Medical Work: Decision-Support Techniques and Medical Practices.* Cambridge, Mass.: MIT Press, 1997.

Berger, Peter L., and Thomas Luckmann. *The Social Construction of Reality: A Treatise in the Sociology of Knowledge.* Garden City, N.Y.: Doubleday, 1966.

Bhabha, Homi K. *The Location of Culture.* New York: Routledge, 1994.

————, ed. *Nation and Narration.* New York: Routledge, 1990.

Bhabha, Jacqueline. "Embodied Rights: Gender Persecution, State Sovereignty, and Refugees." *Public Culture* 9 (1996): 3–32.

Bilson, G. *A Darkened House: Cholera in Nineteenth-Century Canada.* Toronto: University of Toronto Press, 1980.

Blake, P. A., D. T. Allegra, J. D. Snyder, et al. "Cholera a Possible Endemic Focus in the United States." *New England Journal of Medicine* 302 (1980): 305–309.

Boas, Franz. *Race, Language, and Culture.* New York: Free Press, 1940.

Boon Bartolozzi, Lisseth. "Comunidades indígenas del país tomaron el Congreso." *El Diario de Caracas,* 17 July 1992.

————. "Indígenas exigen derecho sobre propiedad de la tierra." *El Diario de Caracas,* 16 July 1992.

Borroto, R. J., and R. Martínez Piedra. "Geographical Patterns of Cholera in Mexico, 1991–1996." *International Journal of Epidemiology* 29 (2000): 764–772.

Bourdieu, Pierre. "Opinion Polls: A 'Science' without a Scientist." In *In Other Words: Essays towards a Reflexive Sociology,* translated by Matthew Adamson, 168–174. Cambridge: Polity, 1990.

————. *Outline of a Theory of Practice.* Translated by Richard Nice. Cambridge: Cambridge University Press, 1977 (1972).

————. "Public Opinion Does Not Exist." In *Communication and Class Struggle,* vol. 1, 124–130. New York: International General, 1979.

Bowker, Geoffrey C., and Susan Leigh Star. *Sorting Things Out: Classification and Its Consequences.* Cambridge, Mass.: MIT Press, 1999.

Bracamonte, Amilcar. "303 casos de cólera detactados en el país." *El Mundo,* 10 August 1991, 7.

Braudel, Fernand. *A History of Civilizations.* Translated by Richard Mayne. New York: A. Lane, 1994.

————. *La historia y las ciencias sociales.* Translated by Josefina Gómez Mendoza. Madrid: Alianza Editorial, 1968.

Breilh, Jaime. *Epidemiología: Economía, medicina y política.* Mexico: Editorial Fontamara, 1986.

————. *Nuevos conceptos y técnicas de investigación.* Serie Epidemiología Crítica, no. 3. Quito: Centro de Estudios y Asesoría en Salud, 1994.

Briggs, Asa. "Cholera and Society in the Nineteenth Century." *Past and Present* 19 (1961): 76–96.

Briggs, Charles L. "Análisis sociolingüístico del discurso Warao: Notas preliminares sobre las formas seculares." *Montalbán* 20 (1988): 103–120.

————. "Conflict, Language Ideologies, and Privileged Arenas of Discursive Authority in Warao Dispute Mediation." In *Disorderly Discourse: Narrative, Conflict, and Social Inequality,* edited by Charles L. Briggs, 204–242. Oxford: Oxford University Press, 1996.

———. "Emergence of the Non-Indigenous Peoples." In *Translating Native Latin American Verbal Art: Ethnopoetics and Ethnography of Speaking,* edited by Kay Sammons and Joel Sherzer, 174–196. Washington, D.C.: Smithsonian Institution Press, 2000.

———. "Generic versus Metapragmatic Dimensions of Warao Narratives: Who Regiments Performance?" In *Reflexive Language: Reported Speech and Metapragmatics,* edited by John A. Lucy, 179–212. Cambridge: Cambridge University Press, 1993.

———. "The Meaning of Nonsense, the Poetics of Embodiment, and the Production of Power in Warao Shamanistic Healing." In *The Performance of Healing,* edited by Carol Laderman and Marina Roseman, 185–232. New York: Routledge, 1996.

———. "Notes on a 'Confession': On the Construction of Gender, Sexuality and Violence in an Infanticide Case." *Pragmatics* 7, no. 4 (1997): 519–546.

———. "The Patterning of Variation in Performance." In *American Dialect Research,* edited by Dennis R. Preston, 379–431. Amsterdam: John Benjamins, 1993.

———. "Personal Sentiments and Polyphonic Voices in Warao Women's Ritual Wailing: Music and Poetics in a Critical and Collective Discourse." *American Anthropologist* 95 (1993): 929–957.

———. "The Politics of Discursive Authority in Research on the 'Invention of Tradition.'" *Cultural Anthropology* 11, no. 4 (1996): 435–469.

———. "'Since I Am a Woman, I Will Chastise My Relatives': Gender, Reported Speech, and the (Re)production of Social Relations in Warao Ritual Wailing." *American Ethnologist* 19 (1992): 337–361.

———. "'You're a Liar—You're Just Like a Woman!' Constructing Dominant Ideologies of Language in Warao Men's Gossip." In *Language Ideologies: Practice and Theory,* edited by Bambi Schieffelin, Kathryn A. Woolard, and Paul V. Kroskrity, 229–255. New York: Oxford University Press, 1998.

Briggs, Charles L., and Richard Bauman. "Genre, Intertextuality, and Social Power." *Journal of Linguistic Anthropology* 2, no. 2 (1992): 131–172.

Briggs, Charles L., and Clara Mantini-Briggs. "'Bad Mothers' and the Threat to Civil Society: Race, Cultural Reasoning, and the Institutionalization of Social Inequality in a Venezuelan Infanticide Trial." *Law and Social Inquiry* 25, no. 2 (2000): 299–354.

———. "'The Indians Accept Death as a Normal, Natural Event': Institutional Authority, Cultural Reasoning, and Discourses of Genocide in a Venezuelan Cholera Epidemic." *Social Identities* 3, no. 3 (1997): 439–469.

Brown, Phyllida. "Latin America Struggles as Cholera Spreads." *New Scientist* 130, no. 1767 (1991): 12.

Bruner, Jerome S. *Acts of Meaning.* Cambridge, Mass.: Harvard University Press, 1990.

Burke, Kenneth. *A Grammar of Motives*. Englewood Cliffs, N.J.: Prentice Hall, 1945.

Burkett, P. "Poverty Crisis in the Third World: The Contradictions of World Bank Policy." *International Journal of Health Services* 21, no. 3 (1991): 471–480.

Bustamante, Miguel E. *The Pan American Sanitary Bureau: Half a Century of Health Activities, 1902–1954*. Washington, D.C.: Pan American Sanitary Bureau, 1953.

Caldera, Rosita. "70% de los caraqueños puede contraer el cólera." *El Nacional*, 4 June 1991, C-4.

Camel Anderson, Eduardo. "Indice de informalidad económica se elevo a 56% de la población activa." *El Nacional* (Web version), 9 March 2001.

Campisi, Jack. *The Mashpee Indians: Tribes on Trial*. Syracuse, N.Y.: Syracuse University Press, 1991.

Caplan, R., and Scott L. Malcomson. "Giving the U.N. the Business." *The Nation* 16, no. 23 (1986): 109–111.

Carrasco, Morita. "Cólera, cultura y poder: La trama discursiva del cólera." In *Cultura, salud y enfermedad: Temas en antropología médica*, edited by Marcelo Alvarez and Victoria Barreda, 145–154. Buenos Aires: Instituto Nacional de Antropología y Pensamiento Latinoamericano, 1995.

Castells, Manuel. *The Information Age: Economy, Society and Culture*, vol. 1: *The Rise of the Network Society*. Oxford: Blackwell, 1996.

CBS News. "Why?" Transcript of text for segment of *60 Minutes*, 4 December 1994, vol. 27, no. 13. Livingston, N.J.: Burrelle's Information Services, 1994.

"Cerrar la frontera piden los caraqueños." *El Nacional*, 29 April 1991, C-1.

Chagnon, Napoleon A. *Yanomamö: The Fierce People*. 3d ed. New York: Holt, Rinehart and Winston, 1983.

Chakrabarty, Dipesh. "Postcoloniality and the Artifice of History: Who Speaks for Indian Pasts?" *Representations* 37 (1992): 1–26.

———. *Provincializing Europe: Postcolonial Thought and Historical Difference*. Princeton, N.J.: Princeton University Press, 2000.

Chase, Susan E. *Ambiguous Empowerment: The World of Narratives of Women School Superintendents*. Amherst: University of Massachusetts Press, 1995.

Chetley, Andrew. *The Politics of Babyfoods: Successful Challenges to an International Marketing Strategy*. London: Francis Pinter, 1986.

Chevalier, Louis. *Le choléra: La première épidémie du XIXe siècle*. Roche-sur-Yon: Imprimerie Centrale de l'Ouest, 1958.

Chirimuuta, Richard C., and Rosalind J. Chirimuuta. *AIDS, Africa and Racism*. Rev. ed. London: Free Association Books, 1989.

Christen, Catherine A. "Rapporteur's Report: May 1, 1998 Conference." In *Infectious Diseases and Social Inequality in Latin America: From Hemispheric Insecurity to Global Cooperation*. Working Paper Series, no. 239. Washington, D.C.: Latin American Program, Woodrow Wilson International Center for Scholars, 1999.

Cicourel, Aaron V. "The Interpenetration of Communicative Contexts: Examples from Medical Encounters." In *Rethinking Context: Language as an In-*

teractive Phenomenon, edited by Alessandro Duranti and Charles Goodwin, 291–310. Cambridge: Cambridge University Press, 1992.

"121 nuevos casos de cólera en zona de Nabasanuka." *Notidiario,* 15 August 1992, 11.

Clifford, James. *The Predicament of Culture: Twentieth-Century Ethnography, Literature, and Art.* Cambridge, Mass.: Harvard University Press, 1988.

Clifford, James, and George E. Marcus, eds. *Writing Culture: The Poetics and Politics of Ethnography.* Berkeley: University of California Press, 1986.

Cohen, Elizabeth. "Programa de ayuda a Waraos ofreció Comunidad Económica Europea." *El Nacional,* 15 September 1992.

———. "Repunte del cólera en países vecinos pone en alerta al MSAS." *El Nacional,* 9 March 1992, D-16.

"Cólera y dengue en Venezuela admite Sanidad." *El Mundo,* 14 November 1991, 1.

Collier, Jane Fishburne, and Sylvia Junko Yanagisako, eds. *Gender and Kinship: Essays toward a Unified Analysis.* Palo Alto, Calif.: Stanford University Press, 1987.

Colloredo-Mansfeld, Rudi. "'Dirty Indians,' Radical *Indígenas,* and the Political Economy of Social Difference in Modern Ecuador." *Bulletin of Latin American Research* 17, no. 2 (1998): 185–205.

———. *The Native Leisure Class: Consumption and Cultural Creativity in the Andes.* Chicago: University of Chicago Press, 1999.

Colwell, Rita R., and William M. Spira. "The Ecology of Vibrio Cholerae." In *Cholera,* edited by Dhiman Barua and William B. Greenough III, 107–127. New York: Plenum Medical, 1992.

Committee on Foreign Affairs, House of Representatives, U.S. Congress. *The Cholera Epidemic in Latin America. Hearing before the Subcommittee on Western Hemisphere Affairs.* Washington, D.C.: Government Printing Office, 1991.

"Continua avanzando el cólera en el estado Delta Amacuro." *Notidiario,* 18 August 1992, 24.

Contreras Altuve, César. "Atribuyen a una falsa política de integración la crisis indígena." *Ultimas Noticias,* 26 August 1994, 14.

"Controlado brote de cólera en el Delta." *El Diario de Monagas,* 18 August 1992, 3.

"Cordón fronterizo contra el cólera." *El Nacional,* 15 February 1991, A-1.

"Cordón sanitario en la frontera para evitar el colera." *El Nacional,* 22 November 1991, C-4.

Coronil, Fernando. *The Magical State: Nature, Money, and Modernity in Venezuela.* Chicago: University of Chicago Press, 1997.

Coronil, Fernando, and Julie Skurski. "Dismembering and Remembering the Nation: The Semantics of Political Violence in Venezuela." *Comparative Studies in Society and History* 33, no. 2 (1991): 288–337.

Crenshaw, Kimberle. "Demarginalizing the Intersection of Race and Sex: A Black Feminist Critique of Antidiscrimination Doctrine, Feminist Theory and Antiracist Politics." *The University of Chicago Legal Forum* (1989): 139–168.

———. "Mapping the Margins: Intersectionality, Identity Politics, and Violence against Women of Color." *Stanford Law Review* 43 (1991): 1241–1299.

"Criollos temen contagiarse del cólera." *Notidiario,* 21 August 1992, 23.

Cristancho, María Victoria. "Se acerca el cólera y avanza el dengue y los médico permanecen en huelga." *El Mundo,* 23 November 1991, 1.

Crosby, Alfred W., Jr. *The Columbian Exchange: Biological and Cultural Consequences of 1492.* Westport, Conn.: Greenwood Press, 1972.

"Cuatro casos de cólera diarios en Venezuela." *El Mundo,* 9 March 1992, 23.

Cueto, Marcos. *El regreso de las epidémias: Salud y sociedad en el Perú del siglo XX.* Lima: Instituto de Estudios Peruanos, 1997.

Culler, Jonathan. *The Pursuit of Signs.* London: Routledge & Kegan Paul, 1981.

Daniel, E. Valentine. *Charred Lullabies: Chapters in an Anthropography of Violence.* Princeton, N.J.: Princeton University Press, 1996.

Das, Veena. "Official Narratives, Rumour, and the Social Production of Hate." *Social Identities* 4 (1998): 109–130.

———. "Suffering, Legitimacy and Healing: The Bhopal Case." In *Critical Events: An Anthropological Perspective on Contemporary India,* 137–174. Delhi: Oxford University Press, 1995.

Davis, Peter, director. *Hearts and Minds.* Film. 1974.

"Decenas de muertos causa epidemia de cólera en Ecuador." *El Nacional,* 16 April 1991, A-2.

"Declarado en emergencia sanitaria Delta Amacuro por brote de cólera." *Notidiario,* 12 August 1992, 3.

"Declarar en emergencia al Delta ante la amenaza de el cólera." *El Diario de Monagas,* 25 February 1992, 15.

de la Cadena, Marisol. *Indigenous Mestizos: The Politics of Race and Culture in Cuzco, Peru, 1919–1991.* Durham, N.C.: Duke University Press, 2000.

Delaporte, François. *Disease and Civilization: The Cholera in Paris, 1832.* Translated by Arthur Goldhammer. Cambridge, Mass.: MIT Press, 1986.

"Delta Amacuro llamando al SAS S.O.S." *Notidiario,* 7 August 1992, 1.

Derrida, Jacques. *Of Grammatology.* Translated by Gayatri Chakravorty Spivak. Baltimore: Johns Hopkins University Press, 1974.

Desrosières, Alain. *The Politics of Large Numbers: A History of Statistical Reasoning.* Translated by Camille Naish. Cambridge, Mass.: Harvard University Press, 1998.

Díaz Hung, Verónica. "El cólera no debería llegar de incógnito." *El Nacional,* 22 May 1991, C-4.

———. "La prevención del cólera disminuyó las diarreas." *El Nacional,* 19 September 1991, C-4.

Díaz Zurita, Isaias. "MSAS: Alarma por el cólera debe continuar hasta finalizar vacaciones y lluvias." *Nuevo País,* 19 August 1992.

"Diez reglas de oro de las OMS para evitar el cólera por los alimentos." *Notidiario,* 4 September 1992, 20.

"17 casos de tuberculosis en el hospital Razetti." *Notidiario,* 8 August 1992, 23.

"1701 casos de cólera con 49 defunciones." *El Diario de Monagas,* 26 January 1993, 1.

Douglas, Mary. *Purity and Danger: An Analysis of the Concepts of Pollution and Taboo.* London: Routledge & Kegan Paul, 1966.

Drasar, B. S., and B. D. Forrest, eds. *Cholera and the Ecology of* Vibrio cholerae. London: Chapman and Hall, 1996.

Duara, Prasenjit. *Rescuing History from the Nation: Questioning Narratives of Modern China.* Chicago: University of Chicago Press, 1995.

Dunn, Frederick L., and Craig R. Janes. "Introduction: Medical Anthropology and Epidemiology." In *Anthropology and Epidemiology,* edited by Craig R. Janes, Ron Stall, and Sandra M. Gifford, 3–34. Dordrecht: Reidel, 1986.

Durey, Michael. *The Return of the Plague: British Society and the Cholera, 1831–32.* Dublin: Gill and Macmillan, 1979.

Dussel, Enrique. "Eurocentrism and Modernity." *Boundary* 2 (1993): 65–76.

"El cólera abre otro frente: El estado Bolívar." *El Nacional,* 20 November 1991, C-4.

"El cólera afecta a todo el continente americano." *El Mundo,* 25 July 1991, 14.

"El cólera alcanzará a Panamá." *El Nacional,* 4 June 1991, A-10.

"El cólera diezma a étnia Warauna." *Notidiario,* 12 November 1992, 23.

"El cólera en el Delta Amacuro está asociado a la baja calidad de la vida." *Notidiario,* 17 August 1992, 15.

"El cólera está matando a los Waraos del Delta." *Notidiario,* 14 August 1992, 12.

"El cólera es una infección típica de las personas de bajos recursos." *El Mundo,* 27 November 1991, 13.

"El cólera llego por el camino del hambre y la contaminación." *Notidiario,* 12 September 1992, 12.

"El cólera: Medio año después." *El Mundo,* 27 August 1991, 5.

Elling, Ray H. "The Capitalist World-System and International Health." *International Journal of Health Services* 11, no. 1 (1980): 21–51.

"El miedo de los Waraos por los cangrejos azules rompe una tradición milenaria." *Notidiario,* 17 August 1992, 11.

"Emergencia nacional por nuevos casos de cólera." *El Nacional,* 12 August 1992, C-4.

"Emergencia sanitaria en Delta Amacuro." *El Diario de Monagas,* 22 November 1991, 1.

"En el Delta Amacuro: Seis muertos por cólera al consumir cangrejos." *El Nacional,* 5 August 1992, D-19.

"Entró el cólera a Delta Amacuro provocando muerte de los indígenas." *Notidiario,* 9 September 1992, 15.

"Epidemia de cólera en Guatemala puede extenderse como en Perú." *El Nacional,* 26 July 1991, A-3.

Epstein, Steven. *Impure Science: AIDS, Activism, and the Politics of Knowledge.* Berkeley: University of California Press, 1996.

Erickson, Frederick, and Jeffrey Shultz. *The Counselor as Gatekeeper: Social Interaction in Interviews*. New York: Academic Press, 1982.

Erikson, Kai. *Everything in Its Path: The Destruction of Community in the Buffalo Creek Flood*. New York: Simon and Schuster, 1977.

Escalante, Luis Manuel. "En 40% ha caído el ingreso turístico." *El Universal*, 10 June 1992, 2–4.

Escalante G., Bernarda, and Librado Moraleda. *Warao a rejetuma*. Caracas: Instituto Caribe de Antropología y Sociología, Fundación La Salle, 1992.

Escobar, Arturo. *Encountering Development: The Making and Unmaking of the Third World*. Princeton, N.J.: Princeton University Press, 1995.

"Establecen puente aéreo entre Tucupita y Caracas." *Notidiario*, 19 August 1992, 3.

Estacio, Pedro. "Guerrilleros y narcos: Barrera contra el cólera." *El Nacional*, 29 June 1991, C-4.

Evans, Richard J. *Death in Hamburg: Society and Politics in the Cholera Years 1830–1910*. Oxford: Clarendon Press, 1987.

Evans-Pritchard, Edward E. *Witchcraft, Oracles and Magic among the Azande*. Oxford: Clarendon Press, 1937.

"Extrema medidas para impedir entrada del cólera." *El Nacional*, 14 February 1991, C-3.

Fabian, Johannes. *Time and the Other: How Anthropology Makes Its Object*. New York: Columbia University Press, 1983.

Fajardo, Victor. "Colapso del paquete económico: Causas, efectos y perspectivas, Venezuela 1989–92." *Cuadernos del CENDES*, no. 20 (1992): 27–52.

Fanon, Franz. "The Fact of Blackness." In *Anatomy of Racism*, edited by David Theo Goldberg, 108–126. Minneapolis: University of Minnesota Press, 1990.

Farmer, Paul. *AIDS and Accusation: Haiti and the Geography of Blame*. Berkeley: University of California Press, 1992.

———. *Infections and Inequalities: The Modern Plagues*. Berkeley: University of California Press, 1999.

"Fedecámaras exhorta a Gobierno y CTV para que mejoren la salud." *El Nacional*, 8 March 1991, C-2.

Fenster, Mark. *Conspiracy Theories: Secrecy and Power in American Culture*. Minneapolis: University of Minnesota Press, 1999.

Fernández Nays, Antonio. "El invierno provoca el éxodo de los Warao." *El Universal*, 20 August 1994.

Ferrándiz, Francisco José. "The Body in Its Senses: The Spirit Possession Cult of María Lionza in Contemporary Venezuela." Ph.D. dissertation, University of California, Berkeley, 1996.

Finelli, Lyn, David Swerdlow, Kristen Mertz, Halina Ragazzoni, and Kenneth Spitalny. "Outbreak of Cholera Associated with Crab Brought from an Area with Epidemic Disease." *Journal of Infectious Diseases* 166 (1992): 1433–1435.

Fineman, Martha. "Images of Mothers in Poverty Discourses." *Duke Law Journal* 1991, no. 1 (1991): 274–295.

Fiske, John. *Television Culture*. London: Routledge, 1989.

Flores, William V., and Rina Benmayor, eds. *Latino Cultural Citizenship: Claiming Identity, Space, and Rights*. Boston: Beacon, 1997.

Foucault, Michel. *The Archaeology of Knowledge*. Translated by A. M. Sheridan Smith. New York: Harper and Row, 1972.

———. *The Birth of the Clinic: An Archaeology of Medical Perception*. Translated by Alan Sheridan. London: Tavistock, 1973.

———. *Discipline and Punish: The Birth of the Prison*. Translated by Alan Sheridan. New York: Vintage, 1977.

———. *The Foucault Effect: Studies in Governmentality*. Edited by Graham Burchell, Colin Gordon, and Peter Miller. Chicago: University of Chicago Press, 1991.

———. *The History of Sexuality: An Introduction*. Translated by Robert Hurley. Vol. 1. New York: Vintage, 1978.

———. *The Order of Things: An Archaeology of the Human Sciences*. New York: Vintage, 1970.

———. *Power/Knowledge: Selected Interviews and Other Writings, 1972–1977*. Translated by Colin Gordon et al. New York: Pantheon, 1980.

Franco, Jean. "Death Camp Confessions and Resistance to Violence in Latin America." *Socialism and Democracy* 2 (1986): 5–17.

Frankenberg, Ronald. "Risk: Anthropological and Epidemiological Narratives of Prevention." In *Knowledge, Power, and Practice: The Anthropology of Medicine and Everyday Life*, edited by Shirley Lindenbaum and Margaret Lock, 219–242. Berkeley: University of California Press, 1993.

Frenk, J., T. Frejka, J. L. Bobadilla, C. Stern, R. Lozano, J. Sepulveda, and M. Jose. "La transición epidemiological en América Latina." *Boletín de la Oficina Sanitaria Panamericana* 111 (1991): 485–496.

Freud, Sigmund. "Screen Memories." In *The Standard Edition of the Complete Psychological Works of Sigmund Freud*, translated by James Strachey, 3: 301–322. London: Hogarth Press, 1962.

Fuenmayor, Ender. "Los indígenas no fueron raptados." *Notidiario*, 23 August 1994, 23.

Gal, Susan. "Between Speech and Silence: The Problematics of Research on Language and Gender." In *Gender at the Crossroads of Knowledge: Feminist Anthropology in the Postmodern Era*, edited by Michaela di Leonardo, 175–203. Berkeley: University of California Press, 1991.

Gall, Norman. *The Death Threat, Part of a Broader Study of Chronic Inflation as Systemic Failure: Latin America and the Polarization of the World Economy*. São Paulo: Fernand Braudel Institute of World Economics, 1993.

Gallegos, Rómulo. *Doña Barbara*. 2d ed. Mexico City: Editorial Orión, 1952.

Gangarosa, Eugene J., and Robert V. Tauxe. "Epilogue: The Latin American Cholera Epidemic." In *Cholera*, edited by Dhiman Barua and William B. Greenough III, 351–358. New York: Plenum Medical, 1992.

García, Argimiro. *Cuentos y tradiciones de los indios guaraunos*. Caracas: Universidad Católica Andrés Bello, 1971.

García, Elsy. "25 nuevos casos de cólera en el Zulia." *El Mundo,* 16 March 1992, 29.

García, Luís R. "Es necesario incrementar la campaña educativa contra el cólera." *El Nacional,* 27 February 1992, C-4.

García Canclini, Néstor. *Culturas híbridas: Estrategias para entrar y salir de la modernidad.* Mexico City: Grijalbo, 1989.

García Márquez, Gabriel. *El amor en los tiempos del cólera.* Bogotá: Editorial Oveja Negra, 1985.

Garrett, Laurie. *The Coming Plague: Newly Emerging Diseases in a World out of Balance.* New York: Farrar, Straus and Giroux, 1994.

Geertz, Clifford. *Local Knowledge.* New York: Basic Books, 1985.

Giddens, Anthony. "Living in a Post-Traditional Society." In *Reflexive Modernization: Politics, Tradition, and Aesthetics in the Modern Social Order,* edited by Ulrich Beck, Anthony Giddens, and Scott Lash, 56–109. Palo Alto, Calif.: Stanford University Press, 1994.

Glass, Robert I., Marlo Libel, and A. David Brandling-Bennett. "Epidemic Cholera in the Americas." *Science* 256 (1992): 1524–1525.

Glass, Roger I., and Robert E. Black. "The Epidemiology of Cholera." In *Cholera,* edited by Dhiman Barua and William B. Greenough III, 129–154. New York: Plenum Medical, 1992.

Glick-Schiller, Nina. "What's Wrong with This Picture? The Hegemonic Construction of Culture in AIDS Research in the United States." *Medical Anthropology Quarterly* 6, no. 3 (1992): 237–254.

"Gobernador de Caracas responsabiliza al gobierno de Delta Amacuro por éxodo de indígenas Waraos." *Correo del Caroní,* 25 August 1994, D-1.

Goffman, Erving. *Stigma: Notes on the Management of Spoiled Identity.* New York: Simon and Schuster, 1963.

Goldwasser, Michele. "The Rainbow Madonna of Trinidad: A Study in the Dynamics of Belief in Trinidadian Religious Life." Ph.D. dissertation, University of California, Los Angeles, 1996.

Gómez, Laura E. *Misconceiving Mothers: Legislators, Prosecutors, and the Politics of Prenatal Drug Exposure.* Philadelphia: Temple University Press, 1997.

Gómez López, José. "Medidas sanitarias y militares en barco procedente del Perú realizan en La Guaira." *El Nacional,* 1 March 1991, D-18.

Gómez V., Raúl. "En peligro étnia waayu por aparición del cólera en el Estado Zulia." *El Mundo,* 5 December 1991, 32.

Gómez Zuloaga, José. "Controlado el cólera en Barrancas." *El Diario de Monagas,* 2 September 1992.

González, Aliana. "Con el cólera en las puertas." *El Nacional,* 15 February 1991, C-2.

———. "Descartarán cólera en placton costero." *El Nacional,* 26 July 1991, C-4.

———. "Juramentado el voluntariado para la lucha anticólera." *El Nacional,* 4 May 1991, C-2.

———. "No hay cólera dice Sanidad." *El Nacional,* 17 May 1991, C-4.

———. "No todo vibrio Cholerau [sic] produce cólera." *El Nacional,* 25 May 1991, C-4.

———. "Tres meses durará alerta por amenaza de cólera." *El Nacional,* 16 February 1991, C-3.

González, Douglas. "Gobierno dice haber controlado el cólera." *El Nuevo País,* 18 August 1992, 2.

Goodman, Louis W., Johanna Mendelson Forman, Moisés Naím, Joseph S. Tulchin, and Gary Bland, eds. *Lessons of the Venezuelan Experience.* Washington, D.C.: Woodrow Wilson Center, and Baltimore: Johns Hopkins University Press, 1995.

Gordon, Avery F. *Ghostly Matters: Haunting and the Sociological Imagination.* Minneapolis: University of Minnesota Press, 1997.

Gotuzzo, E., J. Cieza, L. Estremadoyra, and C. Seas. "Cholera: Lessons from the Epidemic in Peru." *Infectious Disease Clinics of North America* 8 (1994): 183–205.

Gramsci, Antonio. *Selections from the Prison Notebooks of Antonio Gramsci.* Translated by Quintin Hoare and Geoffrey Nowell Smith. New York: International, 1971.

Green, Lawrence W., and Marshall W. Kreuter. *Health Promotion Planning: An Educational and Ecological Approach.* Mountain View, Calif.: Mayfield, 1999.

Gruber, Armando. "El cólera amenaza invadir a Bolívar." *El Nacional,* 17 August 1992, C-3.

"Grupo de socorristas de la Cruz Roja llega a Delta Amacuro." *Notidiario,* 17 August 1992, 23.

Guardia Nacional. *Diálogo intercultural, lideres indígenas–Guardia Nacional.* Mimeograph. Caracas: Guardia Nacional, Comite LV Aniversario, Sub-Comite Actividades Indígenas, 1992.

Guarisma Alvarez, Nolasco. "Indígenas de Mariusa y Winikina volvieron a sus lugares de origen." *Notidiario,* 4 September 1992, 9.

———. "Sub-Comisión congresal visita sectores afectados por el cólera en el Delta." *Notidiario,* 21 August 1992, 2.

Gubrium, Jaber F., and James A. Holstein. *The New Language of Qualitative Method.* New York: Oxford University Press, 1997.

Guerrant, Richard L. "Twelve Messages from Enteric Infections for Science and Society." *American Journal of Tropical Medicine and Hygiene* 51, no. 1 (1994): 26–35.

Guss, David M. *The Festive State: Race, Ethnicity, and Nationalism as Cultural Performance.* Berkeley: University of California Press, 2000.

Hacking, Ian. *The Taming of Chance.* Cambridge: Cambridge University Press, 1990.

Hall, Stuart. "Recent Developments in Theories of Language and Ideology." In *Culture, Media, Language,* edited by Stuart Hall, Dorothy Hobson, Andrew Lowe, and Paul Willis, 157–162. London: Hutchinson, 1980.

Hall, Stuart, Chas Critcher, Tony Jefferson, John Clarke, and Brian Roberts. *Polic-*

ing the Crisis: Mugging, the State, and Law and Order. London: Macmillan, 1978.

Hall, Stuart, and David Held. "Citizens and Citizenship." In New Times: The Changing Face of Politics in the 1990s, edited by Stuart Hall and Martin Jacques, 173–188. London: Verso, 1990.

"Hambre, vomito [sic] y diarrea extingue [sic] la raza warauna." Notidiario, 6 August 1992, 19.

Hanks, William F. Referential Practice: Language and Lived Space among the Maya. Chicago: University of Chicago Press, 1990.

Haraway, Donna. "The Biopolitics of Postmodern Bodies: Determinations of Self in Immune System Discourse." Differences: A Journal of Feminist Cultural Studies 1, no. 1 (1989): 3–43.

———. Primate Visions: Gender, Race, and Nature in the World of Modern Science. New York: Routledge, 1989.

———. "Promises of Monsters." In Cultural Studies, edited by Lawrence Grossberg, Cary Nelson, and Paul Teichler, 295–337. New York: Routledge, 1992.

Harvey, David. The Condition of Postmodernity. Cambridge: Blackwell, 1989.

Hausmann, Ricardo. Dealing with Negative Oil Shocks: The Venezuelan Experience in the Eighties. Working Paper Series, no. 307. Washington, D.C.: Inter-American Development Bank, 1995.

———. Shocks externos y ajuste macroeconómico. Caracas: Banco Central de Venezuela, 1990.

Heinen, H. Dieter. "Adaptive Changes in a Tribal Economy: A Case Study of the Winikina-Warao." Ph.D. dissertation, University of California, Los Angeles, 1972.

———. "Los Warao." In Los aborigenes de Venezuela, vol. 3 of Etnología contemporánea, edited by Walter Coppens, Bernarda Escalante, and Jacques Lizot, 585–689. Caracas: Instituto Caribe de Antropología y Sociología, Fundación La Salle de Ciencias Naturales, 1988.

———. Oko Warao: Marshland People of the Orinoco Delta. Münster: Lit Verlag, 1988.

———, ed. Oko Warao: We Are Marshland People. Münster: Lit Verlag, 1988.

Heinen, H. Dieter, and Kenneth Ruddle. "Ecology, Ritual, and Economic Organization in the Distribution of Palm Starch among the Warao of the Orinoco Delta." Journal of Anthropological Research 30, no. 2 (1974): 116–138.

Heinen, H. Dieter, Werner Wilbert, and Tirso Rivero. Idamo Kabuka: El "Viejo Corto." Caracas: Instituto Caribe de Antropología y Sociología, Fundación La Salle de Ciéncias Naturales, 1998.

Hellinger, Daniel. "Democracy in Venezuela." Latin American Perspectives 12 (1985): 75–82.

Hernández, Teresita. "El asesino a la puerta." El Nacional, 28 April 1991, C-4.

Herzfeld, Michael. The Social Production of Indifference: Exploring the Symbolic Roots of Western Bureaucracy. Chicago: University of Chicago Press, 1992.

Higa, Naomi, Yasuko Honma, M. John Albert, and Masaaki Iwanaga. "Characterization of *Vibrio cholerae* 0139 Synonym Bengal Isolated from Patients with Cholera-Like Disease in Bangladesh." *Microbiology and Immunology* 37, no. 12 (1993): 971–974.

Hill, Jane H. "Junk Spanish, Covert Racism and the (Leaky) Boundary between Public and Private Spheres." *Pragmatics* 5, no. 2 (1995): 197–212.

Hofstadter, Richard. *The Paranoid Style in American Politics and Other Essays.* New York: Random House, 1967.

"Holanda financiará en Venezuela un proyecto masivo de la Comunidad Lucha contra el Cólera." *Notidiario*, 15 October 1992, 20.

Holstein, James A., and Jaber F. Gubrium. *The Self We Live By: Narrative Identity in a Postmodern World.* New York: Oxford University Press, 2000.

Howard-Jones, Norman. *The Pan American Health Organization: Origins and Evolution.* Geneva: World Health Organization, 1981.

———. *The Scientific Background of the International Sanitary Conferences 1851–1938.* Geneva: World Health Organization, 1975.

"Huyendo del cólera." *Notidiario*, 8 August 1992, 1.

Hymes, Dell H. *Ethnography, Linguistics, Narrative Inequality: Toward an Understanding of Voice.* London: Taylor and Francis, 1996.

———. *"In Vain I Tried to Tell You": Studies in Native American Ethnopoetics.* Philadelphia: University of Pennsylvania Press, 1981.

Ileto, R. C. "Cholera and the Origins of the American Sanitary Order in the Philippines." In *Discrepant Histories: Translocal Essays on Filipino Cultures*, edited by Vincent L. Rafael, 51–81. Philadelphia: Temple University Press, 1995.

———. "Outlines of a Non-Linear Emplotment of Philippine History." In *Reflections on Development in Southeast Asia*, edited by L. T. Ghee, 130–159. Singapore: ASEAN Economic Research Unit, Institute of Southeast Asian Studies, 1988.

"Inminente el cólera en Venezuela." *El Nacional*, 9 August 1991, D-4.

"Instalado y juramentado Comité Regional de Lucha Contra el Cólera." *Notidiario*, 14 January 1997.

"Instalan en Tucupita laboratorio de microbiología." *Notidiario*, 19 August 1992, 3.

"Instruye a médicos rurales sobre prevención del cólera." *Notidiario*, 16 May 1991, 5.

Jaén, María Helena. *El sistema de salud venezolano: Desafíos.* Caracas: Ediciones IESA, 2001.

Jakobson, Roman. "Closing Statement: Linguistics and Poetics." In *Style in Language*, edited by Thomas A. Sebeok, 350–377. Cambridge, Mass.: MIT Press, 1960.

———. *Novejsaja russkaja poèzija (Nabrosok pervyj): Viktor Chlebnikov.* Prague, 1921.

———. *Shifters, Verbal Categories, and the Russian Verb.* Cambridge, Mass.: Harvard University Russian Language Project, 1957.

Jameson, Fredric. *The Geopolitical Aesthetic*. Bloomington: Indiana University Press, 1992.

———. *Postmodernism, or, the Cultural Logic of Late Capitalism*. Durham, N.C.: Duke University Press, 1991.

Jauss, H. R. *Toward an Aesthetic of Reception: Theory and History of Literature*. Translated by T. Bahti. Minneapolis: University of Minnesota Press, 1982.

Johnston, Jeffrey, Deborah L. Martin, James Perdue, et al. "Cholera on a Gulf Coast Oil Rig." *New England Journal of Medicine* 309 (1983): 523–526.

Judge, K. "Income Distribution and Life Expectancy: A Critical Appraisal." *British Medical Journal* 311, no. 7015 (1995): 1282–1285.

Kanji, Najmi, et al., eds. *Drugs Policy in Developing Countries*. London: Zed, 1992.

Kaplan, Martha, and John D. Kelly. "Rethinking Resistance: Dialogics of 'Disaffection' in Colonial Fiji." *American Ethnologist* 21 (1994): 122–151.

Kearns, Gerry. "Cholera, Nuisances and Environmental Management in Islington, 1830–55." In *Living and Dying in London*, edited by W. F. Bynum and Roy Porter, 94–125. Medical History, Supplement no. 11. London: Wellcome Institute for the History of Medicine, 1991.

———. "Private Property and Public Health Reform in England, 1830–70." *Social Science and Medicine* 26 (1988): 187–199.

Keusch, Gerald T., and Masanobu Kawakami, eds. *Cytokines, Cholera, and the Gut*. Amsterdam: IOS Press, 1996.

Khan, M., and W. H. Mosley. "The Role of Boatmen in the Transmission of Cholera." *East Pakistan Medical Journal* 11 (1967): 61–65.

Kim, Jim Yong, Joyce V. Millen, Alec Irwin, and John Gershman, eds. *Dying for Growth: Global Inequality and the Health of the Poor*. Monroe, Me.: Common Courage Press, 2000.

Kleinman, Arthur. *The Illness Narratives: Suffering, Healing and the Human Condition*. New York: Basic Books, 1988.

Kleinman, Arthur, Veena Das, and Margaret Lock, eds. *Social Suffering*. Berkeley: University of California Press, 1997.

Kleinman, Arthur, and Joan Kleinman. "The Appeal of Experience, the Dismay of Images: Cultural Appropriations of Suffering in Our Times." *Daedalus* 125, no. 1 (1996): 1–23.

Koo, Denise, Héctor Traverso, Marlo Libel, et al. "El cólera epidemico en América Latina: Implicancias de las definiciones de casos usadas en la vigilancia sanitaria." *Revista Panamericana de Salud Pública* 1 (1997): 85–92.

Koptiuch, Kristin. "Third-Worlding at Home." *Social Text* 9 (1991): 87–99.

Kraut, Alan M. *Silent Travelers: Germs, Genes, and the "Immigrant Menace."* Baltimore: Johns Hopkins University Press, 1994.

Labov, William, and Joshua Waletzky. "Narrative Analysis." In *Essays on the Verbal and Visual Arts*, edited by June Helm, 12–44. Seattle: University of Washington Press, 1967.

"La epidemia de cólera dejará 40,000 muertos." *El Nacional*, 20 April 1991, A-9.

"La epidemia es una vergüenza." *El Nacional,* 1 June 1991, A-6.

"La prioridad son los créditos internacionales para atacar y prevenir epidemia de cólera." *Notidiario,* 29 February 1992, 21.

"La sombra del cólera." *Notidiario,* 6 August 1992, 1.

Latour, Bruno. *The Pasteurization of France.* Translated by Alan Sheridan and John Law. Cambridge, Mass.: Harvard University Press, 1988.

———. *Science in Action.* Cambridge, Mass.: Harvard University Press, 1987.

———. *We Have Never Been Modern.* Translated by Catherine Porter. Cambridge, Mass.: Harvard University Press, 1993.

"La Ummega realizó operativo médico asistencial." *El Diario de Monagas,* 11 February 1992, 11.

Laurell, Asa Cristina. *La política social en la crisis: Una alternative para el sector salud.* Mexico City: Fundación Friedrich Ebert, 1990.

———. *Nuevas tendencias y alternativas en el sector salud.* Mexico City: Universidad Autónoma Metropolitana, 1994.

Lavandero Pérez, Julio, ed. *Ajotejana I: Mitos.* Caracas: n.p., 1991.

———. *Ajotejana II: Relatos.* Caracas: n.p., 1992.

———. *Noara y otros rituales.* Caracas: Universidad Católica Andrés Bello, 2000.

———. *Uaharaho: Ethos narrativo.* Caracas: Hermanos Capuchinos, 1994.

Leavitt, Judith Walzer. *Typhoid Mary: Captive to the Public's Health.* Boston: Beacon, 1996.

Lederberg, Joshua, Robert E. Shope, and Stanley C. Oaks, Jr., eds. *Emerging Infections: Microbial Threats to Health in the United States.* Washington, D.C.: National Academy Press, 1992.

Lefebvre, Henri. *The Production of Space.* Translated by Donald Nicholson-Smith. Oxford: Blackwell, 1991.

Leventhal, Howard, and Linda Cameron. "Persuasion and Health Attitudes." In *Persuasion: Psychological Insights and Perspectives,* edited by Sharon Shavitt and Timothy C. Brock, 219–249. Boston: Allyn and Bacon, 1994.

Levine, M. M., and O. S. Levine. "Changes in Human Ecology and Behavior in Relation to the Emergence of Diarrheal Diseases, Including Cholera." *Proceedings of the National Academy of Sciences* 91 (1994): 2390–2394.

Lévi-Strauss, Claude. *Conversations with Claude Lévi-Strauss.* Edited by Georges Charbonnier. Translated by John and Doreen Weightman. London: Cape, 1969.

———. *The Raw and the Cooked: Introduction to a Science of Mythology.* Translated by John and Doreen Weightman. New York: Harper and Row, 1969.

Lifton, Robert Jay. *Death in Life: Survivors of Hiroshima.* New York: Random House, 1968.

Linares, Yelitza. "No hay suero ni decreto que detenga el cólera." *El Nacional,* 24 December 1991, C-4.

Linde, Charlotte. *Life Stories: The Creation of Coherence.* New York: Oxford University Press, 1993.

Lindenbaum, Shirley. "Images of Catastrophe: The Making of an Epidemic." In *The Political Economy of AIDS*, edited by Merrill Singer, 33–58. Amityville, N.Y.: Baywood, 1998.

———. "Kuru, Prions, and Human Affairs: Thinking about Epidemics." *Annual Review of Anthropology* 30 (2001): 363–385.

Lipsitz, George. *Dangerous Crossroads: Popular Music, Postmodernism, and the Politics of Place*. London: Verso, 1994.

"Llaman a comisión indigenista en zona afectada por cólera." *Notidiario*, 4 September 1992, 1.

Locke, John. *An Essay Concerning Human Understanding*. 2 vols. New York: Dover, 1959 [1690].

"Los casos de cólera que se han presentado están sanos y salvos." *Notidiario*, 18 February 1992, 22.

"Los venezolanos creen que el SAS no tomará las medidas necesarias." *El Nacional*, 15 February 1991, C-3.

Luhmann, Niklas. *The Differentiation of Society*. Translated by Stephen Holmes and Charles Larmore. New York: Columbia University Press, 1982.

Luna Noguera, Rafael. "Entre el hambre, la insalubridad y el cangrejo peludo transcurre la vida en el Delta Amacuro." *Ultimas Noticias*, 17 August 1992, 24.

Lyotard, Jean François. *The Postmodern Condition: A Report on Knowledge*. Translated by Geoff Bennington and Brian Massumi. Minneapolis: University of Minnesota Press, 1984.

Mahalanabis, Dilip, A. M. Molla, and David A. Sack. "Clinical Management of Cholera." In *Cholera*, edited by Dhiman Barua and William B. Greenough III, 253–283. New York: Plenum Medical, 1992.

Mahler, Halfdan. "The Meaning of 'Health for All by the Year 2000.'" *World Health Forum* 3, no. 1 (1981): 5–22.

Mamalakis, Markos. *Poverty and Inequality in Venezuela: Mesoeconomic Dimensions*. Working Paper Series, no. 205. Washington, D.C.: Inter-American Development Bank, 1996.

Marcus, George E. *Ethnography through Thick and Thin*. Princeton, N.J.: Princeton University Press, 1998.

———. "Ethnography in/of the World System: The Emergence of Multi-Sited Ethnography." *Annual Review of Anthropology* 24 (1995): 95–117.

———, ed. *Paranoia within Reason: A Casebook on Conspiracy as Explanation*. Chicago: University of Chicago Press, 1999.

Marcus, George E., and Michael M. J. Fischer. *Anthropology as Cultural Critique: An Experimental Moment in the Human Sciences*. Chicago: University of Chicago Press, 1986.

Marín, Cruz José. *Estampas deltanas*. Tucupita, Venezuela: privately published, 1977.

Marín Rodriguez, Cruz José. *Historia del Territorio Federal Delta Amacuro*. Caracas: Ediciones de la Presidencia de la República, 1981.

Márquez, Gustavo, Joyita Mukherjee, Juan Carlos Navarro, Rosa Amelia González, Roberto Palacios, and Roberto Rigobón. "Fiscal Policy and Income Distribution in Venezuela." In *Government Spending and Income Distribution in Latin America*, edited by Ricardo Hausmann and Roberto Rigobón, 145–213. Washington, D.C.: Inter-American Development Bank, 1993.

Márquez, Patricia C. *The Street Is My Home: Youth and Violence in Caracas.* Palo Alto, Calif.: Stanford University Press, 1999.

Marshall, T. H. "Citizenship and Social Class." In *Class, Citizenship, and Social Development*, edited by Seymour Martin Lipset, 65–122. Westport, Conn.: Greenwood Press, 1964.

Martín, Elías. *En las bocas del Orinoco: 50 años de los misioneros capuchinos en el Delta Amacuro, 1924–1974.* El Hatillo, Venezuela: Ediciones Paulinas, 1977.

Martin, Emily. *Flexible Bodies: Tracking Immunity in American Culture from the Days of Polio to the Age of AIDS.* Boston: Beacon Press, 1994.

———. "Mind-Body Problems." *American Ethnologist* 27, no. 3 (2000): 569–590.

Martínez, Manuel. "No se ha determinado presencia del cólera en el Delta Amacuro." *Notidiario*, 14 January 1997, 16.

Martz, John D., and David J. Meyers, eds. *Venezuela: The Democratic Experience.* New York: Praeger, 1977.

Marwick, Charles. "Like Attacker Probing Defenses, Cholera Threatens U.S. Population from Elsewhere in This Hemisphere." *Journal of the American Medical Association* 267, no. 10 (1992): 1314–1315.

Mausner, Judith S., and Shira Kramer. *Epidemiology: An Introductory Text.* 2d ed. Philadelphia: W. B. Saunders, 1985.

McClure, John A. "Postmodern Romance: Don DeLillo and the Age of Conspiracy." In *Introducing Don DeLillo*, edited by Frank Lentricchia, 99–115. Durham, N.C.: Duke University Press, 1991.

McCord, Colin, and Harold Freeman. "Excess Mortality in Harlem." *New England Journal of Medicine* 322, no. 3 (1990): 173–177.

McGrew, Roderick E. *Russia and the Cholera, 1823–1832.* Madison: University of Wisconsin Press, 1965.

McNeill, William H. *Plagues and People.* New York: Anchor Books, 1976.

Mena Cifuentes, Hernán. "Aviones y barcos procedentes de Perú, Colombia y Ecuador bajo control anticólera." *El Nacional*, 5 April 1991, D-20.

———. "Extreman medidas de control anticólera en Puerto La Guaira y en Maiquetía." *El Nacional*, 7 July 1991, D-6.

Mignolo, Walter. *The Darker Side of the Renaissance.* Ann Arbor: University of Michigan Press, 1995.

———. *Local Histories/Global Designs: Coloniality, Subaltern Knowledges, and Border Thinking.* Princeton, N.J.: Princeton University Press, 2000.

Ministerio de Sanidad y Asistencia Pública. "Cólera." *Boletín Epidemiológico Semanal* 46 (1991): 66–75.

———. "Epidemias en actividad." *Boletín Epidemiológico Semanal* 47 (1992): 267.

———. *Legislación sanitaria nacional: Acuerdos, leyes, decretos, reglamentos y resoluciones sobre sanidad nacional.* Caracas: Editorial Jurídical Venezolana, 1967.

——. *Manual de normas y procedimientos para la prevención y manejo de enfermedades diarréicas y cólera.* Caracas: Division de Enfermedades Transmisibles, Dirección de Epidemiología y Programas, Dirección General Sectorial de Salud, Ministerio de Sanidad y Asistencia Social, 1991.

——. *Medidas de saneamiento ambiental para evitar el cólera.* Caracas: Dirección General Sectorial del Subsistema de Saneamiento Sanitario Ambiental, Ministerio de Sanidad y Asistencia Social, 1991.

——. *Modulo de Instrucción: Cólera.* Caracas: División de Docencia, Dirección de Promoción Social para la Salud, Dirección General Sectorial de Salud, Ministerio de Sanidad y Asistencia Social, 1991.

Ministerio de Sanidad y Asistencia Pública, Departamento de Epidemiología, Estado Delta Amacuro. "Casos de cólera, positivos." Typescript, 1993.

Minkler, Meredith, and Nina Wallerstein. "Improving Health through Community Organization and Community Building." In *Health Behavior and Health Education: Theory, Research, and Practice,* edited by Karen Glanz, Frances Marcus Lewis, and Barbara K. Rimer, 241–268. 2d ed. San Francisco: Jossey-Bass, 1997.

Mishler, Elliot G. *Storylines: Craft Artists' Narratives of Identity.* Cambridge, Mass.: Harvard University Press, 1999.

Montes de Oca, Acianela. "Aún es un enigma origen de casos de cólera en Caracas." *El Nacional,* 22 January 1992, C-4.

——. "El cólera nos acompañará hasta el próximo siglo." *El Nacional,* 26 March 1992, C-1.

——. "Nuevo caso en el Zulia." *El Nacional,* 21 January 1992, C-4.

Moraleda, Librado. *Mawaraotuma, Karata teribukitane naminaki. Primer libro de lectura Warao.* Caracas: Ministerio de Educación, Oficina Ministerial de Asuntos Fronterizos Indígenas, 1979.

Moraleda, Librado, and Basilio Lopez. *Ka jobaji ekuya kujuki. Viajemos por nuestra tierra.* Caracas: Ministerio de Educación, Dirección de Asuntos Indígenas, 1982.

Moreno Durán, Rafael Humberto. *De la barbarie a la imaginación: La experiencia leída.* Bogotá: Tercer Mundo Editores, 1988.

Morley, David. "Changing Paradigms in Audience Studies." In *Remote Control: Television, Audiences, and Cultural Power,* edited by E. Seiter, H. Borchers, G. Kreutzner, and E. Warth, 16–43. London: Routledge, 1989.

Morley, Samuel A., and Carola Alvarez. *Poverty and Adjustment in Venezuela.* Working Paper Series, no. 124. Washington, D.C.: Inter-American Development Bank, 1992.

Morris, J. Glenn, Jr., and the Cholera Laboratory Task Force. "*Vibrio cholerae* 0139 Bengal." In *Vibrio Cholerae and Cholera: Molecular to Global Perspectives,* edited by I. Kaye Wachsmuth, Paul Blake, and Ørjan Olsvik. Washington, D.C.: ASM Press, 1994.

Morris, R. J. *Cholera 1832: The Social Response to an Epidemic.* New York: Holmes & Meier, 1976.

Morsy, Soheir. "Political Economy in Medical Anthropology." In *Medical Anthropology: A Handbook of Theory and Method,* edited by Thomas M. Johnson and Carolyn F. Sargent, 26–46. New York: Greenwood, 1990.

"Muerto por cólera dos indígenas en el Delta." *Notidiario,* 20 January 1997.

Nations, Marilyn K. "Epidemiological Research on Infectious Disease: Quantitative Rigor or Rigormortis? Insights from Ethnomedicine." In *Anthropology and Epidemiology,* edited by Craig R. Janes, Ron Stall, and Sandra M. Gifford, 97–123. Dordrecht: Reidel, 1986.

———. "Illness of the Child: The Cultural Context of Child Diarrhea in Northeast Brazil." Ph.D. dissertation, University of California, Berkeley, 1982.

Nations, Marilyn K., and Cristina M. G. Monte. "'I'm Not Dog, No!': Cries of Resistance against Cholera Control Campaigns." *Social Science and Medicine* 43, no. 6 (1996): 1007–1024.

Nations, Marilyn K., and Linda-Anne Rebhun. "Angels with Wet Wings Can't Fly: Maternal Sentiment in Brazil and the Image of Neglect." *Culture, Medicine, and Psychiatry* 12, no. 2 (1988): 141–200.

Navarro, Vicente. *Crisis, Health and Medicine: A Social Critique.* New York: Tavistock, 1986.

———. "A Critique of the Ideological and Political Position of the Brandt Report and the Alma Ata Declaration." *International Journal of Health Services* 15, no. 4 (1984): 525–544.

———. "Neoliberalism, 'Globalization,' Unemployment, Inequalities, and the Welfare State." *International Journal of Health Services* 28, no. 4 (1998): 607–682.

———. "The Underdevelopment of Health or the Health of Underdevelopment: An Analysis of the Distribution of Human Health Resources in Latin America." *International Journal of Health Services* 4, no. 1 (1974): 5–27.

"Ningún país latinoamericano está ajeno a epidemia del cólera." *El Nacional,* 21 March 1991, 15.

"No hay cólera en Maicao ni en Venezuela." *El Mundo,* 21 November 1991, 32.

"No se ha registrado casos de cólera en Barrancas del Orinoco." *Notidiario,* 17 August 1992, 11.

Nuñez, Mariela. "Delta Amacuro, Sucre, D.F. y Monagas: Focos mas activos del cólera." *El Globo,* 18 August 1992, 45.

———. "Sociedad de Salud Pública pide más vigilancia del SAS ante el cólera." *El Nacional,* 18 February 1991, D-15.

Ocando Hernández, Casto. "Continúan llegando contigentes de indígenas a Caracas." *El Universal,* 21 August 1994, 1, 28.

Ochs, Elinor, and Lisa Capps. *Living Narrative: Creating Lives in Everyday Storytelling.* Cambridge, Mass.: Harvard University Press, 2001.

Oficina Central de Estadística e Informática. *Censo Indígena de Venezuela, 1992.* 2 vols. Caracas: Oficina Central de Estadística e Informática, 1993.

———. *El Censo 90 en Delta Amacuro.* Caracas: Oficina Central de Estadística e Informática, 1995.

———. *El censo 90 en Monagas.* Caracas: Oficina Central de Estadística e Informática, 1995.

Oliver-Smith, Anthony. "The Crisis Dyad: Meaning and Culture in Anthropology and Medicine." In *Nourishing the Humanistic in Medicine,* edited by William R. Rogers and David Barnard. Pittsburgh: University of Pittsburgh Press, 1979.

———. *The Martyred City: Death and Rebirth in the Andes.* Albuquerque: University of New Mexico Press, 1986.

Olsen, Dale A. *Music of the Warao of Venezuela: Song People of the Rain Forest.* Gainesville: University Presses of Florida, 1996.

Omi, Michael, and Howard Winant. *Racial Formation in the United States: From the 1960s to the 1990s.* New York: Routledge, 1994.

Ong, Aihwa. *Flexible Citizenship: The Cultural Logics of Transnationality.* Durham, N.C.: Duke University Press, 1999.

"11 muertos por cólera en Panamá." *El Mundo,* 20 October 1991, 14.

"Operativo de saneamiento en hospital Luís Razetti." *Notidiario,* 4 June 1991, 9.

"ORAI emprende campaña contra el cólera en zonas indígenas." *Notidiario,* 8 August 1992, 23.

Packard, Randall M. *White Plague, Black Labor: Tuberculosis and the Political Economy of Health and Disease in South Africa.* Berkeley: University of California Press, 1989.

Pan American Health Organization. *Basic Documents of the Pan American Health Organization.* 15th ed. Official Document no. 240. Washington, D.C.: Pan American Health Organization, 1991.

———. "Cholera Situation in the Americas." *Epidemiological Bulletin* 12, no. 1 (1991): 1–24.

———. "Cholera Situation in the Americas: An Update." *Epidemiological Bulletin* 12, no. 2 (1991): 1–15.

———. "Cholera Situation in the Americas: An Update." *Epidemiological Bulletin* 12, no. 4 (1991): 11–13.

———. "Cholera Situation in the Americas: An Update." *Epidemiological Bulletin* 15, no. 1 (1994): 13–16.

———. *Pro Salute Novi Mundi: A History of the Pan American Health Organization.* Washington, D.C.: Pan American Health Organization, 1992.

———. "Update: The Cholera Situation in the Americas." *Epidemiological Bulletin* 12, no. 3 (1991): 11–14.

"Pánico en el delta." *Notidiario,* 6 August 1992, 24.

Panos Institute. *AIDS and the Third World.* Philadelphia: New Society, 1989.

"Para evitar el cólera la OMS anuncia diez medidas." *El Nacional,* 20 November 1991, C-4.

"Para evitar el cólera prohiben consumo de alimentos crudos y hielo." *Notidiario,* 22 February 1992, 23.

Parker, Richard. *Beneath the Equator: Cultures of Desire, Male Homosexu-*

ality and Emerging Gay Communities in Brazil. New York: Routledge, 1999.

Pateman, Carole. *The Sexual Contract.* Palo Alto, Calif.: Stanford University Press, 1988.

Patton, Cindy. *Fatal Advice: How Safe-Sex Education Went Wrong.* Durham, N.C.: Duke University Press, 1996.

———. *Inventing AIDS.* New York: Routledge, 1990.

Pearce, N. "Traditional Epidemiology, Modern Epidemiology, and Public Health." *American Journal of Public Health* 86 (1996): 678–683.

Pelling, Margaret. *Cholera, Fever, and English Medicine 1825–1865.* Oxford: Oxford University Press, 1978.

Pestana de Castro, A. F., and W. F. Almeida, eds. *Cholera on the American Continents.* Washington, D.C.: ILSI Press, 1993.

Petrera, Margarita, and Maibí Montoya. *Impacto económico de la epidemia del cólera Peru—1991.* Serie Informes Técnicos, no. 22. Washington, D.C.: Programa de Políticas de Salud, Organización Panamericana de la Salud, 1993.

"Plan de la OPS contra el cólera." *El Nacional,* 11 July 1991, C-5.

Pollak-Eltz, Angelina. *María Lionza: Mito y culto venezolano.* Caracas: Instituto de Investigaciones Históricas, Universidad Católica Andrés Bello, 1972.

Pollitzer, R. *Cholera.* Geneva: World Health Organization, 1959.

Popovic, Tanja, Cheryl Bopp, Ørjan Olsvik, and Kay Wachsmuth. "Epidemiologic Application of a Standardized Ribotype Scheme for *Vibrio cholerae* 01." *Journal of Clinical Microbiology* 31, no. 9 (1993): 2474–2482.

"Por nada del mundo regresaremos a los sitios que dejamos en el Delta." *Notidiario,* 17 August 1992, 12–13.

Porter, Theodore. *Trust in Numbers: The Pursuit of Objectivity in Science and Public Life.* Princeton, N.J.: Princeton University Press, 1995.

Prashad, V. "Native Dirt/Imperial Ordure: The Cholera of 1832 and the Morbid Resolutions of Modernity." *Journal of Historical Sociology* 7 (1994): 243–260.

Pratt, Mary Louise. *Imperial Eyes: Travel Writing and Transculturation.* London: Routledge, 1992.

"Presencia de la Guardia Nacional contribuyó grandemente a combatir el mal." *El Diario de Monagas,* 19 August 1992.

Preston, Richard. *The Hot Zone.* New York: Random House, 1994.

"Prioridad: Atacar el cólera." *2001,* 17 August 1992, 5.

Propp, Vladímir. *The Morphology of the Folktale.* Translated by Laurence Scott. Austin: University of Texas Press, 1968.

"49 casos de cólera registra el SAS de Delta Amacuro." *Notidiario,* 19 August 1992, 3.

Rabbani, G. H., and William B. Greenough III. "Pathophysiology and Clinical Aspects of Cholera." In *Cholera,* edited by Dhiman Barua and William B. Greenough III, 209–228. New York: Plenum Medical, 1992.

Rabinow, Paul. *French Modern: Norms and Forms of the Social Environment.* Cambridge, Mass.: MIT Press, 1989.

Ram, Kalpana, and Margaret Jolly, eds. *Maternities and Modernities: Colonial and Postcolonial Experiences in Asia and the Pacific.* Cambridge: Cambridge University Press, 1998.

Ramos, Alcida Rita. *Sanumá Memories: Yanomami Ethnography in Times of Crisis.* Madison: University of Wisconsin Press, 1995.

Ranger, Terence, and P. Slack, eds. *Epidemics and Ideas.* Cambridge: Cambridge University Press, 1992.

"Reunión de alto nivel discutió migración de indígenas a Caracas." *El Universal,* 12 September 1994.

Reyna, Carlos, and Antonio Zapata. *Crónica sobre el cólera en el Perú.* Lima: Desco, 1991.

Ricoeur, Paul. *Hermeneutics and the Human Sciences.* Translated by John B. Thompson. Cambridge: Cambridge University Press, 1981.

———. *Time and Narrative.* Vol. 1. Translated by K. McLaughlin and D. Pellauer. Chicago: University of Chicago Press, 1984.

Ries, Allen, et al. "Cholera in Piura, Peru: A Modern Urban Epidemic." *Journal of Infectious Diseases* 166 (1992): 1429–1433.

Rimonte, Nilda. "A Question of Culture: Cultural Approval of Violence against Women in the Pacific-Asian Community and the Cultural Defense." *Stanford Law Review* 43 (1991): 1311–1332.

Rivero G., Modesto. "Acerca del cólera." *El Mundo,* 1 June 1991, 4.

Rizk, Marlene. "Alerta en el país por dengue e inevitable entrada del cólera." *El Nacional,* 10 August 1991, C-4.

———. "Confirman primera muerte de cólera en Maracaibo." *El Nacional,* 17 December 1991, C-4.

———. "Controlarán ventas ambulantes." *El Nacional,* 23 April 1991, C-1.

———. "El cólera llegó al país pero el MSAS lo oculta." *El Nacional,* 12 July 1991, C-4.

———. "El 83% de los venezolanos es vulnerable al cólera." *El Nacional,* 29 April 1991, C-1.

———. "Pese al caso de cólera no estamos en emergencia." *El Nacional,* 5 December 1991, C-4.

Riz[k], Marlene, and Graciela García. "El cólera viaja en comidas ambulantes." *El Nacional,* 18 April 1991, C-4.

Roberts, Dorothy. *Killing the Black Body: Race, Reproduction, and the Meaning of Liberty.* New York: Vintage, 1997.

Robertson, Roland. *Globalization: Social Theory and Global Culture.* London: Sage, 1995.

Rockefeller, Abby A. "Civilization and Sludge: Notes on the History of the Management of Human Excreta." *Capitalism, Nature, Socialism* 9, no. 3 (1998): 3–18.

Rodríguez Rivero, P. D. *Epidemias y sanidad en Venezuela.* Caracas: Tip. Mercantil, 1924.

Rosaldo, Renato. "Cultural Citizenship, Inequality, and Multiculturalism." In

Latino Cultural Citizenship: Claiming Identity, Space, and Rights, edited by William V. Flores and Rina Benmayor, 27–38. Boston: Beacon, 1997.

Roseberry, William. *Coffee and Capitalism in the Venezuelan Andes*. Austin: University of Texas Press, 1983.

———. "Images of the Peasant in the Consciousness of the Venezuelan Proletariat." In *Proletarians and Protest*, edited by Michael Hanagan and Charles Stephenson. Westport, Conn.: Greenwood Press, 1986.

Rosenberg, Charles E. *The Cholera Years: The United States in 1832, 1849, and 1866*. Chicago: University of Chicago Press, 1962.

———. *Explaining Epidemics and Other Studies in the History of Medicine*. Cambridge: Cambridge University Press, 1992.

Rousseau, Jean-Jacques. *Discourse on the Origin of Inequality*. Translated by Franklin Philip. Oxford: Oxford University Press, 1994.

Sahlins, Marshall. *Culture and Practical Reason*. Chicago: University of Chicago Press, 1976.

Said, Edward. *Orientalism*. New York: Pantheon, 1978.

Salas, Julio C. *Civilización y barbarie: Estudios sociológicos americanos*. Caracas: Fundación Julio C. Salas, 1998 [1919].

———. *Tierra Firme, Venezuela y Colombia: Estudios sobre ethnología e historia*. Caracas: Fundación Julio C. Salas, 1997 [1908].

Salas, Yolanda. "La dramatización social y política del imaginario popular: el fenómeno del bolivarismo en Venezuela." In *Estudios latinoamericanos sobre cultura y transformaciones sociales en tiempos de globalización*, edited by Daniel Mato, 201–221. Buenos Aires: Consejo Latinoamericano de Ciencias Sociales, 2001.

———. "Narrando y construyendo nuestro pasado: La historia y los heroes según la conciencia colectiva." Paper presented at the V Jornadas de Estudio de la Narrativa Folklórica, Santa Rosa, Argentina, 3–5 August 2000.

Salas de Lecuna, Yolanda. *Bolívar y la historia en la conciencia popular*. Caracas: Instituto de Altos Estudios de América Latina, Universidad Simón Bolívar, 1987.

Santa Ana, Otto. *Brown Tide Rising: Metaphors of Latinos in Contemporary American Public Discourse*. Austin: University of Texas Press, 2002.

Santiago-Irizarry, Vilma. "Culture as Cure." *Cultural Anthropology* 11, no. 1 (1996): 3–24.

Santos Amaral, Desiree. "Tráfico de indígenas convertidos en mendigos investiga el Consejo." *Ultimas Noticias*, 24 August 1994, 19.

Sassen, Saskia. *Globalization and Its Discontents*. New York: New Press, 1998.

———. *Losing Control? Sovereignty in an Age of Globalization*. New York: Columbia University Press, 1996.

———. "Spatialities and Temporalities of the Global: Elements for a Theorization." *Public Culture* 12, no. 1 (2000): 215–232.

Saussure, Ferdinand de. *A Course in General Linguistics*. Translated by Wade Baskin. New York: McGraw-Hill, 1959 [1916].

Scheper-Hughes, Nancy. *Death without Weeping: The Violence of Everyday Life in Brazil.* Berkeley: University of California Press, 1992.

———. "The Madness of Hunger: Sickness, Delirium, and Human Needs." *Culture, Medicine and Psychiatry* 12 (1988): 429–458.

"Se desplaza hacia Monagas brote epidémico de cólera." *Notidiario,* 20 August 1992, 2.

"Se extiende el cólera en el Delta por migración de los indígenas." *Notidiario,* 12 August 1992, 2.

Sen, Amartya. *Commodities and Capabilities.* Amsterdam: North-Holland, 1985.

———. *On Economic Inequality.* Expanded ed. Oxford: Clarendon Press, 1997.

———. *Poverty and Child Health.* Oxford: Radcliff Medical Press, 1996.

"Serán dotados todos los centros asistenciales con servicios de hospitalización." *El Diario de Monagas,* 26 June 1991, 1.

Serbin, Andrés, Andrés Stambouli, Jennifer McCoy, and William Smith, eds. *Venezuela: La democracia bajo presión.* Caracas: Instituto Venezolano de Estudios Sociales y Políticos & Editorial Nueva Sociedad, 1993.

"70% de habitantes de la región capital podría padecer el cólera." *El Mundo,* 1 June 1991, 22.

Shandera, W. X., B. Hafkin, D. L. Martin, et al. "Persistence of Cholera in the United States." *American Journal of Tropical Medicine and Hygiene* 32 (1983): 812–817.

Shohat, Ella, and Robert Stam. *Unthinking Eurocentrism.* New York: Routledge, 1994.

Sikkink, Kathryn. "Codes of Conduct for Transnational Corporations: The Case of the WHO/UNICEF Code." *International Organization* 40, no. 4 (1986): 817–840.

Sklair, Leslie. *Sociology of the Global System.* 2d ed. Baltimore: Johns Hopkins University Press, 1995.

Skurski, Julie. "The Ambiguities of Authenticity in Latin America: Doña Bárbara and the Construction of National Identity." *Poetics Today* 15, no. 4 (1994): 59–81.

Skurski, Julie, and Fernando Coronil. "Savage Capitalism: Redefining Citizenship in Venezuela." Paper presented at Discourses of Genocide, University of California, San Diego, 12–13 April 1996.

Snow, John. *Snow on Cholera, Being a Reprint of Two Papers by John Snow.* New York: The Commonwealth Fund, 1936.

SOCSAL (Servicio de Apoyo Local, A.C.). "Registro sociodemográfico Warao de Punta Pescador." Photocopy. Caracas: SOCSAL [1998].

Soja, Edward W. *Postmodern Geographies: The Reassertion of Space in Critical Social Theory.* London: Verso, 1989.

Sommer, Doris. *Foundational Fictions: The National Romances of Latin America.* Berkeley: University of California Press, 1991.

Sontag, Susan. *Illness as Metaphor and AIDS and Its Metaphors.* New York: Doubleday, 1990.

Spivak, Gayatri Chakravorty. "Can the Subaltern Speak?" In *Marxism and the Interpretation of Culture*, edited by Cary Nelson and Lawrence Grossberg, 271–313. Urbana: University of Illinois Press, 1981.

Stallybrass, Peter, and Allon White. *The Politics and Poetics of Transgression.* Ithaca, N.Y.: Cornell University Press, 1986.

Starrels, John M. *The World Health Organization: Resisting Third World Ideological Pressures.* Washington, D.C.: The Heritage Foundation, 1985.

Stocking, George W., Jr. *Race, Culture, and Evolution: Essays in the History of Anthropology.* New York: Free Press, 1968.

Sturken, Marita. *Tangled Memories: The Vietnam War, the AIDS Epidemic, and the Politics of Remembering.* Berkeley: University of California Press, 1997.

Suárez, Rubén, and Bonnie Bradford. *The Economic Impact of the Cholera Epidemic in Peru.* Washington, D.C.: Environmental Health Project, 1993.

"Suramerica en tiempos del cólera." *El Nacional,* 5 May 1991, A-2.

Swerdlow, David L. "*Vibrio Cholerae* non-01—the Eighth Pandemic?" *The Lancet* 342, no. 8868 (1993): 382–383.

Swerdlow, David L., Eric D. Mintz, Marcela Rodríguez, et al. "Waterborne Transmission of Epidemic Cholera in Trujillo, Peru: Lessons for a Continent at Risk." *The Lancet* 340, no. 8810 (1992): 28–32.

Swerdlow, David L., and Allen A. Ries. "Cholera in the Americas: Guidelines for the Clinician." *Journal of the American Medical Association* 267 (1992): 1495–1499.

Tabuas, Mireya. "Consejo de Caracas investigará la presencia de indígenas." *El Nacional,* 24 August 1994, C-3.

Tacket, C. O., G. Losonksy, J. P. Nataro, S. S. Wasserman, S. J. Cryz, R. Edelman, and M. M. Levine. "Extension of the Volunteer Challenge Model to Study South American Cholera in a Population of Volunteers Predominantly with Blood Group Antigen O." *Trans. Royal Soc. Trop. Med. Hygiene* 89 (1995): 75–77.

Tambiah, Stanley Jeyaraja. *Buddhism Betrayed?: Religion, Politics, and Violence in Sri Lanka.* Chicago: University of Chicago Press, 1992.

Taussig, Michael. *The Magic of the State.* New York: Routledge, 1997.

———. *The Nervous System.* New York: Routledge, 1992.

———. *Shamanism, Colonialism, and the Wild Man: A Study in Terror and Healing.* Chicago: University of Chicago Press, 1987.

Tauxe, Robert V. "Lessons of the Latin American Cholera Epidemic, 1992." *Atlanta Medicine* 66, no. 4 (1992): 41–43.

Tauxe, Robert V., and Paul A. Blake. "Epidemic Cholera in Latin America." *Journal of the American Medical Association* 267, no. 10 (1992): 1388–1390.

Taylor, Charles. *Multiculturalism: Examining the Politics of Recognition.* Edited and introduced by Amy Gutmann. Princeton, N.J.: Princeton University Press, 1994.

Taylor, Paul. "The United Nations System under Stress: Financial Pressures and Their Consequences." *Review of International Studies* 17, no. 4 (1991): 365–382.

Tedlock, Barbara. *Time and the Highland Maya*. Albuquerque: University of New Mexico Press, 1982.

Tedlock, Dennis. *The Spoken Word and the Work of Interpretation*. Philadelphia: University of Pennsylvania Press, 1983.

Terris, M. "Epidemiology and the Public Health Movement." *Journal of Public Health Policy* 7 (1987): 315–329.

Tierney, Patrick. *Darkness in El Dorado: How Scientists and Journalists Devastated the Amazon*. New York: Norton, 2000.

"Todos los casos de diarreas y vómito se tratan como cólera." *Notidiario*, 7 August 1992, 23.

Tompkins, J. P., ed. *Reader-Response Criticism: From Formalism to Post-Structuralism*. Baltimore: Johns Hopkins University Press, 1980.

Treichler, Paula. "AIDS, Africa, and Cultural Theory." *Transitions* 51 (1991): 86–103.

———. "AIDS, Gender, and Biomedical Discourse: Current Contests for Meaning." In *AIDS: Burdens of History*, edited by Elizabeth Fee and Daniel M. Fox, 190–266. Berkeley: University of California Press, 1988.

———. "AIDS, Homophobia, and Biomedical Discourse: An Epidemic of Signification." In *AIDS: Cultural Analysis/Cultural Activism*, edited by Douglas Crimp, 31–70. Cambridge, Mass.: MIT Press, 1988.

"30 mil personas podrían morir en Brasil por el cólera." *El Nacional*, 2 December 1991, C-4.

Trostle, James A. "Early Work in Anthropology and Epidemiology: From Social Medicine to the Germ Theory, 1840–1920." In *Anthropology and Epidemiology*, edited by Craig R. Janes, Ron Stall, and Sandra M. Gifford, 35–57. Dordrecht: Reidel, 1986.

———. "Political, Economic and Behavioral Aspects of the Re-emergence of Cholera in Latin America." Paper presented at the Annual Meeting of the American Anthropological Association, Washington, D.C., November 1995.

Trouillot, Michel-Rolph. "Anthropology and the Savage Slot: The Poetics and Politics of Otherness." In *Recapturing Anthropology: Working in the Present*, edited by Richard G. Fox, 17–44. Santa Fe: School of American Research, 1991.

True, William R. "Epidemiology and Medical Anthropology." In *Medical Anthropology: A Handbook of Theory and Method*, edited by Thomas M. Johnson and Carolyn F. Sargent, 298–318. New York: Greenwood, 1990.

Trumper, Ricardo, and Lynne Phillips. "Cholera in the Time of Neoliberalism: The Cases of Chile and Ecuador." *Alternatives — Social Transformation and Humane Governance* 20, no. 2 (1995): 165–193.

Tsing, Anna. "The Global Situation." *Cultural Anthropology* 15, no. 3 (2000): 327–360.

Tulchin, Joseph S., with Gary Bland, eds. *Venezuela in the Wake of Radical Reform*. Boulder, Colo.: Lynne Rienner. 1993.

United Nations. *Convention on Genocide*. GAOR Resolution 260A (III), 9 December 1948, Article II. Geneva: United Nations, 1948.

United Nations Development Programme. *Human Development Report, 1998.* New York: Oxford University Press, 1998.

Vaughan, Megan. *Curing Their Ills: Colonial Power and African Illness.* Palo Alto, Calif.: Stanford University Press, 1991.

"25 muertos por cólera y 1138 casos en tratamiento." *Notidiario,* 16 September 1992, 3.

Vinogradoff, Ludmila. "El cólera nació en la India." *El Nacional,* 17 April 1991, C-4.

———. "72 barrios de Caracas serían presas del cólera." *El Nacional,* 13 April 1991, C-1.

Vološinov, V. N. *Marxism and the Philosophy of Language.* Translated by Vladislav Metejka and I. R. Titunik. New York: Seminar Press, 1973.

Volpp, Leti. "Blaming Culture for Bad Behavior." *Yale Journal of Law and the Humanities* 12 (2000): 89–116.

———. "(Mis)identifying Culture: Asian Women and the 'Cultural Defense.'" *Harvard Women's Law Journal* 17 (1994): 57–101.

———. "Talking 'Culture': Gender, Race, Nation, and the Politics of Multiculturalism." *Columbia Law Review* 96 (1996): 1573–1617.

Wachsmuth, I. Kaye, Paul A. Blake, and Ørjan Olsvik. *Vibrio cholerae and Cholera: Molecular to Global Perspectives.* Washington, D.C.: ASM Press, 1994.

Wachsmuth, I. Kaye, Gracia M. Evins, Patricia I. Fields, Ørjan Olsvik, Tanja Popovic, Cheryl A. Bopp, Joy G. Wells, Carlos Carrillo, and Paul A. Blake. "The Molecular Epidemiology of Cholera in Latin America." *Journal of Infectious Diseases* 167, no. 3 (1993): 621–626.

Wallerstein, Immanuel. *The Modern World-System.* New York: Academic Press, 1974.

Walt, Gill. "WHO under Stress: Implications for Health Policy." *Health Policy* 24 (1993): 125–144.

Weber, Max. *Economy and Society: An Outline of Interpretive Sociology.* Edited by Guenther Roth and Claus Wittich. New York: Bedminister Press, 1968.

White, Hayden. *Tropics of Discourse: Essays in Cultural Criticism.* Baltimore: Johns Hopkins University Press, 1978.

Wilbert, Johannes. *Folk Literature of the Warao Indians.* Los Angeles: Latin American Center, University of California, 1970.

———. "Genesis and Demography of a Warao Subtribe: The Winikina." In *Demographic and Biological Studies of the Warao Indians,* edited by Johannes Wilbert and Miguel Layrisse, 13–47. Los Angeles: UCLA Latin American Center Publications, 1980.

———. *Mystic Endowment: Religious Ethnography of the Warao Indians.* Cambridge, Mass.: Harvard University Center for the Study of World Religions, 1993.

———. *Textos folklóricos de los indios Warao.* Los Angeles: Latin American Center, University of California, Los Angeles, 1969.

———. *Tobacco and Shamanism in South America.* New Haven, Conn.: Yale University Press, 1987.

———. "Tobacco and Shamanistic Ecstasy among the Warao of Venezuela." In *Flesh of the Gods: The Ritual Use of Hallucinogens,* edited by Peter Furst, 55–83. New York: Praeger, 1972.

———. *Warao Oral Literature.* Monograph no. 9. Caracas: Instituto Caribe de Antropología y Sociología, Fundación La Salle de Ciencias Naturales, 1964.

Wilbert, Johannes, and Miguel Layrisse, eds. *Demographic and Biological Studies of the Warao Indians.* Los Angeles: UCLA Latin American Center Publications, 1980.

Wilbert, Werner. *Fitoterápia Warao: Una teoría pnéumica de la salud, la enfermedad y la terápia.* Caracas: Instituto Caribe de Antropología y Sociología, Fundación La Salle de Ciencias Naturales, 1996.

———. *Infectious Diseases and Health Services in Delta Amacuro.* Acta Ethnologica et Linguistica: Series Americana, no. 10. Vienna-Föhrenau: Engelbert Stiglmyr, 1984.

Wilkinson, Richard G. *Unhealthy Societies: The Afflictions of Inequality.* London: Routledge, 1996.

Williams, Raymond. *Marxism and Literature.* London: Oxford University Press, 1977.

Wills, Christopher. *Yellow Fever, Black Goddess: The Coevolution of People and Plagues.* Reading, Mass.: Addison-Wesley, 1996.

Wohl, Anthony S. *Endangered Lives: Public Health in Victorian Britain.* Cambridge, Mass.: Harvard University Press, 1983.

World Bank. *World Development Report 1998: Investing in Health.* Washington, D.C.: World Bank, 1993.

World Health Organization. "Cholera." *Weekly Epidemiological Record/Relevé épidémiologique hebdomadaire* 66, no. 6 (1991): 40.

———. "Cholera." *Weekly Epidemiological Record/Relevé épidémiologique hebdomadaire* 66, no. 7 (1991): 48–49.

———. "Cholera." *Weekly Epidemiological Record/Relevé épidémiologique hebdomadaire* 66, no. 9 (1991): 61–63.

———. "Cholera in 1991/Le choléra en 1991." *Weekly Epidemiological Record/ Relevé épidémiologique hebdomadaire* 67, no. 34 (1992): 253–260.

———. "Cholera in 1992/Le choléra en 1992." *Weekly Epidemiological Record/ Relevé épidémiologique hebdomadaire* 68, no. 21 (1993): 149–155.

———. "Cholera in 1993/Le choléra en 1993." *Weekly Epidemiological Record/ Relevé épidémiologique hebdomadaire* 69, nos. 28–29 (1994): 205–216.

———. "Cholera in 1994/Le choléra en 1994." *Weekly Epidemiological Record/ Relevé épidémiologique hebdomadaire* 70, nos. 28–29 (1995): 201–211.

———. "Cholera in 1995/Le choléra en 1995." *Weekly Epidemiological Record/ Relevé épidémiologique hebdomadaire* 71, no. 21 (1996): 157–163.

———. "Cholera in 1996." *Weekly Epidemiological Record/Relevé épidémiologique hebdomadaire* 72, no. 31 (1997): 229–235.

———. "Cholera in 1997." *Weekly Epidemiological Record/Relevé épidémiologique hebdomadaire* 73, no. 27 (1998): 201–208.

———. *Education for Health: A Manual on Health Education in Primary Health Care.* Geneva: World Health Organization, 1988.

———. "Epidemic in Peru—Part 1." *Weekly Epidemiological Record/Relevé épidémiologique hebdomadaire* 66, no. 9 (1991): 61–63.

———. *The First Ten Years of the World Health Organization.* Geneva: World Health Organization, 1958.

———. *Guidelines for Cholera Control.* Geneva: World Health Organization, 1993.

———. *Handbook of Basic Documents.* 6th ed. Geneva: Palais des Nations, 1953.

———. "Infected Areas as at 22 February 1996/Zones infectés au 22 février 1996." *Weekly Epidemiological Record/Relevé épidémiologique hebdomadaire* 71, no. 8 (1996): 62–64.

———. *International Health Regulations.* 3d ed. Geneva: World Health Organization, 1983.

———. "Responding to the Threat of a Cholera Outbreak." Geneva: WHO Programme for the Control of Diarrhoeal Disease, n.d.

———. "Revisions of the International Health Regulations: Progress Report, February 2001." *Weekly Epidemiological Record* 76, no. 8 (2001): 61–63.

———. *WHO Guidance on Formulation of National Policy on the Control of Cholera.* Geneva: World Health Organization, 1992.

———. *The World Health Report 1996: Fighting Disease, Fostering Development.* Geneva: World Health Organization, 1996.

Wright, Winthrop R. *Café con Leche: Race, Class, and National Image in Venezuela.* Austin: University of Texas Press, 1990.

Wyatt, Gail Elizabeth. "The Sexual Experience of Afro-American Women." In *Women's Sexual Experience: Exploration of the Dark Continent,* edited by Martha Kirkpatrick, 17–39. New York: Plenum, 1982.

Yépez Colmenares, Germán. "La epidemia de cólera morbus o asiático de 1854 a 1857 y sus efectos sobre la sociedad venezolana." *Anuario del Instituto de Estudios Hispanoamericanos de la Facultad de Humanidades y Educación* 1, no. 1 (1989): 151–180.

Yoyotte, Yira. "Huyendo de condiciones infrahumanas los indígenas acuden a las ciudades." *Ultimas Noticias,* 26 August 1994, 14.

Zambrano, Alonso. "Aumentaron a 67 casos de cólera en la frontera." *El Nacional,* 18 November 1991, D-6.

———. "Doce nuevas víctimas del cólera en Zulia." *El Nacional,* 21 April 1992, C-4.

———. "Donde murió niña guajira crean cordón sanitario." *El Nacional,* 18 December 1991, C-4.

Index

Page numbers in italics indicate photographs, figures, maps, and tables.

acculturation as pathological, 57, 154–57, 194

Action Programme on Essential Drugs (WHO), 273

activists, 128, 132, *172*, *174*, 175, 177, 252, 265, 291, 305, 310, 320, 324, 328; and AIDS, 345n20

Adecos. *See* Partido Acción Democrática

affection for life, *indígenas* as lacking, 208, 316

Agencia EFE, 20

agency: and anthropomorphization of cholera, 21, 22, 282–83; and cholera transmission, 189; and culture, 250, 317; defined, 22; and globalization, 310; and health education, 115; *indígenas* claim, 131, 196; *indígenas* denied, 67, 108, 109, 123, 127, 303–4, 322; and individualization, 290–91; political, 173–74, 177–78; racialization of, 247, 251

Agrodelca Corporation, 130, 132–33

Aguiar, Asdúbul (governor, Caracas), 304

ahotana (beginning), 78, 79, 229

Albert, M. John, 364n96

Alchon, Suzanne Austin, 363n59

alcohol consumption, 63, 81, *82*, 83, 155, 157, 192–93

algae and *Vibro cholerae*, 249

allies, *criollo*, 128, 130, 132

Alonzo, Bernardo (candidate for Delta Amacuro governor), 56, 125, 346n46

Alvarez, José Félix (Mariusan healer), 185, 187, 304

Alvarez, Sonia E., 366n28

Amazonas state, 51, 53, 55, 115, 231, 323, 370n76

American Journal of Tropical Medicine and Hygiene, 284

American Public Health Association, 348n16

Amoco Corporation, 310

anger, 141, 168

animals, stereotypes of *indígenas* as, 31, 108, 115, 116, 131, 132, 156, 168, 203

Aniyar de Castro, Lolita (senator), 31

anthrax, 6

anthropology, 191, 193–95, 226, 252; and cultural reasoning, 203, 218–19, 222, 312–13, 315, 316–17; and epidemiology, 202, 225–26; and representation of *indígenas*, 155, 222

anthropomorphization, 21

antibiotic resistance, 300

antibiotics, 90, 91, 94, 95, 163, 165, 319

"anti-cholera commandos," 34, 35

anti-cholera committee. *See* Comité Regional de Prevención del Cólera

Text: 10/13 Aldus
Display: Aldus
Cartographer: Bill Nelson
Compositor: Integrated Composition Systems
Printer and Binder: Friesens Corporation